EMERGENCY MEDICINE

self-assessment and review

second edition

EMERGENCY MEDICINE
self-assessment and review

second edition

HAROLD A. THOMAS, Jr., M.D., FACEP

Assistant Professor of Emergency Medicine, Oregon Health Sciences University,
Portland, Oregon
Associate Director, Department of Emergency Medicine,
St. John's Hospital,
Longview, Washington

ROBERT O'CONNOR, M.D.

Department of Emergency Medicine, The Medical Center of Delaware,
Wilmington, Delaware
Clinical Instructor, Department of Surgery,
Section of Emergency Medicine, Thomas Jefferson University,
Philadelphia, Pennsylvania

GWEN HOFFMAN, M.D., FACEP

Emergency Medicine Residency Director, Butterworth Hospital,
Grand Rapids, Michigan
Associate Professor of Internal Medicine, College of Human Medicine,
Michigan State University,
East Lansing, Michigan

The C. V. Mosby Company

ST. LOUIS • BALTIMORE • TORONTO   1988

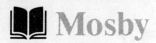 Mosby

Editorial Project Manager: L.G. Cunninghis
Production: The Production House

The C.V. Mosby Company
11830 Westline Industrial Drive
St. Loius, Missouri 63146

0-8016-5058-5
PH/PL/PL 9 8 7 6 5 4 3 2 1

Contents

PART TWO   ANSWERS

EMERGENCY MEDICINE

self-assessment and review

second edition

QUESTIONS

1
Introduction

No questions.

2
Life and Death

No questions.

3
Approach to Patient in Emergency

No questions.

Because Chapters 1, 2, and 3 are of a general nature, no questions were prepared for this material. To assist your review and make it easier to obtain additional information on any topic, the chapter numbers of this book correspond to the chapter numbers in *Emergency Medicine: Concepts and Clinical Practice*, edited by Rosen, Baker, Braen, Dailey, and Levy. Also, the correct answer and rationale for each question includes the page number from the 2-volume text for further consultation.

4

Airway Management

Select the appropriate letter that correctly answers the question or completes the statement.

1. All of the following medications can be given via an endotracheal tube *except*:
    A. Epinephrine
    B. Lidocaine
    C. Sodium bicarbonate
    D. Atropine

2. All of the following statements comparing anatomic differences between the infant airway and the adult airway are true *except*:
    A. The glottic aperture is the narrowest segment of the infant airway.
    B. The infant cricothyroid membrane is too small for cricothyrotomy.
    C. The infant carina angulation of right and left mainstem bronchus is symmetrical, at 55 degrees from the vertical each.
    D. The infant tongue is larger relative to the oral cavity, increasing obstruction potential.

3. Which of the following is *not* true concerning the use of the EOA (esophageal obturator airway)?
    A. It is easy to use and requires less training to acquire and maintain as an active technique.
    B. It is better in the hands of inexperienced personnel than the ET tube in the setting of possible cervical spine trauma.
    C. It prevents aspiration better than a mask alone.
    D. It is contraindicated in the semiconscious patient.

4. A tracheostomy is the emergency airway intervention of choice in which of the following situations?
    A. A 2-year-old who cannot be intubated and is in respiratory arrest
    B. A 60-year-old who is in respiratory arrest and in whom numerous attempts at orotracheal and nasotracheal intubation have failed

5

Intubation and Muscle Relaxation

Select the appropriate letter that correctly answers the question or completes the statement.

1. Under which of the following conditions is blind nasotracheal intubation *not* contraindicated?
    A. Basilar skull fracture involving the cribiform plate
    B. Acute epiglottitis

C. Upper airway foreign body
    D. Possible cervical spine disruption
    E. Coagulopathy anticoagulation

2. Which one of the following statements is false with regard to endotracheal intubation?
    A. Endotracheal intubation may be indicated to protect the airway from aspiration.
    B. A curved laryngoscopic blade (MacIntosh) is inserted into the valeculla during direct laryngoscopy
    C. Bacteremia occurs during nasotracheal intubation in 16% of patients.
    D. High residual volume endotracheal tube cuffs (low-pressure) are less preferable than low residual volume cuffed tubes (high-pressure) because a higher incidence of tracheal ischemia and aspiration with the low-pressure cuffs.
    E. None of the above.

3. A term newborn requires an endotracheal tube of which internal diameter?
    A. 2.5 mm   C. 3.5 mm
    B. 3.0 mm   D. 4.0 mm

4. Which of the following statements is true?
    A. An intubated patient with a vital capacity of 10 to 15 cc/Kg, tidal volume of 3 or 4 cc/Kg, and an inspiratory force of greater than 20–25 cm H_2O should tolerate ventilation weaning and extubation.
    B. A mild sedative may be adminstered to facilitate extubaion.
    C. Sellick's maneuver is indicated to prevent aspiration of gastric contents during active vomiting.
    D. Premedication with lidocaine has been shown to stabilize heart rate and mean arterial pressure during endotracheal intubation.
    E. None of the above.

5. Which of the following neuromuscular blocking agents is most likely to induce hyperkalemia in patients with severe burns, massive muscle trauma, or sepsis?
    A. Vercuronium bromide.
    B. Atracurium besylate.
    C. Pancuronium bromide.
    D. d-tubocurare
    E. Succinylcholine.
    F. None of the above.

6

Cardiac Arrest

Select the appropriate letter that correctly answers the question or completes the statement.

1. Which statement regarding the incidence of cardiac arrest is incorrect?
   A. Over 50% of the fatalities resulting from cardiac arrest occur outside of the hospital.
   B. At least 30 minutes may elapse between cardiac arrest and cerebral death.
   C. Survival following cardiac arrest is improved by early bystander CPR.
   D. Hypothermia and hyperoxemia may delay the onset of cerebral death.

2. Establishing an airway in a patient with a suspected cervical spine injury is best accomplished by;
   A. Head tilt
   B. Abdominal thrust
   C. Jaw thrust
   D. Chin lift

3. The initial step in the treatment of monitored ventricular fibrillation is:
   A. Establishing an airway
   B. Chest compressions and ventilation
   C. Intravenous access
   D. Defibrillation at 200 W-sec
   E. Defibrillation at 360 W-sec

4. Which of the following pharmacologic agents should *not* be given in the treatment of persistent ventricular fibrillation (between defibrillation attempts)?
   A. Atropine 0.5 to 1.0 mg
   B. Epinephrine 0.5 to 1.0 mg
   C. Lidocaine 1.0 mg/kg IV bolus
   D. Oxygen 100% FIO_2

5. Potential complications of excessive sodium bicarbonate administration include all of the following *except*:
   A. Increased tissue binding of oxygen
   B. Hyperkalemia
   C. Hypogosmolality

6. Which of the following is the drug of choice for treating cardiac arrest secondary to hyperkalemia?
   A. Glucose and insulin
   B. Epinephrine and sodium bicarbonate
   C. Calcium chloride
   D. Calcium gluconate

7. All of the following statements regarding isoproterenol are true *except*:
   A. It may cause ventricular fibrillation.
   B. It has nearly pure beta-agonist activity.
   C. It is a potent vasopressor.
   D. It increases myocardial oxygen consumption.

8. Which one of the following statements is true?
   A. In low doses dopamine may cause vasodilation of selected vascular beds.
   B. Norepinephrine selectively increases afterload of the heart.
   C. Norepinephrine decreases myocardial oxygen requirements.
   D. Methoxamine has mixed alpha-and beta-receptor effects.

9. Which of the following antiarrhythmic agents is *not* indicated in digitalis toxicity?
   A. Dilantin
   B. Lidocaine
   C. Procainamide
   D. Bretylium

10. Indications for emergency cardiac pacing include all of the following *except*:
    A. Third-degree A-V block
    B. Mobitz II second-degree block
    C. Asystole
    D. Electromechanical dissociation

11. A 25-year-old man is brought to the emergency department with a gunshot wound of the left anterior chest. The patient had a palpable pulse at the scene but is now apneic and pulseless. Correct initial management includes which one of the following?
    A. Endotracheal intubation and closed chest massage
    B. Endotracheal intubation and open chest cardiac massage
    C. Fluid replacement
    D. Pneumatic antishock trousers and fluid replacement

12. The appropriate endotracheal tube size for a 4-year-old is:
    A. 5.0 to 5.5   C. 6.0 to 6.5
    B. 4.0 to 4.5   D. 3.5 to 4.0

7

Brain Resuscitation

Select the appropriate letter that correctly answers the question or completes the statement.

1. All of the following statements about CPR are true, *except*:
   A. Standard CPR can generate 20–30% of normal cardiac output.
   B. The effectiveness of standard CPR diminishes rapidly after 20 through 25 minutes.
   C. Cerebral blood flow with CPR is not affected by arrest time prior to initiation.

D. No new method of CPR has proven superior to standard CPR in terms of patient survival or neurologic recovery.

2. Which of the following is least important in treatment of a patient with postischemic encephalopathy?
   A. Maintain normal blood pressure
   B. Moderate hyperventilation
   C. Maintain normal pH
   D. Moderate hyperoxia

3. Which of the following is true about postischemic encephalopathy?
   A. Global brain ischemia produces homogeneous histologic damage.
   B. After 4–6 minutes of complete anoxia, irreversible brain damage occurs.
   C. Immediately after resuscitation, there is a period when CNS perfusion is greater than normal.
   D. Anoxic encephalopathy is associated with increased intracranial pressure.

4. As long as cerebral blood flow is maintained above _____, cellular viability is maintained.
   A. 20%   D. 70%
   B. 35%   E. There is no certain
   C. 50%   level

5. All of the following have been proposed to primarily improve neurologic recovery in ischemic encephalopathy *except*:
   A. Naloxone
   B. Desferoxamine
   C. Cardiopulmonary bypass
   D. Phenytoin
   E. Succinylcholine

6. Which of the following is a possible mechanism by which calcium-blocking agents may protect against postischemic encephalopathy?
   A. Increased red blood cell deformability
   B. Decreased vasoconstriction
   C. Improved adenosine triphosphate production
   D. Improved oxygen supply: demand ratio
   E. All of the above

8

Multiple Trauma

Select the appropriate letter that correctly answers the question or completes the statement.

1. A 35-year-old male driver presents following a motor vehicle accident with the following vital signs: BP, 85 systolic; pulse, 122; and respirations, 18 unlabored. He is fully conscious, maintaining a patent airway, the cervical spine is immobilized, and he is able to move all extremities. He complains of neck pain, abdominal pain, and left leg pain. How would you manage this patient hemodynamically?
   A. Start a D5.45 normal saline large-bore IV at 200 cc per hour and follow vital signs.
   B. Start two large-bore IVs D5.45 normal saline at 250 cc per hour total
   C. Start two large-bore IVs of lactated Ringer's; run 2 liters in over 5 minutes. Recheck vitals frequently.
   D. Start two large-bore IVs and run in 4-6 units of packed red blood cells as fast as possible.

2. Following your treatment above, your patient's vital signs are now: BP, 80 systolic; pulse, 128; and respirations the same. How would you respond?
   A. Run 2 liters of lactated Ringer's wide open, start one to two more large-bore IVs.
   B. Run 2–4 units of 0-negative blood in wide open with pressure pack and start one to two more large-bore IVs.
   C. Run lactated Ringer's wide open until 2–4 units of fully crossed-matched blood are available.
   D. Add two more large-bore IVs of lactated Ringer's and run total IV rate at 2 liters per hour.
   E. Start a CVP line and run another 2 liters of lactated Ringer's.

3. Using the same patient scenario as above, which of the following plans is best?
   A. Notify x-ray and the blood bank of this patient.
   B. Notify the surgeon on call.
   C. Perform a peritoneal lavage, then notify the surgeon on call.
   D. Order a trauma profile, including type and cross, order chest x-ray, cervical spine, and left leg films. Ask the surgeon to come in and evaluate the patient.
   E. Notify the surgeon that this patient is in need of an operation.

4. With respect to the concepts put forth in Rosen's, which of the following procedures do you feel are contraindicated in the above patient's situation?
   A. Nasogastric tube placement
   B. Foley catheter
   C. Peritoneal lavage
   D. Venous cut down
   E. Chest x-ray

5. A 57-year-old female presents following a motor vehicle accident. Vital signs are: BP, 162/88; pulse, 66; and respirations of 10 with short periods of apnea. How would you initially manage this patient, provided there is no airway obstruction?
   A. Prepare to nasotracheally intubate.
   B. Bag the patient with 100% oxygen while closely monitoring respiratory status.
   C. 4 liters nasal cannula oxygen and check arterial blood gases in 5 minutes while watching closely.
   D. Bag the patient with 100% oxygen and check arterial blood gases in 5 minutes.

6. Your patient from the above question ceases to breathe as you commence your therapy. Which of the following is the best response?
   A. Continue to bag the patient being careful to watch for good lung filling.
   B. Nasotracheally intubate the patient.
   C. Orotracheally intubate the patient.
   D. Pass an esophageal obturator airway.

7. A 25-year-old male suffering from a single self-inflicted .22 caliber gunshot wound to the posterior pharyngeal wall presents with an adequate blood pressure but no respirations. You attempt orotracheal intubation without success due to the hemorrhage present. Your next step should be which of the following?
   A. Cricothyrotomy
   B. Attempt nasotracheal intubation prior to cricothyrotomy
   C. Attempt nasotracheal intubation guided by the laryngoscope
   D. Tracheostomy

8. You elect to transfer a trauma patient whom you have adequately stabilized to a regional trauma center. Who is responsible for the patient in transit?
   A. The trauma center, following their acceptance of transfer
   B. The transferring physician and the receiving center
   C. The transferring physician alone
   D. The transferring hospital alone

9. A 2-year-old male, back-seat occupant, wearing his seat belt, presents following a motor vehicle accident. He was carried by a paramedic while crying unconsolably. He is fully alert and no obvious trauma is present. He is moving all extremities well. His vital signs are: BP, 96 systolic; pulse, 110; and respiratory rate, 31. How would you respond?
   A. Establish IV access and run lactated Ringer's wide open.
   B. As above, but limit to 500 cc bolus and recheck vitals.
   C. As in B, but obtain a trauma screen and type and cross-match.
   D. Complete physical exam and observe for any deterioration in vitals.

10. Which of the following should be given to patients who have received multiple units of blood and IV fluid in the emergency department?
    A. Heparin
    B. Clotting factor concentrate
    C. Fresh frozen plasma
    D. Dextran
    E. All of the above
    F. B and C

11. Which of the following is the proper order of priorities for the management of multiple trauma patients?
    A. Airway, treat shock, and cervical spine control
    B. Airway, breathing, control hemorrhage, and treat shock
    C. Control hemorrhage, airway, breathing, and treat shock
    D. Cardioversion, airway, breathing, and treat shock

12. Which of the following is true regarding multiple trauma?
    A. Vital signs can be a poor indication of intravascular volume.
    B. It is preferred to await a positive lavage before infusing greater than 2 liters of lactated Ringer's into mildly hypotensive patient.
    C. Venous cutdowns are reserved for patients with blood pressures below 60.
    D. All of the above.
    E. A and C.

13. In a unconscious patient, which of the following can indicate significant spinal cord injury?
    A. Priapism
    B. Loss of rectal tone
    C. Absent deep tendon reflexes
    D. Diaphragmatic breathing
    E. All of the above
    F. A, B, and C.

14. Which of the following portable films should always be obtained on multiple trauma victims while resuscitation is underway?
    A. Lumbar spine
    B. Pelvis
    C. Skull
    D. All of the above
    E. B and C.

15. Complications of massive blood transfusions include all of the following, except:
    A. Thrombocytopenia
    B. Hypothermia
    C. Decreased Factor V
    D. Decreased Factor VIII
    E. All of the above

16. A 25-year-old patient is involved in a head-on collision at high speed. On examination his blood pressure is 80/68, and he has bilateral jugular vein distention and muffled heart sounds. Which of the following should be done?
    A. Two large-bore IVs lactated Ringer's wide open frequently monitoring vital signs
    B. No. 14-gauge needle placed at the second intercostal space
    C. Pericardiocentesis
    D. Nasotracheal intubation

17. Open thoracotomy is recommended for patients who have:
    A. Blunt trauma who arrest in the emergency department.
    B. Penetrating trauma who arrest en route to the hospital.
    C. Penetrating trauma with no signs of life at the scene.
    D. Blunt trauma with no signs of life before arrival at the emergency department.
18. The minimum urine output in children is:
    A. 0.3–0.5 ml/kg/hour
    B. 0.5–1.0 ml/kg/hour
    C. 1.0–1.5 ml/kg/hour
    D. 1.5–2.0 ml/kg/hour

9

Hemorrhagic Shock

Select the appropriate letter that correctly answers the question or completes the statement.

1. In defining shock which of the following is *not true*?
   A. Shock is a clinical syndrome involving dysfunction at the cellular and microcellular level.
   B. In the shock state, all cells in body respond in a similar fashion.
   C. Substances released into the blood may be responsible for promoting the shock state.
   D. A model for the shock state has been conceptualized using hydraulic systems as an anology.

2. Epinephrine and norepinephrine combine to cause an increase in total peripheral resistance. Which of the following is *false*?
   A. Peripheral vascular resistance is increased at the expense of cardiac output.
   B. The functional volume of the vascular compartment is reduced.
   C. An increase in the end diastolic volume results in a decrease in cardiac output.
   D. It is possile to compensate for a small blood loss without other changes in physiologic condition.

3. Concerning sympathetically mediated arteriolar constriction in response to hemorrhagic shock:
   A. Arteriolar constriction occurs to a greater extent in essential organs.
   B. In the kidney urinary output is increased.
   C. Renal salt and fluid retention is stimulated.
   D. It occurs in a homogenous fashion.
   E. Blood flow to the muscles are sustained.

4. With continued blood loss the physiologic condition of the patient begins to decompensate. Which best reflects the body's response to this process?
   A. Ischemia causes a change from anaerobic to aerobic metabolism associated with less available amounts of ATD.
   B. The sodium-potassium membrane pump fails, resulting in efflux of sodium into the interstitium.
   C. Capillary leaks occur secondary to lysozomal rupture and persist for days following successful resuscitation.
   D. As cardiac output is increased, injured mitochondria retain the ability to increase oxygen consumption.

5. Systemic metabolic acidosis related to the shock state:
   A. Shifts the oxyhemoglobic dissociation curve to the right, resulting in less affinity of hemoglobin for oxygen.
   B. Increases the sensitivity of the body to catecholamines.
   C. Increases cardiac output.
   D. Have a detrimental effect on peripheral oxygen delivery.

6. In severe shock:
   A. Myocardial oxygen extraction increases.
   B. Stroke volume increases.
   C. Hemorrhagic necrosis occurs in myocardial tissues.
   D. Stroke volume and contractility decreases while myocardial oxygen extraction increases.

7. Which of the following is *not* a complication of shock?
   A. Gastrointestinal hypermotility
   B. Immunologic blockage
   C. Bleeding diasthesia
   D. ARDS
   E. Centrolobar hepatic congestion

8. Which of the following is *not true* of hypovolemic shock?
   A. Sympathetic blockage brought on by medications or diabetic neuropathy renders a patient more susceptible to hypovolemia.
   B. Hypovolemia may present as syncope.
   C. Hypovolemia may present as primary cardiac arrest with characteristics of nodal or idioventricular rhythms.
   D. Hypovolemia presents with initial episode of bleeding from placenta previa.

9. Characteristics of compensated shock include all, *except*:
   A. Normal mean aortic pressure in the supine position
   B. Mild tachycardia, hyperventilation, and moist cool skin
   C. Increased peripheral vascular resistance, increased heart rate, and increased contractility in response to assuming an upright position
   D. Slight decrease in systolic and diastolic blood pressure

10. A patient being evaluated for hypovolemic shock with a tilt test exhibits no alteration in pulse or blood pressure but becomes dizzy on standing. The tilt test is therefore considered:
    A. Negative
    B. Positive
    C. Indeterminant
11. Bradycardia in the setting of the shock state may be secondary to all of the following, *except*:
    A. Well-conditioned athlete
    B. Preterminal event
    C. Head injury
    D. Vagal stimulation
    E. Beta blocker
12. Whole blood contains:
    A. Albumin and serum proteins in an isotonic medium.
    B. Elevated levels of clotting factors.
    C. Significant amounts of leukocytes and platelets.
    D. Diminished levels of potassium.
13. Concerning blood and blood products, which of the following is true?
    A. Blood should ideally be typed and cross-matched prior to transfusion, a process that usually takes 20 minutes.
    B. Stored blood contains elevated levels of 2,3 DPG, which diminishes oxygen delivery to peripheral tissues.
    C. It is uncommon for a major allergic reaction to occur after the administration of type-specific, un-cross-matched blood to a trauma victim.
    D. Autotransfusion with blood from the chest cavity is beneficial because of increased compatibility and decreased coagulopathy.
14. Which of the following statements is true regarding Ringer's lactate?
    A. Dextrose-Ringer's lactate is the crystalloid fluid of choice in trauma victims.
    B. It should not be used in the presence of significant overdose.
    C. Even in hypotensive patients, the liver converts lactate to bicarbonate rapidly.
    D. It should not be used in the setting of ARDS.
15. A 21-year-old patient arrives in the emergency department suffering from profound hemorrhagic shock. Initial fluid management would include in order of priority:
    A. Lactated Ringer's O-negative blood, low-dose dopamine, whole blood
    B. Lactated Ringer's O-negative blood, type-specific blood, fresh-frozen plasma
    C. Lactated Ringer's, cross-matched blood, fresh-frozen plasma, dopamine
    D. Lactated Ringer's, fresh-frozen plasma, type-specific blood, dopamine

16. All of the following statements concerning CVP measurements in trauma patients are true, *except*:
    A. A low CVP effectively rules out cardiac tamponade.
    B. Serial CVP measurements are helpful in monitoring the resuscitation process.
    C. In the young healthy patient the CVP is well correlated with left ventricular pressure.
    D. A normal pulse, blood pressure, and CVP does not guarantee adequate volume replacement.
17. Which of the following is *not true*?
    A. Citrate contained in stored blood may bind calcium present in the patient's own blood.
    B. A potential deleterious effect of administering bicarbonate during trauma resuscitation is shifting the oxyhemoglobin curve to the left, which diminishes oxygen delivery to peripheral tissues.
    C. Tetanus toxoid should be given in the previously immunized patient with a tetanus prone wound only if the patient's last booster was more than 5 years earlier.
    D. Mannitol and Lasix should be given as early as possible in order to prevent acute tubular necrosis.

10
Anaphylaxis

Select the appropriate letter that correctly answers the question or completes the statement.

1. Which one of the following is an example of an anaphylactoid reaction?
   A. Urticaria
   B. Contact dermatitis
   C. Angioedema
   D. Radiopaque contrast media reaction
2. All of the following modify the course of anaphyolaxis by increasing cAMP levels, *except*:
   A. Solbutamol
   B. Theophylline
   C. Atropine
   D. Epinephrine
3. Stimulation of histamine receptors causes all of the following, except:
   A. Increased vascular permeability
   B. Intestinal smooth muscle relaxation
   C. Gastric acid secretion
   D. Airway mucus production
4. Which one of the following is the leading cause of fatal anaphylaxis?
   A. Bee stings   C. Penicillin
   B. Sulfa drugs   D. Radiopaque contrast media

5. Local measures to decrease the absorption of an antigen include all of the following, *except*:
   A. Extremity elevation
   B. Ice
   C. Loose tourniquet
   D. Stinger removal

6. Which one of the following is most helpful in differentiating vasovagal syncope from anaphylaxis?
   A. Mental status
   B. Blood pressure
   C. Heart rate
   D. Respiratory rate

7. A 5.0-kg infant presents with mild anaphylaxis (urticaria, rhinitis, conjunctivitis, mild bronchospasm). Which of the following is the correct dose and route of administration of epinephrine?
   A. 0.5 cc of 1:10,000 solution SQ
   B. 0.5 cc of 1:1,000 solution IM
   C. 0.5 cc of 1:1,000 solution SQ
   D. 0.05 cc of 1:1,000 solution SQ

8. Epinephrine modifies anaphylaxis in all of the following ways, *except*:
   A. Inhibits further mediator release
   B. Reverses bronchospasm
   C. Decreased myocardial oxygen consumption
   D. Increased cardiac output

9. Protection against anaphylaxis can be conferred by hyposensitization immunotherapy by a rise in which of the following?
   A. Compliment
   B. IgE
   C. IgG
   D. IgM

10. All of the following are correct advice to give a patient sensitive to hymenopteran stings, *except*:
    A. Wear shoes outdoors
    B. Wear loose-fitting clothing
    C. Wear white, gray, or red clothing
    D. Avoid scented soaps and cosmetics

11. Predisposing risk factors for an anaphylactoid reaction to radiopaque contrast media include all of the following, *except*:
    A. Increasing age
    B. Renal dysfunction
    C. Dehydration
    D. Black race

12. Patients who have reacted adversely to past administrations of radiopaque contrast media should have all of the following precautionary measures, *except*:
    A. Prednisone, 50 mg orally for three doses
    B. Benadryl, 50 mg intramuscularly one hour before the procedure
    C. Epinephrine, 0.3 cc of a 1:1,000 solution subcutaneously at the time of the procedure
    D. Nonionic radiopaque contrast media

11
Blood and Blood Component Therapy

Select the appropriate letter that correctly answers the quetion or completes the statement.

1. The use of O-negative blood is most appropriate for which of the following patients?
   A. A patient with active bleeding from a thigh laceration whose blood pressure is 98/50
   B. A patient with a penetrating chest wound and recently extinguished vital signs
   C. A tachycardic woman with brisk third trimester bleeding and a blood pressure of 100/70
   D. All of the above patients should get O-negative blood initially

2. So-called universal donor blood is:
   A. Any O-type blood
   B. Any O-type Rh-negative blood
   C. Any O-type Rh-negative blood with anti-A and anti-B titers greater than 1:200 in saline
   D. Any O-type Rh-negative blood with anti-A and anti-B titers less than 1:200 in saline

3. Orthostatic hypotension is a sensitive indicator of acute blood loss. What is the minimum volume of acute loss that would produce orthostatic hypotension in a 70-Kg adult?
   A. 500 ml   C. 1,000 ml
   B. 750 ml   D. 2,000 ml

4. All of the following statements about stored blood are true *except*:
   A. Granulocytes lose functional capacity within 24 hours.
   B. Platelets have normal function for up to 3 to 5 days.
   C. Factor VIII levels fall to 50% activity within one week.
   D. Factor V levels fall to 50% activity within 3 to 5 days.

5. Factor VIII deficiency and its correction can be monitored in the emergency department by:
   A. Protime (PT)
   B. Activited partial thromboplastin time (aPTT)
   C. Both PT and aPTT are required
   D. Platelet count

9

6. A 38-year-old woman who is taking warfarin (Coumadin) following treatment for deep venous thrombosis comes to the emergency department after an intentional overdose of her anticoagulant. She has gross hematuria and is complaining of flank pain. Therapy at this point should be:
   A. Immediate intravenous vitamin K replacement
   B. Vitamin K plus whole blood
   C. Protamine sulfate
   D. Fresh frozen plasma, 2 to 3 ml/kg, and vitamin K

7. Salt-poor 25% albumin has:
   A. The same osmotic load as human plasma
   B. Approximately 20 to 50 mEq/L of sodium
   C. Almost no sodium content
   D. 100 to 160 mEq/L sodium

8. A patient with a history of simple febrile transfusion reactions develops fever and malaise during transfusion. You should:
   A. Stop the transfusion immediately
   B. Order 50 mg of IV diphenhydramine plus 650 mg of acetaminophen by mouth and observe for any progression of symptoms while transfusing
   C. Continue the transfusion and observe for further symptoms without giving any medications
   D. Obtain an immediate hematology consultation

9. A 48-year-old alcoholic with liver failure is receiving a third unit of rapidly infused whole blood because of a massive upper GI bleeding. He has had many transfusions in the past. He is afebrile but develops muscle tremors. You should:
   A. Stop the transfusions and administer 1 mg epinephrine IV (1:10,000 dilution)
   B. Perform a transfusion reaction work-up after cessation of the transfusion
   C. Obtain an EKG immediately
   D. Infuse 10 mg of vitamin K

10. Cryoprecipitate is useful in the treatment of:
    A. Factor II, VII, and X deficiencies
    B. Factor VIII and fibrinogen deficiencies
    C. Thrombocytopenia
    D. All of the above

11. All of the following statements are true *except*:
    A. Normal platelet count ranges from 150,000/mm^3 to 400,000/mm^3.
    B. Platelet counts less than 90,000/mm^3 are considered thombocytopenic.
    C. Spontaneous bleeding occurs in the range of 40,000 to 50,000/mm^3 platelets.
    D. Platelets must be transfused within 24 hours of collection, because function deteriorates with storage.

12. One unit of platelet concentrate given to a 70-Kg adult raises the platelet count by:
    A. 50,000/mm^3 C. 5,000/mm^3
    B. 10,000/mm^3 D. 1,000/mm^3

13. Which one of the following is not a complication of massive blood transfusion?
    A. Hypercolcemia
    B. Hemolysis
    C. Hyperkalemia
    D. Acidosis
    E. Hypokalemia

14. A patient with cirrhosis needs a transfusion. To reduce the risk of citrate toxicity, which of the following should be done?
    A. Pretreatment with 10% calcium chloride
    B. Administration of packed RBCs
    C. Packed RBCs plus fresh-frozen plasma
    D. Administration of whole blood
    E. Pretreatment with sodium bicarbonate

12
Coma

Select the appropriate letter that correctly answers the question or completes the statement.

1. All of the following are true about intracranial pressure (ICP) *except*:
   A. Normal ICP ranges from 0 to 15 mm Hg.
   B. Signs of elevated ICP include increased systolic blood pressure, tachypnea, and tachycardia.
   C. The Cushing reflex is more pronounced in children than in adults.
   D. Cerebral perfusion pressure (CPP) is defined as the difference between mean arterial pressure (MAP) and intracranial pressure (ICP).

2. Which of the following treatments most effectively lowers elevated intracranial pressure?
   A. Dexamethasone 10 mg initially and then 6 mg every 6 hours
   B. Pentobarbital 2 to 5 mg/kg every 2 hours
   C. Hyperventilation that produces a PaCO$_2$ of 25 to 28 mm Hg and adequate PaO$_2$
   D. Mannitol 0.5 to 2.0 g/kg initially, then 0.15 to 0.30 g/kg every 1 to 2 hours
   E. Hyperventilation producing a PaCO$_2$ of less than 20 mm Hg with adequate PO$_2$

3. All patients presenting with coma should routinely receive all of the following *except*:
   A. 50 g of 50% dextrose
   B. Dexamethasone 10 mg
   C. Naloxone 0.8 to 4.0 mg
   D. Thiamine 50 to 100 mg

4. Which of the following statements about the ocular reflexes is true?
   A. A normal oculocephalic reflex entails conjugate eye movement in the same direction as head rotation.

B. Deeper levels of coma may blunt the oculovestibular reflex while the oculocephalic reflex is preserved.

C. The corneal reflex tests the integrity of the fifth and third cranial nerves.

D. Noxious cutaneous stimulation produces bilateral pupillary dilatation (ciliospinal reflex).

5. Which of the following statements about testing the oculovestibular reflex is true?

A. The test is conducted with the patient lying flat.

B. Water used for irrigation must be at least 25° below body temperature.

C. After testing the response, one must wait at least 5 minutes before performing contralateral irrigation.

D. After irrigation with cold water, horizontal nystagmus is seen with the fast component toward the irrigated ear.

6. The Glasgow coma scale assesses all of the following *except*:

A. Eye opening

B. Pupillary response

C. Motor response

D. Talking

7. Which of the following statements regarding the herniation syndromes is incorrect?

A. Uncal herniation may cause ipsilateral pupillary dilatation and ipsilateral hemiparesis.

B. Contralateral ocular reflexes may remain intact despite ipsilateral pupillary dilatation and hemiparesis.

C. Apnea precedes loss of the corneal reflex during herniation.

D. Uncal herniation may cause ipsilateral pupillary dilatation and contralateral hemiparesis.

8. A 32-year-old female presents with a 6-hour history of unresponsiveness. The patient is unresponsive to deep pain and has stable vital signs. She resists eye opening and snaps her eyes shut when released. Cold water calorics induced nystagmus bilaterally. The most likely diagnosis is:

A. Akinetic Mutism

B. Barbiturate overdose

C. Neuroleptic malignant syndrome

D. Conversion reaction

E. Locked-in syndrome

13
Chest Pain

For the five questions below select the best answer from those listed below:

A. Acute myocardial infarction

B. Aortic dissection

C. Both

D. Neither

1. Which may have acute ECG changes suggesting ischemia?

2. Which present with new onset aortic insufficiency?

3. Which may have a low hematocrit?

4. For which is hypertension a major risk factor?

5. Which usually has premonitory symptoms before the acute event?

Select the appropriate letter that correctly answers the question or completes the statement.

6. Chest pain that may be relieved with nitroglycerin includes all the following *except*:

A. Princemetal's variant angina

B. Esophageal spasm

C. Neural compression

D. Mitral valve prolapse

E. All of the above

7. Which of the following is not true about diagnostic test for chest pain?

A. The CPK-MB fraction may not be elevated for 12 hours after the onset of symptoms of an acute myocardial infarction.

B. A completely normal EKG is very unusual in a patient with an acute myocardial infarction.

C. Therapeutic challenges with local anesthetics or antiacids can help confirm an esophageal origin.

D. Conditions other than cardiac may be reflected in the electrocardiogram.

E. None of the above.

8. Recognizing that myocardial ischemia can cause any pattern of pain, which of the following is the least typical of coronary ischemia?

A. Burning type pain

B. Radiation to right arm

C. Brief stabbing pain

D. Pain worsened by recumbency

E. Pain brought on by emotion

9. Chest pain that is relieved by sitting up and leaning forward is most typically due to:

A. Esophageal spasm

B. Pericarditis

C. Mitral valve prolapse

D. Aortic dissection

E. Costochondritis

10. A patient who has S-T segment elevation during an episode of chest pain with return to normal after the pain episode subsides most likely has:

A. Princemetal's variant angina

B. Mitral valve prolapse

C. Pericarditis

D. Pulmonary emboli

E. Subendocardial infarction

14
Headache

Select the appropriate letter that correctly answers the question or completes the statement.

1. Which one of the following cranial structures is not sensitive to pain?
   A. Fascial planes of scalp and neck
   B. Major arteries at base of brain
   C. Great venous sinuses and their tributaries
   D. Pia mater and superficial brain parenchyma

2. Headaches of acute onset are likely to be caused by all of the following *except*?
   A. Subarachnoid hemorrhage
   B. Stroke
   C. Hypertension
   D. Tumor

3. Headaches that tend to awaken people from sleep include which of the following?
   A. Cluster headaches
   B. Headaches associated with vascular accidents
   C. Headaches associated with intracranial masses
   D. All of the above

4. What does the finding of tenderness of scalp musculature suggest?
   A. Arteriovenous malformation
   B. Epidural abscess
   C. Muscle contraction headache
   D. All of the above

5. What are the most commonly affected cranial nerves in increased intracranial pressure?
   A. III and VI
   B. I and V
   C. XI and XII
   D. All of the above are affected with equal frequency

6. The headache caused by elevated blood pressure is not likely to occur until the diastolic pressure is greater than:
   A. 95
   B. 115
   C. 130

7. All of the following are characteristic of temporal arteritis *except*:
   A. Patients over 50 years old
   B. Women affected more commonly than men
   C. Dull, unilateral headache at time of acute exacerbation
   D. Systemic complaints of low-grade fever and muscle pain

8. What laboratory test will most likely confirm the diagnosis of temporal arteritis?
   A. CBC   B. ESR
   C. LDH   D. CK isoenzyme (BB band)

9. Which of the following is *not* characteristic of classic migraine headache?
   A. Transient motor deficit contralateral to headache
   B. Throbbing bilateral headache initially
   C. Maximum intensity in 1 to 4 hours
   D. Associated nausea, vomiting, and photophobia

10. By which of the following is an ophthalmoplegic migraine characterized?
    A. Suddenly visual dimming sometimes progressing to transient blindness
    B. Miosis, ptosis, and esotropia
    C. Mydriasis, diplopia, and external strabismus
    D. Extreme pain over one eye similar to that of acute angle closure glaucoma

11. Ergot alkaloids are contraindicated with all of the following *except*:
    A. Pregnancy
    B. Peripheral vascular disease
    C. Insulin dependent diabetes mellitus
    D. Angina pectoris

12. Characteristics of cluster headaches include which one of the following?
    A. More commonly affect females; chronic; awaken patients
    B. Pain usually bilateral; considered vascular type
    C. Awaken patients after 2 to 3 hours of sleep; have characteristic prodrome
    D. More common in males; awaken patients; last 30 to 90 minutes

13. A rheumatoid arthritis patient complains of a suboccipital headache. The description sounds like a muscle contraction headache, except that pain is relieved by lifting the head and is exacerbated by flexion. You should:
    A. Advise the patient to rest and get follow-up in 12 hours if headache does not get better with routine analgesics.
    B. Apply cervical collar and get C-spine x-ray series.
    C. Give patient soft collar, analgesics, and order follow-up with rheumatologist.
    D. Obtain lumbar puncture after CT scan (if normal)

14. A 24-year-old right-handed man is seen in the emergency department with severe headache and an acute left hemiparesis. Funduscopic examination reveals *no* papilledema but discloses retinal hemorrhages of the right eye. The most likely diagnosis is:
    A. Thrombotic CVA
    B. Hemiplegic migraine
    C. Subarachnoid hemorrhage
    D. Acute subdural hematoma

15. A 65-year-old woman has acute-onset left-sided headache accompanied by ipsilateral diminished visual acuity. Which of the following statements is true?
    A. The acute onset rules out temporal arteritis.

B. One must wait for temporal artery biopsy before initiating therapy for temporal arteritis.
C. The intraocular pressure should be measured.
D. Untreated cases of temporal arteritis result in blindness of the ipsilateral eye only.

16. Which of the following statements regarding migraine headaches is incorrect?
A. Ophthalmoplegia or hemiplegia are rare components of classic migraine headaches.
B. Patients with ophthalmoplegic migraines may safely be sent home following an acute attack despite incomplete recovery.
C. Only 10% of all migraines are classic.
D. Ergot alkaloids are often successful in the treatment of the acute attack, especially if given during the prodrome.

15
Pain Control: Anesthesia and Analgesia

Select the appropriate letter that correctly answers the question or completes the statement.

1. All of the following are contraindications to the use of nitrous oxide except:
A. Myocardial infarction
B. Pneumothorax
C. Bowel obstruction
D. Head injury

2. The use of local anesthetics containing epinephrine is contraindicated in all of the following anatomic areas except:
A. Fingers and toes
B. Skin flaps
C. Penis
D. Mucous membranes

3. All of the following have mixed agonist-antagonist opiate activity except:
A. Nalbuphine   C. Proproxyphene
B. Pentazocine   D. Butorphanol

4. Which of the following local anesthetics should be used for infiltration anesthesia in someone who reacted with articaria to procaine in the past?
A. Novocain   C. Chlorprocaine
B. Lidocaine   D. Cocaine

16
Fever

Select the appropriate letter that correctly answers the question or completes the statement.

1. The beneficial effects of fever are thought to include all of the following except:
A. Increased phagocytic activity of lymphocytes
B. Inhibition of certain viruses such as coxsackie and polio
C. Increased gastric acid secretion
D. Decreased levels of circulating iron

2. A higher index of suspicion and consideration for possible hospitalization is needed in which of the following pediatric patients?
A. An 18-month-old child with a fever of 38.8°C who appears well and has no obvious source of infection
B. A 5-week-old infant with a temperature of 38.4°C and a normal WBC count
C. A 4-year-old child with a fever of 40.0°C, a runny nose and cough, and a normal WBC count
D. A 6-month-old infant with fever of 39.2°C and evidence of exudative pharyngitis

Match the items on the right with their associated items on the left.

Causes of elevated temperature		Pathophysiology
3. Infection, tissue injury, allergic reaction		a. Environmental heat load exceeds heat loss
4. Hypothalamic stroke, tumor, CNS stimulants (e.g., amphetamines)		b. Defective heat loss mechanism with normal heat load
5. Hyperthyroidism, aspirin overdose, malignant hyperthermia		c. Endogenous pyrogen causes an increase in hypothalamic set point— "true fever"
6. Hot environment—sauna, hot tub, industrial exposure		d. Direct action on thermoregulatory center to raise set point
7. Burns, heat stroke, anticholinergic drugs or phenothiazine		e. Heat production exceeds heat loss

8. At rest, the most important mechanism of heat loss is:
A. Radiation
B. Convection
C. Vaporization
D. Respiration

9. A relative leukocytosis with an increase in band forms (left shift) is seen with which one of the following conditions?
A. Epinephrine
B. Addison's disease
C. Cushing's syndrome
D. Burns

17
Poisoning

Select the appropriate letter that correctly answers the question or completes the statement.

1. Which of the following is *not* indicated in the initial resuscitation of a comatose patient?
A. 50 gm dextrose IV
B. Orotracheal intubation if gag reflex is absent *Nonintubated*
C. Oxygen
D. Narcan 2.0 mg IV
E. Fluid bolus for hypotension

2. Select the most appropriate associations:
A. Bradycardia—mushrooms, organophosphates
B. Tachycardia—cocaine, digoxin
C. Bradycardia—tricyclic antidepressants, pilocarpine
D. Tachycardia—amphetamines, musarinic agonists

3. Each of the following may cause tachypnea, *except*:
A. Salicylates
B. Benzodiazepines
C. Hydrocarbons
D. Caustics
E. Strychnine

4. The combination of horizontal and vertical nystagmus is characteristic of:
A. Cholinesterase inhibitors
B. Phencyclidine *only drug*
C. Opiates
D. Barbiturates
E. Cocaine

5. Which of the following associations is correct?
A. Vesiculobullous lesions—barbiturates
B. Hyperhidrosis—atropinism
C. Hypoactive bowel sounds—organophosphates *Hyperactive*
D. Urinary retention—barbiturates *Atropine*

6. Laboratory tests that should be routinely included on a STAT basis of a comatose patient include:
A. Glucose, drug screen, liver function tests
B. Arterial blood gases, drug screen, glucose

C. Electrolytes, glucose, drug screen
D. Electrolytes, liver function tests, arterial blood gases

7. In cholinergic toxicity which of the following does not apply?
A. Urinary retention
B. Parasympathetic stimulation *SLUDE*
C. Diaphoresis
D. Urination
E. Miosis

8. The efficacy of induced emesis in the recovery of drugs versus that of gastric lavage has been substantiated. True or false?
A. True
B. False

9. Which of the following is true of activated charcoal?
A. Several absolute contraindications exist
B. Useful in treatment of ferrous sulfate *Not*
C. Repeated doses useful in treatment of phenobarbital and theophylline
D. No complications if aspirated

10. Forced diuresis enhances the elimination of all of the following drugs, *except*:
A. Phencyclidine
B. Phenobarbital
C. Salicylate
D. Acetaminophen
E. Lithium

11. Which of the following drug antidote combinations is *not* true?
A. Organophosphates—atropine *PAM*
B. Methanol—ethanol
C. Opiates— naloxone
D. Anticholinergics—pralidoxime *Physostigmine*
E. Cyanide—sodium thiosulfate

12. Which of the following is customary therapy for the condition listed?
A. Extrapyramidal syndrome—thorazine
B. Methemoglobinemia—methylene blue
C. Lithium toxicity—EDTA
D. Nitroprusside—deferoxamine

18
Treatment of Wounds

Select the appropriate letter that correctly answers the question or completes the statement.

1. The goal of emergency department treatment of wounds is to restore function and tissue integrity with good cosmetic result while at the same time minimizing risk of infection. Greatly increased risk of infection is present in all of the following, *except*:

A. Blunt or crush mechanism
B. Primary repair of most lacerations greater than 2 hours old
C. Distal extremity injury
D. Anesthesia with epinephrine

2. You have just sutured a large antecubital laceration on a premiere halfback for a local college using 2-layer technique. He questions you about his return to practice and game situations. You instruct him in the following manner:
   A. Give the wound 3–4 weeks to heal then return to full contact.
   B. Give the wound 3–4 weeks to heal then return to light contact and if feeling well, full contact over 1–2 weeks.
   C. With 1–2 months of no contact your chances of reinjury are very low with full contact.
   D. Advise him that with his major laceration he should not return to full contact this season.

3. History-taking is important prior to repair of lacerations. When asking about history of reaction to local anesthetics, a patient tells you "the dentist said I shouldn't receive Novocain but I don't know why." You should then:
   A. Use tetracaine in substitution
   B. Not use any local anesthetic as ester and amide families exhibit cross-reactivity
   C. Use cardiac lidocaine without fear of reaction
   D. Ignore this history as allergies to Novocain are exceedingly rare

4. All of the following are effective means of wound cleansing, except:
   A. Antiseptic soak for 20 to 30 minutes
   B. High-pressure irrigation using normal saline and 35 cc syringe and 19- or 20-gauge angiocath
   C. 1% Povidone-iodine solution
   D. Nonionic detergents such as Shur-Clens

5. The following are situations involving a laceration. Which could be safely closed using appropriate cleansing, debridement, and primary closure?
   A. 3-cm laceration extending to but not through an olecranon bursa
   B. A clean 2-cm laceration of the face approximately 12 hours old
   C. Stellate lesion (i.e., jagged laceration) of the foot that appears to be contaminated
   D. 6-cm laceration on the forearm approximately 12 hours old that appears clean

6. Suture materials used for laceration repair often differ with respect to individual preference. Needle types are poorly described and therefore poorly understood. Which of the following is an inappropriate use of either suture or needle?

A. PDS for subcutaneous closure
B. Conventional cutting needle for skin repair
C. Interrupting sutures in areas of high tensile strength
D. Subcutaneous sutures in deep lacerations of hand to increase static and dynamic tension

7. There is little evidence to support prophylactic antibiotic usage in traumatic lacerations, even if contaminated. Nevertheless, all of the following circumstances may warrant antibiotics, except:
   A. A patient with mitral valve prolapse
   B. Wound greater than 8 hours old that appears contaminated
   C. Crush injury on a distal extremity
   D. Grossly contaminated wound

8. Wound care instruction sheets are vital to proper care and follow-up. When discussing these with the patient all of the following are appropriate instructions, except:
   A. Elevate the wound for 24 to 48 hours
   B. Maintain immobilization until sutures are out
   C. Do not cleanse scab with hydrogen peroxide as it helps healing
   D. Facial sutures should remain in place for minimum of 5 days regardless of past recommendations

19
Head Trauma

Select the appropriate letter that correctly answers the question or completes the statement.

1. A 67-year-old male driver presents to the emergency department unconscious following an accident. No one was with him at the time. He has a laceration over his forehead and his vitals are adequate. Which of the following should be considered and ruled out as etiologic factors in this case?
   A. Narcotic overdose
   B. Hypoglycemia
   C. Airway obstruction
   D. Acute psychosis
   E. A and B
   F. B and C

2. Which of the following can be found during uncal herniation?
   A. Dilated contralateral pupil
   B. Dilated ipsilateral pupil
   C. Contralateral weakness
   D. Ipsilateral weakness
   E. All of the above
   F. B and C

3. "Cushing" reflex refers to which of the following?
   A. Tachycardia, hypertension, and a rising intracranial pressure
   B. Tachycardia, hypotension, and a rising intracranial pressure
   C. Bradycardia, hypotension, and a falling intracranial pressure
   D. Bradycardia, hypertension, and a rising intracranial pressure
4. Cushing's reflex:
   A. Refers to a rise in pulse and fall in blood pressure in response to increased intracranial pressure.
   B. Is an indication for immediate mannitol therapy.
   C. Is the first sign of increasing intracranial pressure.
   D. All of the above
   E. None of the above
5. What is the Glasgow coma score for a patient that does not open his eyes, makes no noise, and has no motor response to pain?
   A. 0   C. 14
   B. 3   D. 16
6. A 16-year-old male has fallen, striking his head. He is brought to the emergency department. In addition to mechanism of trauma, which of the following historical information is *most* important?
   A. History of loss of consciousness
   B. Change in the level of consciousness
   C. History of drug or alcohol ingestion
   D. Seizure activity
   E. Past medical history
7. On examination, the patient in the question above talks nonsensibly, pushes away noxious stimuli but does not follow simple commands, and opens his eyes on loud verbal command. What is his Glasgow Coma Scale?
   A. 15   C. 9
   B. 3   D. 11
8. All of the following are true regarding the Glasgow Coma Scale, *except*:
   A. Has prognostic significance in head injured patients
   B. Is simple to use because it is scored on specific responses affected only by head injury
   C. Is most valuable with constant repetition of exams
   D. Can be used by a variety of health care personnel
   E. None of the above (all statements are true)
9. A patient is brought to the emergency department with head and facial trauma with oral and nasal bleeding. His airway is adequate but he is confused and has been drinking. Which is correct?
   A. If patient denies cervical pain, may sit up and expectorate blood into basin
   B. Cervical immobilization with collar, supine on backboard
   C. Oral intubation with inline traction to prevent aspiration

   D. Prophylactic cricothyroidotomy
   E. None of the above
10. A 24-year-old motorcycle accident victim with head trauma is in respiratory arrest at the scene. Preferred immediate management is:
    A. Nasotracheal intubation
    B. Incisional cricothyroidotomy
    C. Oral intubation with as little movement of neck as possible
    D. Esophageal obturator airway
    E. Needle cricothyroidotomy
11. A 19-year-old male presents to you with some neck stiffness following a diving incident. What next?
    A. Order a cross table lateral C-spine film
    B. Palpate the neck for tenderness
    C. Perform passive range of motion for neck pain or limitation
    D. Immobilize C-spine
12. What should you do if a patient with cervical collar starts to vomit?
    A. Nasotracheal intubation to guarantee protection of the airway
    A. Log-roll victim to one side while suctioning
    B. Turn head and suction immediately
    C. Suction out the pharynx and then pass an NG tube
    D. Remove collar and orotracheally intubate
13. Which of the following prevertebral soft tissue findings on lateral cervical spine radiography are indicative of possible cervical spine injury?
    A. Greater than 4 mm at C_2-C_4 in the adult
    B. Greater than 5 mm at C_6
    C. Greater than 6 mm at C_2-C_4
    D. Greater than 2 mm at C_2-C_4 in child
14. A 24-year-old motorcycle accident victim has sustained obvious head trauma. He is unconscious with a blood pressure of 70/40, pulse of 140, and a respiratory rate of 24. He has had some jerking movement of his left arm and leg. Which of the following is appropriate?
    A. Nasotracheal intubation, hyperventilation
    B. Mannitol 1-2 g/kg to prevent herniation
    C. Cervical spine and skull x-rays
    D. Furosemide intravenously
    E. All of the above
15. What is the most effective way to initially control a rising intracranial pressure in a head trauma patient?
    A. Maintain $PaCO_2$ and pO_2 in normal ranges
    B. Osmotic diuresis with mannitol 20% solution 1–2 g/kg
    C. Decadron 10 mg IV bolus
    D. Maintain $PaCO_2$ 25–30 mm/Hg
16. Posttraumatic seizures are most likely in which of the following types of head injury?
    A. Epidural hematoma
    B. Concussion

C. Temporal lobe contre coup injury
D. Basilar skull fracture
E. Depressed skull fracture

17. All of the following regarding seizure control in head trauma vistims are true, *except*:
A. Dilantin is the second line treatment behind phenobarbital
B. Valium is the drug of choice for status epilepticus
C. Phenobarbital alters the mental status
D. Phenobarbital is the third drug of choice behind Dilantin and Valium
E. Loading doses should be adjusted according to what antiseizure medication the patient is already on

18. In which sinus is x-ray evidence of blood a sign of basilar skull fracture?
A. Maxillary
B. Sphenoid
C. Frontal
D. Sphenopalatine

19. Your only finding in a head trauma patient is CSF rhinorrhea. Which of the following is true?
A. Prophylactic antibiotics may be beneficial.
B. Lumbar puncture is indicated to rule out infection.
C. Conservative management is indicated since it will likely stop with intervention.
D. Major risk is loss of spinal fluid volume from dural tear.
E. A and C

20. Which of the following sequences occurs with epidural hemorrhage?
A. Minor trauma, delayed loss of consciousness
B. Immediate and persistent unconsciousness
C. Loss of consciousness, alert state, then signs of increased intracranial pressure   *Most common*
D. None of the above
E. All of the above

21. Contrasting subdural hemorrhage and epidural hemorrhage, which of the following is true?
A. Mortality is less for acute subdurals.   *More*
B. Bleeding is usually caused by venous interruption in subdurals.
C. Epidurals are more common.
D. None of the above
E. All of the above

22. All of the following are causes of epidural hematomas *except*:
A. Transected middle meningeal artery
B. Torn communicating vein
C. Torn sinus
D. Torn calvarial arteriole

23. All of the following regarding subdural hematomas are true, *except*:
A. May be an indication of child abuse in infants

B. Become hypodense on CT scan between 7 and 21 days
C. May manifest as only personality change
D. Delayed deterioration may occur if the clot enlarges from rupture of an organizing vessel
E. None of the above (all are true)

24. A 2-year-old has sustained a dog bite to the scalp. Which of the following is true?
A. Scalp vessels in this age group do not bleed as readily as in older patients.
B. The wound should be repaired in single-layer closure, with the galea left open.
C. The injury may involve underlying depressed skull fracture.
D. *A* and *C*
E. *B* and *C*

25. Patients with basilar skull fracture:
A. Will have blood in the maxillary sinus
B. May have normal x-rays
C. Should recieve antibiotics prophylactically
D. A and B
E. B and C

26. A motorcycle accident victim was not wearing a helmet. He has normal vital signs and adequate airway, but opens eyes with pain only, moans, and does not localize noxious stimuli (GCS = 8). He has a nasal fracture, but no CSF rhinorrhea. The GU exam is normal. Lateral cervical spine, chest, and pelvis x-rays are normal. All of the following are appropriate, *except*:
A. Orotracheal intubation   *- after complete C-spine*
B. Nasogastric tube
C. Foley catheter
D. Peritoneal lavage
E. Intravenous normal saline
F. None of the above (all are appropriate)

27. A 74-year-old lady presents with falling episodes, personality change, and headaches. There is a possible history of remote (2–3 weeks) head trauma. Which would be the preferred initial study?
A. NMR
B. Plain CT scan   *2nd CT c̄ contrast*
C. Skull x-ray
D. Cerebral angiography
E. Lumbar puncture

28. Subdural hemorrhage is caused by rupture of which of the following:
A. Bridging veins
B. Cortical arterioles
C. Delayed hemorrhage from damaged parenchyma
D. All of the above
E. None of the above

29. Ensuring which of the following is most important when you discharge a head injured patient?
    A. He understands pupillary inequality
    B. Has not vomited within 1 hour
    C. Has adequate analgesia for posttraumatic headache
    D. Will be in the care of a responsible adult
    E. B and D
30. J.H., a known alcoholic and emergency department abuser, was found in an alley with bruises and abrasions to the head and face. He smells of alcohol and is lethargic but has normal vitals, equal and reactive pupils, and moves all four extremities to pain. Which of the following is appropriate?
    A. Alcohol level STAT, CT if less than 250 mg/dl
    B. Alcohol level STAT, observe with q 30-minute neurologic checks
    C. Cervical spine and skull x-ray (or CT with bone window)
    D. None of the above
31. Which of the following are true regarding concussion?
    A. No gross brain damage
    B. Diagnosis requires loss of consciousness
    C. Potential long term sequelae
    D. A and C
    E. A, B, and C

20
Facial Trauma

Select the appropriate letter that correctly answers the question or completes the statement.
1. Hemorrhage with facial trauma should initially be controlled with:
    A. Cautery   C. Direct pressure
    B. Ligation   D. Clamping
2. All of the following are associated with facial trauma, *except*:
    A. Closed head injury
    B. Cervical spine injury
    C. Hemorrhagic shock
    D. Airway compromise
3. Facial nerve motor function is evaluated by all of the following, *except*:
    A. Forehead wrinkling
    B. Extraocular muscle movements
    C. Eye closing
    D. Baring the teeth
4. When evaluating extraocular muscles, the patient should be questioned about:
    A. Feeling pain

B. Seeing double
C. Seeing flashing lights
D. Limited eye movements
5. Which of the following is the best radiologic view for zygomatic arch fractures?
    A. Panoramic view
    B. Water's view
    C. Submental view
    D. Posteroanterior view
6. Clean facial wounds can be closed primarily up to how many hours postinjury?
    A. 6   C. 18
    B. 12   D. 24
7. Lidocaine with epinephrine is appropriate for facial lacerations involving the following areas, *except*:
    A. Lip   C. Cheek
    B. Eyebrow   D. Nose
8. Abrasions with material embedded into the dermis require vigorous scrubbing to prevent:
    A. Recurrent infections
    B. Traumatic tattooing
    C. Hypertrophic scarring
    D. Dermal excoriation
9. Which one of the following should be looked for in association with a nasal fracture?
    A. Malocclusion
    B. Infraorbital anesthesia
    C. Septal hematoma
    D. Diplopia
10. Debridement of eyebrow lacerations should be minimal and done:
    A. After shaving the hair around the laceration
    B. Perpendicular to the skin
    C. Perpendicular to the hair follicles
    D. Parallel to the hair follicles
11. Which would least likely be injured in an injury just anterior to the ear?
    A. Trigeminal nerve
    B. Parotid gland
    C. Parotid duct
    D. Facial nerve
12. CSF rhinorrhea is unusual in which one of the following facial fractures?
    A. LeFort I   C. LeFort III
    B. LeFort II   D. Nasoethmoid
13. Which one of the following is *not* seen in an orbital floor fracture?
    A. Enophthalmos
    B. Diplopia
    C. Infraorbital hypoesthesia
    D. Malar flattening
14. In which direction does the mandible dislocate in a temporomandibular joint dislocation?
    A. Forward and superior
    B. Forward and inferior

C. Backward and superior
D. Backward and inferior

15. After complete traumatic tooth avulsion, which of the following is *not* an appropriate way to transport a tooth?
    A. Under the tongue
    B. In a glass of milk
    C. Held by the root after being wiped clean
    D. In a wet handkerchief

16. Only a 5% survival rate is likely if an avulsed tooth is not replaced in how many hours?
    A. 1   C. 3
    B. 2   D. 4

17. Posterior nosebleeds are difficult to manage at times. The source of bleeding should be known in regard to specific anatomy. Of the following, which would be the most common site of a posterior bleed:
    A. Anteroinferior portion of nasal septum
    B. Superior to the middle turbinate
    C. Posterior to inferior and middle turbinates
    D. No commonly encountered site, rather diffuse

18. Of the following, which is not a contributing factor to anterior nosebleeds in children:
    A. Allergies and nasal polyps
    B. Acute febrile illness
    C. Septal perforation
    D. Rupture of internal carotid artery aneurysm

19. When posttraumatic bleeding persists despite appropriate therapy, the following should be considered and ruled out:
    A. Fluctuating hypertension leading to intermittent bleeding
    B. Basilar skull fracture
    C. Lower levels of bleeding manifesting intranasally
    D. Commonly encountered and should merely be observed

20. When using silver nitrate cautery sticks to stop an identifiable nosebleed in the emergency department, you are unable to successfully cauterize the vessel. You should next:
    A. Attempt better identification of the vessel with suction handy
    B. Assume septal perforation has occurred
    C. Use electrocautery if a coagulopathy is found
    D. Pack with petroleum jelly gauze

21. Admission criteria for nosebleeds include all of the following, *except*:
    A. All posterior packs
    B. Bilateral anterior packs
    C. Coagulopathy association
    D. Suspected basilar skull fracture

21
Neck Injuries

Select the appropriate letter that correctly answers the question or completes the statement.

1. Prehospital care of neck injuries includes rigin protocols regarding stabilization and treatment. Of the following, which is incorrect in regard to appropriate prehospital management:
   A. Rapid stabilization and expedient transport is the most basic fundamental.
   B. All neck injuries must be rigidly stabilized until properly assessed in the hospital setting.
   C. Nasotracheal intubation is the preferred method of airway management unless massive facial trauma or apnea is present.
   D. Supplemental oxygen and large-bore intravenous lines should be implemented, although time is crucial in regard to venous access.

2. Initial management in the emergency department often dictates future morbidity and mortality in regard to neck injury. All of the following are appropriate maneuvers in management, *except*:
   A. Percutaneous transtracheal ventilation (PTV) is an acceptable alternative to airway management in cases of complete airway obstruction.
   B. Early intubation is preferred if impairment of ventilation, depressed mental status, likelihood of aspiration, or expanding hematoma is present.
   C. Nasotracheal, orotracheal intubation, then cricothyrotomy is the preferred sequence of airway management. Special circumstances may eliminate one or more of these options.
   D. Penetrating neck injuries requiring intubation should first receive rapid-sequence induction anesthesia prior to intubation.

Match the following neck injuries with the appropriate symptoms listed below:

3. Phrenic nerve injury
4. Cervical sympathetic nerve injury
5. Cranial nerve XI, XII injury
6. Laryngeal fracture

A. Ptosis, miosis, anhidrosis (Horner's syndrome)
B. Subcutaneous air
C. Elevated hemidiaphragm
D. Motor dysfunction of trapezius and tongue

7. A 35-year-old black male presents to your emergency department after a one-car motor vehicle accident. He is in mild-to-moderate respiratory distress and you notice a 2-cm abrasion and swelling 2 cm inferior to the thyroid as well as subcutaneous emphysema. Appropriate steps in management include all of the following, *except*:
   A. Endotracheal intubation
   B. Antibiotics are not recommended in this situation; therefore, they are withheld
   C. Obtain cervical spine series, chest x-ray, lateral soft tissue film of neck
   D. Steroids may be considered

8. A patient presents with a cervical hyperextension injury and no neurologic deficit. He complains of acute onset severe pain substernally and is found to be drooling. As well, crepitus is noted in the neck. You suspect esophageal injury, but neck films are negative as well as Gastrografin swallow and esophagoscopy. Your next step is:
   A. Barium swallow
   B. Discharge with referral to a gastroenterologist for follow-up
   C. Observation in the department for 2 to 4 hours then discharge
   D. Treatment with antacids and H_2 blockers for symptoms of reflux

9. A motor vehicle accident victim presents to your emergency department, having been brought in by bystanders of the accident. He has multiple puncture wounds and lacerations of the face and neck. Vital signs are stable and no neurologic deficit is found. You suspect vascular injury and your examination should include:
   A. Gentle probing of the more open lacerations to identify vital stuctures
   B. Lateral neck film followed by suturing of lacerations since healing the neck is very good; then, if no cervical spine injury, discharge
   C. Recheck of neurologic exam in 2 hours and, if no deficit, it may be assumed that carotid artery injury is more than likely not present
   D. Auscultation of the neck to detect carotid bruit

10. Arteriography including a major four-vessel study is very useful in cases of neck injury. Classification of penetrating neck injuries may be subdivided into three separate zones. Of the following, an injury to the neck mandates arteriography in which cases:
    A. Zone I   C. Zones I, II, III
    B. Zones I, II   D. Zones I, III

11. Neck lacerations can be primarily closed in all cases except grossly contaminated wounds without regard to time, since the excellent regional blood supply lends itself to rapid healing. True or False?
    A. True   B. False

12. Of the following statements regarding near-hanging and strangulation injuries, which is false?
    A. Greatest likelihood of arterial occulsion occurs when the point of suspension is over the occiput.
    B. Tardieu's spots are subcutaneous hemorrhages found at the area of compression of the neck.
    C. All patients should be observed a minimum of 24 hours to detect delayed airway compromise.
    D. Cervical spine films are usually not indicated unless the injury involves a significant drop of at least 6 feet.

13. Management of strangulation victims should include all of the following, *except*:
    A. Meticulous respiratory care and management
    B. Hyperventilation and mannitol for signs of increased intracranial pressure
    C. Dilantin
    D. Steroids

22
Spinal Injury

Select the appropriate letter that correctly answers the question or completes the statement.

1. Spinal cord injuries are caused by more than one mechanism. Of the following, which does not fall into categories of commonly seen mechanisms?
   A. Primary vascular damage seen with compression secondary to extradural hematoma, bleeding disorders, anticoagulation therapy, felty syndrome
   B. Disruption of vertebral column with transection of neural elements
   C. Embolism involving spinal arteries and/or arterioles
   D. Cervical osteoarthritis and spondylosis with extension injury and subsequent ligamentum flavum compression of cord

2. With blunt spinal trauma all of the following are pertinent points for the emergency medicine physician's fund of knowledge in recognition and treatment, *except*:
   A. Maximal neurologic deficit is encountered immediately with usual slow return of function.
   B. Ultrastructural changes occur leading to vessel damage, protein extravasation, and spinal cord edema.
   C. Although efficacy has not been fully established and usage is controversial, dexamethasone may be given either intravenously or intramuscularly.
   D. Cryotherapy or surgical decompression yield best results if performed in less than 4 hours.

3. Choose the following true statement concerning anatomy of and/or injury to the spinal cord:
   A. Posterior column disruption is seen occasionally and felt to be due to posterior longitudinal ligament disruption.
   B. Mechanically stable injuries rarely exhibit neurologic deficits.
   C. Fracture fragments, herniated discs, and epidural hematomas are evidence of spinal cord vascular compromise and should be suspect for neurologic instability.
   D. Incidence of spinal cord injuries occurring with vertebral injuries is 50% or greater. *14%*

4. Which of the following would yield greatest chance of encountering neurologic deficit: *27%*
   A. Dislocation with fracture of posterior elements
   B. Dislocation with fracture of vertebral body *5%*
   C. Fracture of posterior elements and vertebral body *11*
   D. Fracture of posterior element alone *19*

5. In the radiographic examination of cervical spine, C_7 and T_1 are occasionally not well visualized. In this case, of the following, select the alternative view for an acceptable radiograph: *C A D B*
   A. Swimmer's view (or transaxillary view)
   B. CT scan
   C. Repeat lateral with slow steady traction on arms
   D. Tomography

6. The following are normal variants on pediatric cervical spine films except for:
   A. Predental space of 4 mm *< 5 mm*
   B. Base of spinous process of C_2 4-mm behind posterior cervical line *(2 mm)*
   C. Anterior border of C_2 to posterior wall of pharynx distance of 5 mm *< 7 mm*
   D. Anterior border of C_6 to posterior wall of trachea distance of 10 mm *14 mm < 15 yo ? < 22 mm*

7. In evaluation of the odontoid you note a fracture and malalignment of the odontoid with the lateral masses of C_1. Your next step bould be which of the following: *unstable*
   A. Evaluate carefully with flexion and extension views under your supervision
   B. Obtain tomographic cuts or CT scan as next step in evaluation
   C. Attempt to elicit pain on motion after carefully removing protective collar
   D. Obtain immediate neurosurgical consultation

8. A 26-year-old male presents to the emergency room with complaint of right posterior neck pain of sudden onset while swinging a bat very hard. His neck is held in extension with deviation to right involving a rotational component. No neurologic deficit is found. After exam, which of the following would you order to help differentiate torticollis from a unilateral facet dislocation?

A. Tomograms
B. Neurology consultation
C. Oblique films of the cervical spine to go along with AP, lateral, and odontoid views
D. No tests required; give him muscle relaxers and discharge

9. In flexion injuries of the cervical spine, of the following, which would be considered a false statement?
   A. Flexion wedge fracture is usually stable, whereas flexion teardrop injury is considered unstable.
   B. Clay Shoveler's fracture is usually unstable because of the force exerted to cause the injury. *stable from direct blow to spinous process*
   C. Widening of the intervertebral space posteriorly may be the only finding of subluxation and is only occasionally seen on flexion or extension views.
   D. Displacement of a superior vertebral body greater than 50% on a lower vertebral body suggests bilateral facet dislocation and is considered extremely unstable neurologically.

10. A car accident victim presents to your emergency room with a history of having driven into a tree at 45 MPH without wearing a seat belt. Paramedics give a history of broken steering wheel and windshield. Vital signs are stable on admission. Disregarding thoracic and/or abdominal injury, you become concerned with the C-spine film showing C_2 bilateral pedicle fractures. Your next concern should be: *Hangman's Fx unstable but ok to widest area thru which cord passes*
    A. Evolvement and progression of neurologic deficit
    B. Respiratory compromise secondary to phrenic nerve involvment
    C. Quickly reviewing text on extension teardrop fracture
    D. Respiatory obstruction secondary to swelling

11. Concerning verticle compression injuries, which of the following is a false statement?
    A. They occur most commonly in thoracic vertebrae.
    B. They are usually stable fractures.
    C. A Jefferson fracture of C_1 is extremely unstable, although rare in occurrence.
    D. All ligaments usually remain intact.

12. Levels of C-spine injury can often be ascertained by simple observation of the patient. Of the following, which would be an improper conclusion?
    A. Spontaneous muscle fasciculations of the trapezius suggests injury about the C_6 area.
    B. Horner's syndrome usually suggests injury in C_7-T_2 area.
    C. Burning hands in an athletic individual could be consistent with an extension injury in C_{6-7} level.
    D. Abdominal breathing with absence of thoracic breathing is usually not a helpful finding in assessing cervical spine injury. *C3-4 phrenic nerve*

13. Frequent neurologic exams, both motor and sensory, should be performed periodically in patients exhibiting a neurologic deficit. Which of the following is the most sensitive indicator of deterioration?
    A. Paralyzed muscles with intact deep tendon reflexes
    B. Cephalad progression of hyperesthesia
    C. Islands of sparing of sensation with or without motor paralysis
    D. Muscle paralysis with absent deep tendon reflexes

14. Of the following, which is not a correct association regarding the sensory exam:
    A. S_1— perianal region
    B. C_7—index finger
    C. T_4—nipple line
    D. L_4—knee

15. In differentiating incomplete from complete spinal cord lesions, the following are all consistent with incomplete lesions, *except*:
    A. Buckle injury of ligamentum flavum into cord causing upper extremity neurologic deficit greater than lower extremity deficit
    B. After 24 hours further neurologic recovery is not expected
    C. Ipsilateral motor paralysis and contralateral sensory hyperesthesia
    D. Occasionally secondary to thrombosis of anterior spinal artery or protrusion of fracture fragments into canal

16. All of the following are true of placement of tongs except:
    A. Little danger exists concerning penetration of inner table
    B. 2–5 lbs. per interspace or inital 5–10 lbs. of traction weight should be used
    C. X-ray studies are necessary to assure proper alignment of vertebre and in monitoring results of therapy
    D. Clean and shave small area just anterior and superior to pinna for tong insertion

17. A patient presents to the emergency department in transfer from a smaller, less well-equipped emergency department. He has documented evidence of spinal cord injury occurring about 2 hours ago and on presentation is noted to be in respiratory arrest. The preferred next step in treatment would be:
    A. Nasotracheal intubation
    B. Obtain immediate blood gas and routine laboratory screen
    C. Cricothyrotomy
    D. Detailed sensory/motor exam including deep tendon reflexes

18. All of the following are consistent with spinal shock, *except*:
    A. Tachycardia

B. Hypotension
C. Normal to slight decreased CVP
D. Rapid response to Trendelenburg position or fluid bolus of 500–1000 cc crystalloid

19. Appropriate preventative measures in spinal trauma patients, used to prevent known complications of spinal injuries, include all of the following, *except*:
    A. Antacids and H_2 blocking agents
    B. Mannitol
    C. Decadron
    D. Periodic bladder catheterization

23
Pulmonary and Chest Wall Injuries

Select the appropriate letter that correctly answers the question or completes the statement.

1. Treatment of fractured ribs includes all of the following, *except*:
    A. Stress deep breathing
    B. Narcotics for pain relief
    C. Use of binders, belts
    D. Intercostal block with bupivacaine if needed

2. All are true about pulmonary contusion, *except*:
    A. It is parenchymal damage with edema.
    B. There is hemorrhage.
    C. It is accompanied by pulmonary laceration.
    D. It occurs most commonly from motor vehicle accidents.
    E. There is increased pulmonary membrane permeability.

3. Pulmonary contusion is differentiated from adult respiratory distress syndrome by all of the following, *except*:
    A. Occurs within minutes
    B. Localized to a segment or lobe
    C. Lasts 48-72 hours
    D. Apparent on x-ray because it is diffuse

4. All of the following are associated with rib fractures 1–2, *except*:
    A. Brachial plexus injury
    B. Horner's syndrome
    C. Aortic arch aneurysm, rupture
    D. Hiatal hernia

5. Which of the following is true concerning flail chest?
    A. Three or less adjacent ribs are fractured at one point
    B. Commonly associated with pulmonary contusion
    C. Respiration is not adversely affected
    D. Flail segment moves inward on expiration and outward on inspiration

6. The most reliable indicator of pulmonary contusion is:
   A. Widening alveolar-arterial oxygen difference
   B. Low PaO_2
   C. X-ray
   D. Patient complaint

7. All of the following are true of pulmonary lacerations, *except*:
   A. Result from penetrating chest injuries
   B. May be injured by inward protrusion of a fractured rib
   C. Avulsion of a pleural adhesion
   D. Frequently produce a hemothorax/pneumothorax
   E. Frequently life-threatening   47%

8. A police officer shows up in your emergency room for evaluation following a shootout. The officer was wearing a bulletproof vest. You would suspect all of the following, *except*:
   A. Heart injury   C. Spleen injury
   B. Liver injury   D. Renal contusion

9. All of the following are complications of tube thoracostomy, *except*:
   A. Hemothorax
   B. Pulmonary edema   *all correct*
   C. Empyema
   D. Ipsilateral pneumothorax

10. Pulmonary contusion can result from which of the following?
   A. Motor vehicle accidents
   B. Blunt chest trauma
   C. Single energy shock waves of an explosion in air or water
   D. High velocity missiles
   E. All of the above

24

Vascular and Cardiac Injuries

Select the appropriate letter that correctly answers the question or completes the statement.

1. Which of the following conditions known to be associated with cardiac contusion is most likely to be present at the initial trauma evaluation:
   A. Pericardial effusion
   B. Transmural or coronary arterial thrombosis
   C. Sinus tachycardia
   D. Retrosternal chest pain   *usually delayed*

2. Which is true regarding myocardial contusion?
   A. Usually subendocardial
   B. Right ventricular
   C. Complicated by coronary thrombosis

D. Complicated by mural thrombi
   E. All of the above

3. The most common presenting symptoms of aortic rupture is:
   A. Retrosternal or interscapular pain   25%
   B. Dyspnea with tracheal compression or deviation
   C. Dysphagia caused by esophageal compression
   D. Ischemic pain of the extremities
   E. Stridor from compression of the recurrent laryngeal nerve

4. Which of the following are the set of most reliable physical findings in traumatic disruption of ascending aorta?
   A. Muffled heart sounds, JVD, and hypotension
   B. Tachycardia, precordial heave, and pallor
   C. Heart murmur, JVD, hypertension, chest wall ecchymoses
   D. Tachypnea, tachycardia, hypotension, chest wall ecchymoses

5. Hypertension involving both upper and lower extremities in an individual with an aortic injury:
   A. Rarely exists
   B. Precludes the diagnosis of pseudocoarctation
   C. Most likely is related to preexisting disease
   D. Results from stretching of sympathetic fibers in the area of the aortic isthmus

6. Given the varied nonspecific spectrum of clinical presentations of myocardial contusion, which is the clinical finding most frequently present?
   A. Dysrhythmias or ST changes
   B. Retrosternal chest pain, anginal in character
   C. Sinus tachycardia   70%
   D. Elevation of the CPK-MB isoenzymes

7. In one study of traumatic cardiac rupture, 20% of patients survived 30 minutes, long enough to benefit from surgical intervention if the diagnosis had been made early. Which initial intervention would be the most helpful in identifying potential myocardial rupture in patients with severe trauma?   *cardiac tamponade*
   A. Central venous pressure monitor
   B. Vital signs: systemic blood pressure, pulse, and respiration
   C. Electrocardiographic monitor
   D. Chest x-ray

25

Acute Pericardial Tamponade

Select the appropriate letter that correctly answers the question or completes the statement.

1. In a normotensive patient, what is usually the earliest response to acute pericardial tamponade?
   A. Tachycardia
   B. Increase in diastolic pressure
   C. Progressive rise in CVP
   D. Increase in pulmonary artery wedge pressure

2. Which diagnostic maneuver should be considered in a situation in which cardiac tamponade is suspected and the patient is gradually yet steadily deteriorating?
   A. EKG, looking for electrical alternans
   B. Chest x-ray, looking for increased cardiac silhouette
   C. Ultrasound
   D. Pericardiocentesis

3. A 20-year-old male is brought to the emergency department with a single stab wound to the epigastrium; he is unresponsive, with a pulse of 130 and an unobtainable blood pressure. Your first intervention would be:
   A. Alert the cardiac bypass team
   B. Insert large-bore IVs
   C. Perform an emergency thoracotomy
   D. Intubate the patient

26

Esophageal and Diaphragmatic Injuries

Match the items on the left with the associated esophageal site of injury.

1. Esophageal obturator airway
2. Endoscopic perforation
3. Foreign body in 2-year-old child
4. Boerhaave's syndrome
5. Nasotracheal tube and Ewald tube

A. Caustic burn site
B. Distal left posterior
C. Mid-esophagus
D. Level of crossing mainstem bronchus and aortic arch
E. Pyriform sinus
F. Cricopharyngeal narrowing

Select the appropriate letter that correctly answers the question or completes the statement.

6. An intoxicated 50-year-old man is eating a steak when he suddenly begins coughing, gagging, and retching. On exam 4 hours later he complains of gagging and localized retrosternal chest pain increased with swallowing. His vital signs are normal and he has a normal CXR. Which of the following is most likely?
   A. Pulmonary aspiration
   B. Dissecting aortic aneurysm
   C. Spontaneous esophageal rupture (Boerhaave's syndrome)
   D. Esophageal foreign body
   E. Acute myocardial infarction

7. Signs that differentiate spontaneous pneumomediastinum from esophageal perforation include:
   A. Pericardium distinctly raised from heart border on x-ray
   B. Hamman's crunch
   C. Low-grade fever
   D. Air fluid levels in the mediastinum on x-ray

8. All of the following are true regarding esophageal perforation, *except*:
   A. Negative intrathoracic pressure on inspiration tends to promote drainage of gastrointestinal contents into the mediastinum.
   B. Esophageal perforation from a foreign body usually occurs in the lower third in the absence of preexisting disease
   C. The single most reliable symptom of this syndrome is pleuritic-type pain localized along the course of the esophagus, which often moves upward in the chest.
   D. The most common cause is iatrogenic.

9. Which of the following is *false* regarding diaphragmatic injury?
   A. Small defects are more likely to result in obstruction and strangulation than large ones.
   B. The diagnosis is often missed in the initial workup.
   C. The CXR is usually specific for the injury.
   D. The most common associated intraabdominal injury is a ruptured spleen.

10. Due to the nature and presentation of patients with diaphragm injuries, the diagnosis is often missed in favor of all of the following, *except*:
    A. Gastritis
    B. Renal colic
    C. Peptic ulcer disease
    D. Gall bladder disease
    E. Angina

11. All of the following are *true* regarding diaphragmatic injuries, *except*:
    A. Left-sided injuries predominate in both penetrating and blunt trauma.
    B. Asymptomatic defects should be managed conservatively since 85% will heal spontaneously.
    C. The most common delayed presentation is that of nonspecific abdominal pain, which is worse after meals and when supine.
    D. Suspect a diaphragmatic hernia in any patient with obstruction who has not had prior abdominal surgery.

12. Which of the following is _false_ regarding the diagnosis of diaphragmatic injury?
    A. Inability to pass a nasogastric tube may be an early sign.
    B. The CXR is normal initially 20–40% of the time.
    C. A dilated hollow viscous in the chest may simulate a pneumothorax.
    D. The presence of a diaphragmatic hernia may increase the false-positive rate of peritoneal lavage.

27
Abdominal Trauma

Select the appropriate letter that correctly answers the question or completes the statement.

1. How does blunt trauma compare to penetrating abdominal trauma in relation to mortality?
    A. Blunt trauma has a greater mortality than penetrating trauma.
    B. Blunt trauma has a lower mortality than penetrating trauma.
    C. Blunt trauma has the same mortality as penetrating trauma.
    D. There are no consistent data comparing the two.

2. A 23-year-old male was stabbed with a 3-inch switchblade to the anterior abdomen. He presents with stable vital signs, alert, and oriented, and laboratory values are unremarkable except for free intraperitoneal air on x-ray. After initial stabilization, what would be the next step in management?
    A. Admission and serial observations
    B. Exploration of the wound
    C. Peritoneal lavage
    D. CT scan of the abdomen
    E. Laparotomy

3. In a patient with stable vital signs, how does the management of stabbing trauma of the anterior abdomen compare to gunshot trauma?
    A. Stabbing trauma has a higher mortality rate.
    B. Stabbing trauma has a less stringent criteria to claim a positive peritoneal lavage.
    C. Stabbing trauma has a lower incidence of intraperitoneal injury, therefore the physician may be more selective in performing immediate laparotomies.
    D. Peritoneal lavage in stabbing trauma is less accurate due to the low incidence of intraperitoneal injury.

4. In a patient with blunt abdominal trauma who is alert, oriented, and verbally responsive, what are the most consistently expressed physical findings associated with internal injury?

A. Rebound tenderness and rigidity
B. Rebound tenderness and guarding
C. Abdominal tenderness and guarding
D. Pain on rectal examination
E. Blood on rectal examination

5. Which is the most commonly involved organ injured in penetrating abdominal trauma?
    A. Stomach
    B. Liver
    C. Pancreas
    D. Colon
    E. Spleen

6. A 17-year-old female stabbing victim presents to the emergency room with stable vital signs, alert, oriented, with a pair of scissors still impaled in her abdomen. Which would be the management of choice?
    A. Remove the scissors in the emergency room and explore the wound
    B. Remove the scissors in the emergency room and perform a peritoneal lavage
    C. Leave the scissors in place, and perform a peritoneal lavage in the emergency room
    D. Bring the patient to the operating room for removal of scissors and possible laparotomy

7. A 40-year-old male presents to the emergency room with a gunshot to the abdomen. Which is _not_ an appropriate management course?
    A. Perform immediate laparotomy for a site of missile entrance at the right flank
    B. Perform immediate laparotomy for free intraperitoneal air on x-ray
    C. Perform immediate laparotomy for a patient whose peritoneal lavage returns with 17,000 RBCs/mm^3
    D. Local exploration of anterior abdominal wounds in a patient with stable vital signs
    E. Peritoneal lavage for a patient with stable vital signs and unsure missile path

8. What is the organ most commonly injured in blunt abdominal trauma?
    A. Liver
    B. Spleen
    C. Small bowel
    D. Kidneys
    E. Bladder

9. Which is true about the incidence of specific injuries in patients in motor vehicle accidents restrained by a combination lap and shoulder belt?
    A. High incidence of head injuries and abdominal injuries
    B. High incidence of head injuries and rib fractures
    C. High incidence of abdominal injuries and rib fractures
    D. Low incidence of abdominal injuries and high incidence of rib fractures

10. A 42-year-old male painter fell three stories off a scaffold. He presents with lethargy, hypotension, multiple cranial contusions, and an obvious left tibia fracture. After initial stabilization and cervical spine clearance, the management of choice for determining hypotension etiology is:
    A. CT scan of head since an intracranial hemorrhage is the most likely cause
    B. Complete neurologic evaluation and consultation since the symptoms are neurogenic cause
    C. Peritoneal lavage since you must assume intraperitoneal hemorrhage unless proven otherwise
    D. Chest x-ray since the symptoms are most likely caused by aortic pathology
11. Which is true regarding the amylase level in trauma?
    A. It is a reliable screening test for pancreatic injury (both a sensitive and specific marker).
    B. It is a sensitive, but not a specific marker for pancreatic injury.
    C. It is a specific, but not a sensitive marker for pancreatic injury.
    D. It is neither a sensitive nor a specific marker for pancreatic injury.
12. Rupture of the retroperitoneal duodenum is characterized most by which of the following abdominal flat plate findings?
    A. Free air in the peritoneal cavity
    B. Kidney clearly outlined by surrounding air
    C. Displacement of the kidney
    D. Shifting of the stomach bubble
13. The use of ultrasound as a safe and noninvasive test has been shown to be helpful in the diagnosis of all of the following conditions, *except*:
    A. Fetal viability in trauma to a pregnant female
    B. Abdominal aortic aneurysm
    C. Thoracic aortic aneurysm
    D. Pancreatic pseudocyst
    E. Hepatic and splenic ruptures
14. A 14-year-old bicycle accident victim complains of sensation of pain to testicles with no obvious evidence of trauma. What is the most likely source of this referred pain?
    A. Diaphragmatic injury
    B. Large-bowel injury
    C. Small-bowel injury
    D. Urogenital or duodenal injury
    E. Pelvic fracture
15. The incidence of maternal death compared to fetal death in a gunshot trauma to the abdomen of a 33-weeks-pregnant female would be:
    A. Both maternal and fetal death are very high.
    B. Maternal death is high and fetal death is low.
    C. Maternal death is low and fetal death is high.
    D. Both maternal and fetal death are rare.

16. A 22-year-old female, 31 weeks pregnant, was in a low-speed motor vehicle accident and presents on a backboard and with a cervical collar. After clearance of C-spine and back, vitals are noted to be BP 110/75, HR 72, RR 19, and fetal heart rate 98 and regular. What is the next step in management?
    A. Immediate cesarean section
    B. Trendelenburg position
    C. Turn on left side
    D. Amniocentesis to determine fetal maturity
    E. Pelvic and bimanual exam
17. A 28-weeks-pregnant female with significant intraperitoneal hemorrhage from blunt abdominal trauma would most likely present with which of the following vital sign changes with imminent maternal shock?
    A. Maternal tachycardia
    B. Maternal bradycardia
    C. Maternal hypotension
    D. Fetal tachycardia
    E. Fetal bradycardia
18. A 37-year-old unrestrained motor vehicle accident driver presents with mild dizziness and mild hypotension. The patient is on a backboard, two IVs are running, and patient is in mild Trendelenburg position. On abdominal palpation, the patient begins having left shoulder pain. Which is the most likely organ involved?
    A. Liver   C. Pancreas   *Kehr's sign*
    B. Spleen   D. Stomach
19. In lower chest stab wounds, a positive peritoneal lavage has a red blood cell count lowered to 5000/mm^3 to detect what kind of injury?
    A. Splenic   C. Renal
    B. Diaphragmatic D. Stomach

28
Genitourinary Trauma

Select the appropriate letter that correctly answers the question or completes the statement.
1. The ratio of blunt trauma to penetrating trauma in renal injury is approximately which of the following:
    A. 1:1   D. 10:1
    B. 3:1   E. 50:1
    C. 5:1

2. Which of the following renal injuries is not represented by the appropriate IVP findings?
   A. Renal contusion (Class I)/normal IVP
   B. Cortical laceration (Class II)/extravasation of dye through cortical laceration
   C. Caliceal laceration (Class III)/intrarenal and extrarenal extravasation of dye
   D. Complete tear or fracture (Class IV)/separation of parenchyma from pelvicaliceal system to the capsule with intrarenal and extrarenal dye extravasation
   E. Vascular pedicle injury (Class IV)/kidney not visualized
3. Which of the following renal injuries are often seen without hematuria?
   A. Renal vascular thrombosis resulting from blunt trauma
   B. Renal contusion
   C. Renal pedicle trauma
   D. A and C
   E. B and C
4. Which of the following is the correct dose of renographin for an IVP in an adult following trauma?
   A. 1 ml/kg of 30% solution
   B. 2 ml/kg of 10% solution
   C. 1 ml/kg of 10% solution
   D. 2 ml/kg of 30% solution
5. There is increased risk of developing contrast material nephropathy with which of the following?
   A. Preexisting renal disease
   B. Dehydration
   C. Shock
   D. Multiple myeloma
   E. All of the above
6. Which of the following is *not* indication for an IVP following trauma?
   A. Fractured pelvis with hematuria
   B. Abdominal pain, nausea, emesis, and positive peritoneal lavage
   C. CVA tenderness and flank mass
   D. Fracture of lower ribs, vertebrae, or transverse processes
7. Which radiographic finding is suspicious of renal injury?
   A. Scoliosis with the spine concave toward the injured side
   B. Unilateral enlargement of kidney shadow
   C. Absence of the psoas margin
   D. Displaced bowel secondary to hemorrhage or urine extravasation
   E. All of the above
8. Which of the following is a contraindication for selective renal arteriography?
   A. Vascular pedicle injury with patient unstable
   B. Nonvisualization of a kidney

   C. Gross renal distortion
   D. Suspected renal tumor as well as trauma
9. Patients with cortical lesions (Class II) are treated in all of the following ways, *except*:
   A. Hospitalization
   B. Restriction to bedrest
   C. Antibiotics
   D. Sent home with daily follow-up with a urologist
   E. C and D
10. Which of the following renal injuries do not require immediate surgery?
    A. Shattered kidney
    B. Small cortical laceration
    C. Small calyceal laceration
    D. Deep renal parenchymal and collecting system lacerations
    E. B and C
    F. B, C, and D
11. Which of the following is the most common preexisting renal abnormality noted during work-up of trauma patients with renal injury?
    A. Hydronephrosis
    B. Hypernephroma
    C. Polycystic kidney disease
    D. Solitary kidney
    E. None of the above
12. What percent of penetrating trauma involves the kidneys?
    A. 1%   C. 10–20%
    B. 5–10%   D. 20–30%
13. All of the following are reasons why children have a greater risk for renal injuries, *except*:
    A. Less ptosis than adults
    B. Less perirenal fat
    C. Kidneys are relatively smaller
    D. Children have a weaker rib cage
    E. All of the above
14. If the ureter is damaged by external trauma, which of the following associated injuries is the most common?
    A. Small intestine
    B. Colon
    C. Major abdominal vasculature
    D. Fractures of the bony pelvis
15. Which of the following is *true* regarding ureteral injuries?
    A. In almost all cases of blunt injury, the ureter is avulsed at the pelvic brim.
    B. Penetrating ureteral injuries are usually in the upper one-third.
    C. They seldom occur without hematuria.
    D. They present with symptoms of ureteral colic, which greatly aids in the diagnosis.
    E. B, C, and D

16. Which of the following is *false* concerning ureteral injuries?
    A. Contrast extravasation often has a ground-glass or hazy appearance because of the contrast dilution in the urine.
    B. If any question remains about injury after excretory pyelogram, retrograde ureterography can be performed.
    C. If the ureteral injury is only a small laceration, it may be treated with hospitalization, observation, and antibiotics.
    D. The must be considered in the emergency department with recent history of trauma, fever, and flank mass with or without tenderness.
17. Which of the following is *false* regarding bladder trauma?
    A. Degree of hematuria is not correlated with the severity of injury.
    B. Sterile urine permeating undrained tissue causes serious necrosis.
    C. The peritoneal surface is the weakest part of the bladder.
    D. Intraperitoneal bladder rupture if not detected will close itself and the urine will be easily reabsorbed.
    E. A and D
18. Which of the following are flat-plate signs associated with bladder injury?
    A. Displaced obturator fat line
    B. Ileus
    C. Pelvic fracure
    D. Intravesicular gas
    E. All of the above
19. Cystography is performed by placing which of the below water-soluble contrast materials through the urethral catheter by gravity or syringe injection?
    A. 500ml of 10% solution
    B. 150–300ml of 10% solution
    C. 500–300ml of 20% solution
    D. 150–300ml of 20% solution
20. A urethrogram is indicated for which of the following?
    A. Meatal blood
    B. If no blood is present, but soft rubber catheter is not easily passed
    C. If blood is present, and soft rubber tube not easily passed
    D. A and B
    E. A and C
21. Posterior urethral tears are characterized by which of the following?
    A. Bloody urine on voiding
    B. High-riding boggy prostate
    C. Not usually accompanied by pelvic fracture
    D. Does not involve transection
    E. B and C

22. Which of the following does not characterize anterior urethral tears?
    A. Straddle injury
    B. Crushing mechanism
    C. Blood at the meatus
    D. No urinary stream
    E. Considerable perineal pain
23. Which of the following are associated with posterior urethral tears?
    A. Urethral stricture
    B. Incontinence
    C. Impotence
    D. A and C
    E. A, B, and C
24. Reanastomosis of a severed penis is possible up to what time postinjury?
    A. 6 hours   C. 12 hours
    B. 3 hours   D. 90 minutes
25. Which of the following is *not* true regarding traumatic rupture of the corpus cavernosum?
    A. Tunica albuginea is torn
    B. Occurs when penis is erect and may hear a cracking sound
    C. Always treated surgically
    D. 10% will develop permanent deformity, suboptimal coitus, or impaired erections
26. Which of the following are *true* regarding traumatic lymphangitis?
    A. No antibiotic therapy needed
    B. Most often secondary to straddle-type injuries
    C. The cordlike structure is extremely tender
    D. Treatment is abstinence from intercourse
    E. B and C
27. Which of the following characterizes Peyronie's disease?
    A. Is a complication of traumatic lymphangitis
    B. Is a complication of dorsal vein thrombosis
    C. Causes painful curved erections
    D. Is induration of the corpora cavernosa with a fibrous chardie
    E. C and D
28. In testicular dislocation, where is the testicle usually found?
    A. In the abdominal cavity
    B. In the abdominal wall
    C. In the bladder
    D. Obscured by hematoma
    E. In the other hemiscrotum
29. Which of the following matches the injury with the correct order of urologic investigation?
    A. Pelvic fracture: IVP, cystogram
    B. Pelvic fracture: cystogram, IVP
    C. Lower rib fracture: cystogram, IVP
    D. Flank mass: cystogram, IVP
    E. B, C, and D

29
Thermal Injury (Burns)

Select the appropriate letter that correctly answers the question or completes the statement.

1. A 26-year-old male presents with flash burns sustained while lighting a natural gas furnace. His face, neck, and hands are red, weeping, and blistered. His eyebrows and hair are singed. There is no bleeding, charring, or visible thrombosis of blood vessels. How would you classify this injury?
   A. 1st degree   C. 3rd degree
   B. 2nd degree   D. 4th degree
2. Shock in burn patients is primarily due to:
   A. Neurogenic factors
   B. Hypovolemia
   C. Acute erythrocyte hemolysis
   D. Myocardial depression factor
   E. All of the above
3. Hospitalization would be appropriate in all of the following cases except:
   A. 18-year-old female with 2nd degree burns to one-half of her back
   B. 3-year-old male with burn to abdomen and anterior thighs
   C. 45-year-old male with electrical burns to upper body
   D. 65-year-old female with IDDM and 10% TBSA 2nd degree burns
   E. 24-year-old male with 2nd degree burns to both hands
4. B.J., a 43-year-old laborer, presents with tar burns on his hands and forearms. You correctly assess him as 6% TBSA 2nd degree burn and decide to admit him. What is the best agent to use for removal of the tar?
   A. Kerosene   D. Acetone
   B. Silvadene cream E. Neosporin ointment
   C. Alcohol
5. The following are all true of inhalation injuries except:
   A. Dry hot air causes more severe injury than humid hot air.
   B. Respiratory complications account for greater than 50% of mortalities in thermal injuries.
   C. Chemical as well as thermal injury often occurs with smoke inhalation.
   D. Direct visualization with bronchoscopy is the best method to evaluate upper airway injury.
   E. All potential inhalation injuries require oxygen therapy.
6. Escharotomy in the emergency department is indicated in:
   A. Circumferential chest wall burn
   B. Decreasing sensation distal to circumferential burn of an extremity
   C. Peripheral cyanosis distal to circumferential burned extremity
   D. All of the above
   E. None of the above
7. Complications of silver sulfadiazine therapy include all except:
   A. Early leukopenia
   B. Rash
   C. Metabolic acidosis
   D. Hyperosmolality
8. The organism most commonly isolated from infected burns is:
   A. Staphylococcus aureus
   B. Staphylococcus epidermidis
   C. Escherichia coli
   D. Pseudomonas aeruginosa
9. The half-life of carboxyhemoglobin is:
   A. 4.5 hours in room air (21% FiO_2)
   B. 1.5 hours in 100% FiO_2
   C. 30 minutes in 3 atm hyperbaric oxygen
   D. All of the above
   E. None of the above

30
Inhalation Injuries

Select the appropriate letter that correctly answers the question or completes the statement.

1. A 30-year-old synthetic factory worker is brought comatose with 6% BSA 1st degree burns following an industrial fire exposure. His vitals are blood pressure 90/60, pulse 100, respirations 6, and temperature 99.6°. An emergency room nurse noted the odor of bitter almond; however, you do not. Appropriate therapy should include all of the following, except:
   A. Amyl nitrite pearls, then intravenous Na thiosulfate
   B. Intubation, hyperventilation with 100% oxygen
   C. Intravenous normal saline, cardiac monitor
   D. Hyperbaric oxygen treatment
   E. Sodium nitrite
2. Which of the following lab profiles are compatable with acute cyanide poisoning?
   A. Plasma lactate level 0.4 mEq/L (normal 0.5–1.5 mEq/L)
   B. Plasma lactate level 1.8 mEq/L (normal 0.5–1.5 mEq/L)
   C. Na 135, K 4.0, CI 90, HCO_3 10
   D. Na 130, K 4.5, CI 105, HCO_3 20

3. Lab evaluation of suspected carbon monoxide poisoning should include all of the following, *except*:
   A. Chest x-ray
   B. ABGs
   C. Carboxyhemoglobin level
   D. Cardiac enzymes
   E. Electrocardiogram

4. Factors that are critical to the production of toxic byproducts of combustion include all of the following, *except*:
   A. Material composition
   B. Flash point
   C. Oxygen availability
   D. Temperature
   E. Heating rate

5. Which of the following patients does not require admission after carbon monoxide exposure?
   A. Headache and nausea that cleared after face-mask oxygen therapy
   B. Passed out at scene of fire
   C. Self-limited seizure prehospital
   D. Found in garage with car running
   E. Abnormal chest x-ray on evaluation

6. The most significant damage secondary to inhalation injury of polyvinyl chloride pyrolysate is due to:
   A. HCL gas fumes
   B. Anhydrous HCL aerosol
   C. Phosgene
   D. Toluene
   E. Chlorine

7. Regarding laboratory evaluation of carbon monoxide poisoning, which of the following statements is false?
   A. CO levels correlate poorly with clinical presentation.
   B. Elevated anion gap acidosis is suspicious of CO poisoning.
   C. Oxygen saturation as calculated by blood gas analyzers is adequate.
   D. pO_2 measurements determine only that oxygen dissolved in plasma and is unaffected by hemoglobin saturation.

8. Accepted explanations for the adverse physiologic effects of carbon monoxide exposure include all of the following, *except*:
   A. Reduced transport of oxygen by reduced oxygen saturation of hemoglobin
   B. Myoglobin saturation results in hypotension and decreased tissue perfusion
   C. Anion gap metabolic acidosis
   D. Rightward shift of oxyhemoglobin dissociation curve
   E. Binding of cytochrome A_3 oxidase system

9. Prior to hyperbaric oxygen therapy for carbon monoxide overdose, which of the following is not indicated?
   A. Chest x-ray to rule out pneumothorax
   B. Electrocardiogram to rule out myocardial ischemia
   C. High-dose steroids to reverse cerebral edema
   D. Dopamine/dobutamine for hypotension
   E. Consider bicarbonate for severe metabolic acidosis

31
Frostbite

Select the appropriate letter that correctly answers the question or completes the statement.

1. Chilblain is characterized by all of the following *except*:
   A. Red patchy swelling on the dorsum of hands and feet
   B. It is a cutaneous manifestation of a vascular disorder
   C. A higher incidence in young men
   D. Patients with Raynaud's disease, collagen diseases, and macroglobulinemia are predisposed to develop it
   E. Itching and burning sensation

2. The following are true statements about immersion foot, *except*:
   A. It is a freezing type of cold injury.
   B. There are three phases: ischemic, hyperemic, recovery.
   C. Injured parts are hypersensitive to cold after recovery.
   D. Depigmentation may occur in the recovery phase.
   E. Pain with weight-bearing is common after recovery.

3. Each of the following are predisposing factors to frostbite injury, *except*:
   A. Improper clothing
   B. Race
   C. Injury or accident
   D. Alcoholic intake or mental instability
   E. Acclimatization

4. Frostnip is characterized by all of the following, *except*:
   A. Skin blanching
   B. Anesthesia of skin or loss of cold sensitivity
   C. Tingling or rewarming
   D. No loss of superficial tissue
   E. Blister formation

5. F.M., a 52-year-old alcoholic, is brought to the emergency department by the police, who found him in an alley on a cold January night. His skin is cold to touch, he smells strongly of alcohol, and he complains of not being able to feel his feet. You suspect superficial frostbite of the feet. If correct, the physical exam should show all of the following *except*:
   A. White, nonblanching skin on both feet
   B. Soft, resilient tissue under the white skin
   C. A waxy appearance to the skin
   D. Absence of bullae formation for at least 24 hours
   E. Anesthesia in the injured area
6. For the patient in the previous question, you diagnose superficial frostbite and begin treatment. You choose to:
   A. Rewarm his feet in a water bath at 112–115°F
   B. A water bath at 104–108°F
   C. A water bath at 98–102°F
   D. Slow and gradual rewarming at room temperature to decrease pain
   E. Partially rewarm his feet before transfer to a larger hospital
7. After initial therapy of this same patient, you reexamine his feet and find they are flushed and edematous. Large blisters are developing on the dorsal surfaces and his fourth and fifth toes on the left foot are cold, mottled, and gray. You decide to:
   A. Release him to the police with instructions to keep his feet warm and covered
   B. Amputate his deeply frostbitten left fourth and fifth digits before gangrene develops
   C. Admit him to the hospital for observation and protective isolation
   D. Rupture all of his blisters, begin prophylactic antibiotics, and cover the ruptured blebs with antibiotic ointment
   E. Allow the patient to smoke a cigarette
8. Which of the following treatment modalities has proven efficacy in the treatment of frostbite?
   A. Rapid rewarming of the frozen tissue
   B. Low molecular weight dextran infusion
   C. Operative sympathectomy
   D. Heparinization and oral anticoagulation
   E. All of the above
9. The most common late sequelae of frostbite is:
   A. Skin pigmentation changes
   B. Hyperhidrosis
   C. Pain
   D. Cold sensitivity
   E. Bone growth abnormalities

32
Chemical Injuries to Skin

Select the appropriate letter that correctly answers the question or completes the statement.
1. All of the following are true of chemical injuries to the skin, *except*:
   A. Skin damaged by chemicals may demonstrate erythema, blistering, or full thickness loss.
   B. The full extent of injury is always apparent within 30 minutes of exposure.
   C. Injury usually occurs by biochemical means and not directly by heat.
   D. The pathophysiology of chemical burns from agent to agent is remarkably similar.
2. Prehospital therapy for chemical injuries to the skin include all of the following, *except*:
   A. Check for specific antidotes
   B. Remove all contaminated clothing
   C. Water lavage for at least 15 minutes
   D. Debridement of any solid chemical particles
   E. Avoid self contamination
3. Emergency department treatment of chemical burns includes:
   A. Copious lavage
   B. Tetanus immunization
   C. Washing with green soap to remove caked compounds and oils
   D. Close follow-up with rechecks at 24 hours, 72 hours, and 7 days
   E. All of the above
4. Chemical burns generally requiring hospital admission include:
   A. Burns in high-risk patients
   B. Burns involving hands, feet, eyes, ears, or perineum
   C. 1st degree burns greater than 15% of body surface
   D. Most 2nd and 3rd degree burns
   E. All of the above

Match the following chemical agents with their specific treatments.

____ 5. Polyethylene glycol 300 and industrial spirits
____ 6. Calcium gluconate
____ 7. Copper sulfate
____ 8. Copious water irrigation
____ 9. Dry debridement before water lavage

a. Hydrofluoric acid
b. Mace and tear gas
c. Epoxy glue
d. Phenol
e. Quick lime
f. Phosphorus

10. The amount of 10% calcium gluconate to be injected subcutaneously for a hydrofluoric acid skin burn measuring 5 cm x 2 cm is:
    A. 0.5 cc
    C. 10.0 cc
    B. 5.0 cc
    D. 50.0 cc

11. Acceptable substitutes for polyethylene glycol 300 and industrial methylated spirits in a 2:1 mixture for phenol exposure include:
    A. Cresol
    B. PEG 300 and 400
    C. Glycerol
    D. Carboxylic acid
    E. B and C

12. After copious water lavage, residual phosphorus in tissue can be identified by application of:
    A. PEG 300/IMS
    B. Calcium gluconate
    C. Chloracetopherase
    D. Copper sulfate

13. Which two of the following metals may ignite spontaneously in the air?
    A. Sodium
    D. Lithium
    B. Calcium
    E. Potassium
    C. Aluminum

14. An EMT calls the emergency department from the scene of an industrial accident, where a workman has a burning piece of sodium imbedded in his arm that cannot be easily removed. Your initial recommendation should be:
    A. Copious lavage with water
    B. Cover with calcium oxide
    C. Extinguish the burning metal with a Class D fire extinguisher
    D. Transport to the emergency department without field treatment

15. A 3-year-old child presents to the emergency department with his right eye glued shut with a fast setting epoxy glue. You should:
    A. Trim the eyelashes
    B. Dissolve the glue with acetone
    C. Forcibly separate the eyelids
    D. Swab the eyelids with vegetable oil

33
Electrical Injuries

Select the appropriate letter that correctly answers the question or completes the statement.

1. All of the following are false regarding electrical injuries, *except*:
    A. Electrical currents less than 50 V are harmless.
    B. Electrical currents of greater than 150 cp are generally less dangerous than those of 60 cp.
    C. Being struck by lightning is uniformly fatal, and victims without vital signs and with fixed, dilated pupils should never be resuscitated.
    D. Higher voltage correlates better with severity of injury than does higher amperage.
    E. Lightning injury results in ventricular fibrillation more frequently than asystole.

2. All of the following are true regarding electrical injuries, *except*:
    A. Amputation due to severe musculoskeletal injury is necessary in 33-60% of cases.
    B. The best estimation of necessary fluid resuscitation is urine output.
    C. Cervical and thoracic spine injuries must be ruled out.
    D. Motor deficits occur more frequently than sensory deficits.
    E. GI complaints are generally of no significance.

3. Based on incidence statistics, which of the following persons is most likely to suffer an electrical injury?
    A. A 35-year-old woman
    B. A 10-year-old boy
    C. A 3-year-old girl
    D. A 39-year-old lawyer
    E. A 7-year-old boy

4. Which of the following electrical sources is the most likely to produce tetanic muscle contractions sufficient to prevent voluntary release when touched?
    A. A 20,000 V powerline at 200 cp
    B. A 12 V battery
    C. A 1,000,000 V transformer at 200 cp
    D. A 110 V/60 cp household extension cord
    E. A live sparkplug wire

5. The extent of the wound of entrance or exit of an electric current will be determined by the resistance of the skin and the area of contact in which of the following manners?
    A. The smaller the resistance the larger the wound.
    B. The larger the area of contact the larger the wound.
    C. The larger the resistance the smaller the wound.
    D. The smaller the victim the smaller the wound.
    E. The smaller the area of contact the larger the wound.

6. Oral commissure electrical injuries have which of the following characteristics?
    A. Most commonly occur in children 3 to 5 years of age
    B. Are usually caused by high tension electrical current
    C. Frequently involve delayed labial artery bleeding
    D. Usually have associated palatal injuries
    E. Often cause late speech impairment from tongue injury

7. Which of the following injury patterns would make you most suspect a true conductive electrical injury in an unconscious victim?
   A. A fracture of a lumbar vertebrae body
   B. A fracture of the proximal humerus
   C. An injury current on EKG
   D. A flexion crease burn
   E. A burn on the palm

8. Which of the following is associated with alternating current injuries?
   A. Arborescent pattern in entrance and exit wounds
   B. More likely to result in ventricular fibrillation than asystole
   C. High-voltage lightning strikes
   D. Usually cause less injury than clinically apparent
   E. Frequently caused by defibrillation paddles

9. Renal involvement resulting from conductive electrical injuries is largely caused by which of the following?
   A. Direct electrical trauma to the kidneys
   B. Scarring of the uterus resulting in obstructive uropathy
   C. Thrombosis of the renal veins
   D. Hypovolemic shock and acute tubular necrosis
   E. Myoglobinuria

10. Ophthalmologic injuries including the development of cataracts occur in what percentage of electrical injuries?
    A. Less than 10%
    B. Between 1 and 10%
    C. Between 10 and 20%
    D. Between 20 and 30%
    E. Over 30%

11. A 40-year-old plumber is brought to the emergency department after suffering an electrical injury while working on a water heater. He is unresponsive with blood pressure of 80 palpable and labored respirations. The best estimation of necessary fluid resuscitation in this patient would be based on:
    A. The Parkland formula
    B. The Brooke formula
    C. The systolic blood pressure
    D. The urine output   1 cc/kg/hr
    E. The central venous pressure

12. Which of the following are more likely to be present in true electrical burns than in simple thermal burns?
    A. Blood pH less than 7.2
    B. Charred skin and hair
    C. Carbonaceous sputum
    D. Eschar formation
    E. Paresthesias and paralysis

13. Each of the following are features of electrical flash burns, _except_:
    A. They represent true conductive electrical injuries.
    B. They result from radiant energy released from electrical arcs.
    C. They are actually simple thermal injuries.
    D. They do not include the body as part of the circuit.
    E. They characteristically have a central blanched area with surrounding erythema and sharply refined borders.

34

Lightning Injuries

Select the appropriate letter that correctly answers the question or completes the statement.

1. The following statements compare injuries sustained from lightning to injuries from industrial high-voltage exposure. Which statement(s) is/are correct?
   A. Lightning strikes transfer less energy to the patient.
   B. Lightning strikes are more likely to cause asystole than ventricular fibrillation.
   C. Lightning strikes are less likely to cause skin burns.
   D. All of the above

2. All of the following are physical findings that might be expected in a patient after lightning injury, _except_:
   A. Ruptured TM
   B. Myoglobinuria
   C. Blue-mottled, cold often pulseless extremities
   D. Linear, punctate, or feathering superficial burns
   E. Confusion, amnesia

3. The initial approach to a patient with witnessed or suspected lightning injury should include all of the following, _except_:
   A. EKG and conventional treatment for arrhythmia
   B. X-ray to rule out cervical, skull, or long-bone fractures
   C. Detailed neurologic exam and peripheral vascular exam
   D. Vigorous hydration for anticipated internal burns
   E. Preparation for admission for monitoring and observation

35
Radiation Injuries

Select the appropriate letter that correctly answers the question or completes the statement.

1. A 43-year-old nuclear technician was accidentally exposed to radiation from a linear accelerator at the college where he works. He appears to have suffered no ill effects and his boss tells you that he was decontaminated in the special shower facility at the site. The clothes he was wearing are in a plastic bag and still register heavily on the Geiger counter. You have the patient reshower but his skin still shows high levels of radioactivity. The most likely type of radiation involved would be:
   - A. X-rays
   - B. Gamma rays
   - C. Neutrons
   - D. Alpha particles
   - E. Beta particles

2. A patient presents to the emergency department 20 minutes after an intense radiation exposure. He is confused but able to complain of headache, tinnitus, vertigo, and numbness in his leg. What is the minimum dose of radiation that will produce these symptoms at this time after exposure?
   - A. 50 rad
   - B. 600 rad
   - C. 2400 rad
   - D. 4800 rad
   - E. 12,000 rad

3. The median lethal dose of radiation exposure for humans is:
   - A. 50 rad
   - B. 150 rad
   - C. 250 rad
   - D. 350 rad
   - E. 450 rad

4. Delayed death following radiation exposure is most likely due to failure of which of the following systems?
   - A. Hematopoietic system
   - B. Cardiovascular system
   - C. Respiratory system
   - D. Central nervous system
   - E. Urologic system

5. Characteristics of alpha particles include:
   - A. They are emitted by radiation therapy machines.
   - B. They are emitted by plutonium.
   - C. They readily penetrate the skin.
   - D. They generally travel farther than beta particles.
   - E. They are only emitted by particle accelerators.

6. A 33-year-old power plant worker is accidentally exposed to high levels of radiation. He has no apparent symptoms when seen in the emergency department 1 hour later. Which of the following procedures should be done first for this patient?
   - A. Immediate gastric lavage to rid the stomach of radioactive material
   - B. Immediate cardiac monitoring and placement of 2 large-bore IV lines
   - C. Immediate placement of protective facemask on the patient
   - D. Immediate removal of all clothing and cleansing hair and skin
   - E. Immediate administration of ipecac to rid the stomach or radioactive material

7. The best laboratory test to determine a patient's prognosis for survival following a high level radiation exposure is:
   - A. Absolute lymphocyte count at 48 hours postexposure
   - B. Absolute thrombocyte count at 24 hours postexposure
   - C. Total white cell count at 24 hours postexposure
   - D. Total red cell count at 48 hours postexposure
   - E. Qualitative prothrombin time at 72 hours postexposure

36
Near-Drowning

Select the appropriate letter that correctly answers the question or completes the statement.

1. What percentage of all drowning victims are less than 4 years of age?
   - A. 10%
   - B. 20%
   - C. 40%
   - D. 60%
   - E. 80%

2. A 3-year-old boy is found by his parents floating upside down in the backyard pool. The boy has vital signs on scene when the paramedics arrive but arrests in transit and does not respond to resuscitative efforts. The correct terminology concerning this child's death is:
   - A. Drowning
   - B. Near-drowning
   - C. Secondary drowning
   - D. Immersion syndrome
   - E. Drowning syndrome

3. Which of the following statements regarding aspiration of water during drownings is *false*?
   - A. If less than 22 ml/kg of fluid is aspirated, life-threatening electrolyte abnormalities do not occur.
   - B. Most victims who drown will aspirate enough fluid to significantly alter serum electrolytes.
   - C. Aspiration of sea water pulls protein-rich fluids into the pulmonary alveoli and interstitial spaces.
   - D. Aspiration of fresh water may result in hemoglobinuria secondary to red blood cell lysis.
   - E. Aspiration of fluid may result in pulmonary infections and pulmonary insufficiency hours to days after the initial resuscitation.

34

4. In comparing the potential metabolic effects of fresh-water drowning versus salt-water drowning when significant fluid aspiration occurs, which of the following is correct?
   A. Salt-water drowning raises serum calcium.
   B. Fresh-water drowning lowers serum potassium.
   C. Salt-water drowning lowers serum potassium.
   D. Fresh-water drowning raises serum chloride.
   E. Salt-water drowning lowers serum magnesium.

5. A 25-year-old surfer is brought to the emergency department, having been submerged in the ocean for 2 minutes after his surfboard hit him in the head. He is in severe respiratory distress and witnesses report that he aspirated a lot of sea water. Which of the following statements regarding this patients condition is *false?*
   A. He should be intubated if he isn't already.
   B. His serum sodium is probably elevated.
   C. His serum magnesiun is probably elevated.
   D. A cervical spine injury should be ruled out.
   E. His blood volume is probably elevated.

6. Which of the following is uncommon in near-drowning?
   A. Acidosis   D. Intrapulmonary shunting
   B. Hypoxemia   E. Elevated serum potassium
   C. Shock

7. An 11-year-old girl with epilepsy is brought in by ambulance after having had a seizure while swimming. Observers say she was under for 5 minutes. She was lethargic at the scene but now is alert with normal vitals and normal ABGs, CXR, and physical exam. Her anticonvulsant level was low but has been corrected. Proper management of this patient would be:
   A. Immediate discharge with close follow-up
   B. Admission to Pediatric ICU and monitoring hemodynamically for 24 hours
   C. Admission to a general pediatric floor
   D. Observation for 5 hours and if okay then discharge with close follow-up
   E. Order a ventilation-perfusion scan to determine the need for admission

8. In the definitive management of a near-drowning victim with possible pulmonary complications, which of the following statements is not correct?
   A. One-hundred percent oxygen should be initially administered.
   B. A normal chest x-ray does not rule out significant pulmonary problems.
   C. Positive pressure ventilation with PEEP or CPAP is indicated in patients requiring intubation.
   D. Broad spectrum prophylactic antibiotics should be administered to prevent pulmonary infections.
   E. Steroids should probably not be given.

9. A 6-year-old boy has fallen through the ice while ice skating; he is recovered from the water 45 minutes later and is pulseless and apneic. Which of the following statements is correct?
   A. The mammalian diving reflex may help preserve his neurologic and cardiac function by facilitating the release of oxygen from hemoglobin at the tissue level.
   B. Severe hypothermia may increase his metabolic demands and result in severe cerebral hypoxia.
   C. The severe hypothermia may have a cardiac protective effect by preventing ventricular fibrillation.
   D. As a child, his chances of surviving neurologically intact are greater than that of an adult with an equally prolonged period of submersion.
   E. Prolonged resuscitation efforts are not indicated since survival with neurologic recovery following extended cold-water submersion is unlikely.

37
Diving Injuries

Select the appropriate letter that correctly answers the question or completes the statement.

1. Of the gases listed below, which is the most likely to have a toxic effect at increasing depths when an individual is sport diving?
   A. Oxygen
   B. Carbon dioxide
   C. Nitrogen
   D. None of the above

2. The toxic effect of the gas in question number one:
   A. Causes a syndrome known as "rapture of the deep" which is due to pulmonary overinflation
   B. Causes a syndrome called "the no panic syndrome"
   C. Occurs because of hyperventilation by a diver prior to descent
   D. Occurs because of the anesthetic effect of the gas on nerve tissue

3. Mechanical effects from changes in ambient pressure cause bodily injury because:
   A. Of the fact that as pressure increases on a gas its volume changes inversely as the temperature rises
   B. The nonviscous strictures of the body can adapt to changes in ambient pressure
   C. Of Boyle's law
   D. During descent mucosal vessels leak fluid into viscous air-filled structures

4. A 24-year-old male presents to your emergency department after his first FSW dive. He complains of headache and left ear pain, and he noted blood from his left nostril. Treatment should consist of:
    A. Instructing the patient to clear his ears using Valsalva's maneuver the next time he dives
    B. An antibiotic if a rupture of the tympanic membrane is present
    C. Evaluation of the patient for other squeeze syndromes
    D. *B and C*

5. Pulmonary overinflation syndrome can manifest in a variety of ways. Which of the following scenarios would most likely not involve pulmonary overinflation syndrome after a routine dive?
    A. A 20-year-old inexperienced diver who continues to complain of chest pain after a normal PA and lateral chest x-ray
    B. A 30-year-old diver with chest pain after a routine dive—he is noted to have a crunching noise on chest auscultation
    C. A 50-year-old experienced salvage diver complaining of chest pain, nausea, and dyspnea 30 minutes after diving
    D. None of the above

6. Which of the following is *not* true concerning decompression sickness (DCS)?
    A. DCS may occur when the gas dissolved in body fluids separates to form bubbles.
    B. Dissolved gases come out of solution and form bubbles when there is an increase in ambient pressure.
    C. Slow ascent will allow equilibration among tissue nitrogen, blood, nitrogen, and alveolar nitrogen.
    D. The bubbles formed in tissue or blood may cause DCS or may be absorbed without adverse effects.
    E. Nitrogen is metabolically inert.

7. All of the following predispose to the development of DCS, *except*:
    A. Cold
    B. Obesity
    C. Exercise during the dive
    D. Youth
    E. Previous recent dives

8. All are true concerning decompression sickness (DCS), *except*:
    A. A patient with "the bends" will generally have a normal physical exam.
    B. Erysipelas rash and cutis marmorata marbleization may herald the onset of more severe DCS.
    C. Type I DCS should prompt a thorough neurologic exam since more than 75% of patients with Type I will develop Type II DCS.
    D. Joints of the knee, shoulder, and elbow are most the commonly affected by the bends.
    E. No cases of Type I DCS involving the spine, ster-

num, or cranium have been reported.

9. A 30-year-old male presents to the emergency department, 5 hours after a dive, complaining of substernal chest pain, cough, and shortness of breath. Based on the most likely diagnosis, all are true, *except*:
    A. Physical examination is usually unremarkable.
    B. The symptoms may persist up to 1 week.
    C. The chest pain may be pleuritic initially.
    D. The cough is usually deep but nonproductive.
    E. He should receive recompression therapy as soon as possible.

10. Which is true concerning Type II decompression sickness?
    A. Aviators have predominantly spinal cord DCS.
    B. Divers have predominantly cerebral DCS.
    C. The cause of spinal cord DCS is obstruction of the anterior spinal artery by air bubbles.
    D. People with a history of migraine headaches are more likely to develop cerebral DCS.
    E. Physical exam is usually normal.

11. All are true concerning decompression sickness, *except*:
    A. Shock may be vasovagal or the more serious delayed or secondary type.
    B. Leukocytosis and marked hemoconcentration may be present.
    C. All patients with DCS except those with erysipelas rash should receive recompression therapy.
    D. If treatment is started within 6 hours of the first symptoms, almost no morbidity occurs.
    E. Recompression therapy is of little value after 24 hours and is not recommended after this time.

38
Accidental Hypothermia

Select the appropriate letter that correctly answers the question or completes the statement.

1. Hypothermia is defined as a core temperature below:
    A. 36°C   D. 33°C
    B. 35°C   E. 32°C
    C. 34°C

2. The last reflex to disappear with hypothermia and the first to reappear with rewarming is:
    A. The knee-jerk reflex   D. The biceps reflex
    B. The jaw-jerk reflex   E. The cremasteric reflex
    C. The plantar reflex

3. Assuming a normal basal metabolic rate and no immersion, which of the following accounts for the greatest percentage of body heat loss?
    A. Conduction   D. Radiation

B. Convection   E. Respiration
C. Evaporation

4. Which one of the following conditions *does not* predispose to hypothermia?
   A. Myxedema   D. Grave's disease
   B. Addison's disease   E. Malnutrition
   C. Cushing's disease

5. Which of the following medications do not predispose to hypothermia?
   A. Phenothiazines   D. Glutethimide
   B. Tricyclic antidepressants   E. None of the above
   C. Ethanol

6. In the hypothermic patient arterial blood gases can be corrected for body temperature. Which of the following statements concerning the method of correction is true?
   A. The uncorrected pH is higher than corrected pH
   B. The uncorrected PaO_2 is lower than the corrected PaO_2
   C. The uncorrected $PaCO_2$ is higher than the corrected PaO_2
   D. All of the above

7. A 6-year-old female was nearly drowned in a frigid lake. Her core temperature is 31°C. The pH on her ABGs says 7.2, uncorrected for temperature. Which of the following is closest to the true pH?
   A. 7.3   D. 7.1
   B. 7.2   E. 7.0
   C. 7.5

8. Which of the following EKG changes are highly characteristic of hypothermia?
   A. Shortened PR interval with bradycardia
   B. Osborn waves between the QRS complex and the ST segment
   C. Jenner waves at the junction of the QRS and the T wave
   D. Bradycardia with diastole-prolonged systole
   E. Bucholtz waves in the QRS complex

9. The only certain criterion for death in hypothermia is:
   A. Loss of corneal reflexes
   B. Loss of Doll's eyes and corneal reflexes
   C. Documented asystole of over 20 minutes duration
   D. Irreversible cardiac arrest when the patient is warm
   E. Loss of all deep tendon reflexes and Doll's eyes

10. A 34-year-old male is found wandering in the woods by hunters on a cold winter night. His car had broken down and he had no warm clothing. He is noted to be confused and when paramedics arrive his oral temp is below 35°C. Which of the following prehospital stabilization procedures are indicated?
    A. Active rewarming with skin rubbing
    B. Giving the patient a hot cup of coffee
    C. Giving the patient a shot of whiskey
    D. Active rewarming with humidified oxygen

E. Amphetamines to increase metabolism

11. An 80-year-old female is found unconscious in an unheated home. The initial rhythm is ventricular fibrillation and is unresponsive to countershocks. The patient arrives at the emergency department in the same rhythm despite lidocaine bolus and drip. She is intubated and has been given epinephrine and bicarbonate at appropriate intervals; CPR is ongoing. Her core temperature is 26°C. Your next step in the management of this patient is:
    A. Bolus with lidocaine and countershock twice
    B. Fluid bolus of lactated Ringer's
    C. Rapid active rewarming to 28°C then countershock
    D. Double the epinephrine and bicarbonate dosage
    E. Bretylium drip at 2 mg/min then countershock

12. Passive external rewarming may:
    A. Be sufficient treatment for an alert patient whose temperature is 35°C
    B. Be ineffective in changing core temperature at all below 30°C
    C. Lead to a drop in core temperature after initiation of therapy
    D. All of the above

39
Heat Illness

Select the appropriate letter that correctly answers the question or completes the statement.

1. The wet bulb thermometer temperature at which the body's heat load exceeds its maximal cooling mechanisms and the incidence of heat stroke skyrockets is:
   A. 33°C   D. 36°C
   B. 34°C   E. 37°C
   C. 35°C

2. The most efficient mechanism for body heat dissipation at environmental temperatures over 37°C is which of the following?
   A. Conduction   D. Evaporation
   B. Convection   E. Respiration
   C. Radiation

3. A 17-year-old male football player endures "two-a-day" practice sessions during an unseasonably hot August day. Which of the following metabolic changes is *not* likely to occur under these conditions?
   A. Decreased peripheral vascular resistance
   B. Increased renal blood flow
   C. Increased respiratory rate
   D. Microscopic hematuria
   E. Decreased plasma volume

4. Which of the following is *not* a characteristic factor in the pathophysiology of heat cramps?
   A. Cramps occur in the most exerted muscles.
   B. Cramps can occur during and after exertion.
   C. Copious sweating occurs during exertion.
   D. Copious hypertonic fluid ingestion occurs during exertion.
   E. Sedentary workers are rarely affected.

5. Which of the following is found in heat stroke but never in heat exhaustion alone?
   A. Delirium
   B. Orthostatic hypotension
   C. Elevation of CPK
   D. Core body temperature over 39°C
   E. Total body salt depletion

6. A 20-year-old army recruit collapses during a training drill at Paris Island in July. He is very confused and thinks he is back home in Cleo, Iowa. His vitals are: temperature 41.5°C, pulse 112, blood pressure 93/45, and respirations of 28. Which of the following most accurately characterizes this patient's illness?
   A. Exertional heat fatigue   D. Classic heat exhaustion
   B. Malingering   E. Exertional heat stroke
   C. Classic heat stroke

7. Which of the following treatment regimens would *not* be appropriate in the above patient?
   A. IV hydration with cool normal saline
   B. Placement of a CVP line and Foley catheter
   C. Cold inhaled air by IPPB and ice water enemas
   D. Warm water mist/dry air fan evaporation technique
   E. Supplemental oxygen at 5 to 10 l/min

8. Which of the following organs is rarely ever directly affected by heat stroke?
   A. Liver   D. Brain
   B. Pancreas   E. Heart
   C. Kidney

9. Which of the following laboratory abnormalities are *not* characteristic of acute heat stroke?
   A. Elevated serum calcium
   B. Elevated prothrombin time
   C. Metabolic acidosis
   D. Elevated SGOT level
   E. Decreased serum phosphorus

40
Orthopedic Injuries

Select the appropriate letter that correctly answers the question or completes the statement.

1. A 28-year-old woman comes to the ED with left wrist pain and swelling after falling onto her outstretched hand. She has tenderness and swelling over the distal aspect of her left radius, with tenderness over the anatomic snuffbox and decreased range of motion of the involved wrist and fingers. Radiographs of the left ulna, radius, wrist, and hand are negative for fracture or dislocation. The emergency room physician should:
   A. Suspect a sprain and apply an elastic bandage
   B. Suspect a fracture and apply a circular short arm plaster cast
   C. Suspect a fracture and apply a circular long arm plaster cast
   D. Suspect a fracture and apply a plaster splint

2. A 48-year-old man arrives in the ED with tingling and swelling in the toes of his left foot. He has a short leg plaster cast on his left leg. The patient explains that his original injury occurred 3 weeks ago, but the cast had just been replaced 8 hours earlier in the orthopedist's office. The emergency physician should:
   A. Cut plaster on one side to relieve pressure
   B. Cut plaster on both sides, remove half of the cast, then replace both halves with bias cut stockinette to hold it together
   C. Cut plaster and inner padding on both sides, remove half of the cast, then replace both halves with bias cut stockinette to hold it together
   D. Remove entire cast and wrap ankle with an elastic bandage
   E. Remove entire cast and reapply a new circular plaster short leg cast

3. Which of the following statements is true?
   A. A greenstick fracture is a type of comminuted fracture.
   B. Usually it is unnecessary to x-ray a dislocation until after a reduction is performed.
   C. Type IV Salter fractures often cause growth arrest.
   D. First degree sprains exhibit at least some joint instability or abnormal joint movement.

4. Appropriate management of open or compound fractures in the emergency department includes all of the following *except*:
   A. Parenteral antibiotics
   B. Copious irrigation followed by reduction
   C. Culturing of wounds
   D. Immobilization in position of deformity

5. The following radiograph depicts:
   A. Dorsal displacement of distal radius
   B. Dorsal angulation of distal radius
   C. Dorsal angulation of distal ulna
   D. Dorsal angulation and displacement of distal radius

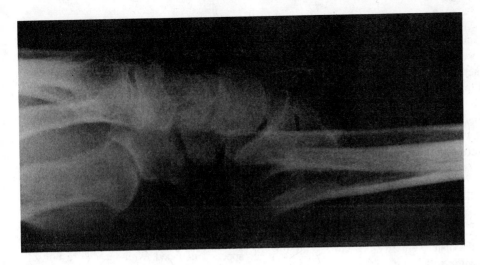
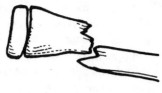

41
Shoulder

Select the appropriate letter that correctly answers the question or completes the statement.

1. Which injury is most likely to result in neurovascular damage?
   A. Posterior glenohumeral dislocation
   B. Fracture and displacement at the humeral surgical neck
   C. Humeral greater tuberosity fracture
   D. Fracture of the middle third of the clavicle

2. Which type of fractures require open reduction and internal fixation?
   A. One-part humeral fractures
   B. Two-part humeral fractures
   C. Three-part humeral fractures
   D. Glenohumeral subluxations

3. A 24-year-old man arrives in the emergency department complaining of right shoulder pain. He is reluctant to move his shoulder and holds his right arm tightly against his chest. The shoulder appears square and the acromion process appears prominent. What is the most likely diagnosis?
   A. Anterior dislocation
   B. Fractured humerus
   C. Posterior dislocation
   D. Luxatio erecta

4. All of the following are true concerning posterior shoulder dislocations *except*:
   A. They are much less common than anterior shoulder dislocations.
   B. External rotation and abduction of the affected shoulder usually cannot be performed.
   C. The subacromial position is the most common type of posterior dislocation.
   D. The axillary nerve is often involved in this injury.

5. Which one of the following statements is incorrect?
   A. The posterior rim of the glenoid is often fractured in cases of posterior dislocations.
   B. 98% of posterior dislocations are subacromial.
   C. The Hill-Sachs deformity occurs with anterior shoulder dislocations predominantly.
   D. Posterior dislocations are visualized on A-P shoulder radiographs.

6. Which of the following fractures of the scapula is the most common?
   A. Fractures of the body of the scapula
   B. Fracture of the neck of the scapula
   C. Fracture of the acromion process
   D. Fracture of the coracoid process

42
Humerus and Elbow

Select the appropriate letter that correctly answers the question or completes the statement.

1. What is the diagnosis according to the x-ray film in Fig. 42–1?
   A. A Colles fracture
   B. Interarticular fracture
   C. A Smith's fracture
   D. A normal elbow x-ray

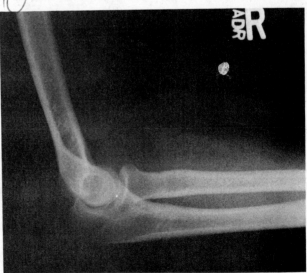

Fig. 42–1.

2. Which structures are most likely to be injured in a supracondylar distal humeral fracture?
   A. Brachial artery and ulnar nerve
   B. Brachial artery and median nerve
   C. Brachioradialis tendon and ulnar nerve
   D. Brachioradialis tendon and median nerve
3. All of the following injuries are seen more commonly in children than in adults.*except*:
   A. An epicondylar humeral fracture with avulsion of the medial epicondyle and posterior dislocation of the elbow
   B. Supracondylar humeral fractures
   C. A dislocation of the radial head without an associated fracture of the ulna
   D. An intercondylar fracture of the distal humerus
4. Pathologic fractures of which of the following could indicate metastatic carcinoma:
   A. Olecrannon
   B. Supracondylar humerus
   C. Humeral shaft
   D. Head of radius

43
Forearm and Wrist

Select the appropriate letter that correctly answers the question or completes the statement.
1. A 35-year-old woman with an undisplaced fracture of the proximal radius in a posterior splint arrives in the ED with deep forearm pain and decreased sensation in her fingers. What complication should be considered at this point?
   A. Compartment syndrome
   B. Displacement of the fracture
   C. Neuropathy
   D. A second fracture
2. If the complication described in Question 1 is left untreated, what deformity might result?
   A. Nonunion
   B. Volkmann's ischemic contracture
   C. Osteonecrosis
   D. Osteomyelitis
3. Which of the following statements is true?
   A. Both-bone fractures are almost never displaced.
   B. Undisplaced fractures of the proximal radius usually require open reduction and internal fixation.
   C. Most both-bone fractures of the forearm heal satisfactorily when treated with closed reduction.
   D. Loss of reduction is not infrequent in displaced proximal ulnar shaft fractures.
4. Which type of carpal dislocation or fracture dislocation is the most common?
   A. Lunate
   B. Perilunate
   C. Scaphoid
   D. Scaphoid-lunate
5. Dorsal shear stresses may cause chip fractures from

the dorsal portion of the carpal bones. Which is the most commonly involved carpal bones?
   A. Lunate
   B. Scaphoid
   C. Triquetrium
   D. Hamate

44
Hand

Select the appropriate letter that correctly answers the question or completes the statement.
1. A 25-year-old comes to the ED with a "sore finger." He has also noticed a "sore" at the corner of his mouth and wonders if the two sores are related. On physical exam his finger appears reddened, with serous crusting discharge at the ungual border. The sore near his mouth is a blister, and you also notice a type of ulcer on his oral mucous membrane. Your treatment at this time would be to:
   A. Excise a crescent-shaped block of subcutaneous tissue just proximal to the nailfold to allow drainage; apply a dressing and put the patient on an antistaphylococcal antibiotic.
   B. Put the patient's finger in a splint to diminish discomfort and give him a prescription for a topical antibiotic ointment.
   C. Warm soaks to his finger 4 times a day; put him on an antistaphylococcal antibiotic and explain to him that he should keep his fingers out of his mouth as it is possible to spread infection in this way.
   D. Make a fish mouth incision in the distal finger to allow drainage, apply a dressing, and give him a prescription for a topical antibiotic.
2. An infection of the terminal pulp space of a digit (a "felon") is best treated by all of the following measures *except*:
   A. An antibiotic that covers *Staphylococcus* and *Streptococcus*
   B. A fish mouth incision to allow for adequate drainage of the pus, and insert a petrolatum gauze pack
   C. Immobilization in a splint
   D. An anterior-midline incision in the fingertip with insertion of a petrolatum gauze pack
3. All of the following statements about infections of the hand with regard to antibiotic therapy are true *except*:
   A. Antibiotic therapy is not necessary with adequate incision and drainage of paronychia and carbuncles on the hand.
   B. Treatment of herpetic whitlow with a topical antibiotic ointment to prevent secondary bacterial infection is adequate antibiotic therapy.
   C. Patients with lymphangitis should be given an oral antibiotic covering *Staphylococcus* and *Strep-*

tococcus, told to elevate the arm, and come in to be checked the next day.

   D. Tenosynovitis is best treated with prompt surgical drainage to prevent tendon damage, because once the tendon is involved in an infection it may be beyond the reach of any antibiotic coverage.

4. A patient comes to the ED after a fall on the ice in which he extended his hand to break the fall. He is tender, swollen, and ecchymotic over the distal interphalangeal joint of his ring finger and also at the base of the ring finger on the volar side. He is able to flex his DIP, PIP, and MP joints simultaneously with trouble, but can't flex the DIP joint when the MP and PIP joints are in extension. X-ray films show only soft tissue swelling. This patient should:

   A. Have his ring finger buddy taped to his middle finger, given a nonsteroidal antiinflammatory drug, and told to call an orthopedist if his hand does not improve in 1 week's time
   B. Be referred to an orthopedic surgeon for repair of his tendon
   C. Be put in a short arm cast with an outrigger to immobilize his ring finger
   D. None of the above

5. All of the following are true statements *except*:

   A. Posterior (dorsal) dislocations of the PIP joint are more common than anterior (volar) dislocations.
   B. All fractures of the metacarpal neck—regardless of the amount of angulation—should be reduced before immobilization.
   C. Acute partial tears of the collateral ligament of the PIP joint are best treated with immobilization.
   D. An attempt at closed reduction should be made on all dislocations of the MP joints.

45

Cervical Hyperextension Injuries and Low-Back Pain

Select the appropriate letter that correctly answers the question or completes the statement.

1. Which statement is *false* with regard to cervical hyperextension injuries?

   A. It is the most common soft tissue neck injury.
   B. The injury is limited to ligamentous structures of the neck.
   C. Legal advice may be sought by more than 50% of the patients.
   D. It occurs when an immobile vehicle is rear-ended.

2. Which one of the following is least likely to cause cervical hyperextension injury?

   A. A vehicle crushed between two cars
   B. Contact sports (i.e., tackling in football)
   C. A person struck on the head by a falling object
   D. A vehicle struck from behind

3. Vigorously shaken abused children are least likely to present with which one of the following?

   A. Acute subdural hematoma
   B. Acute epidural hematoma
   C. Torn bridging veins
   D. Retinal hemorrhage

4. Which one of the following would be the least likely presenting complaint in the shaken baby syndrome?

   A. Failure to thrive
   B. Lethargy
   C. Seizures
   D. A history of shaking

5. Which one of the following would not be a finding on computed tomography of shaken children?

   A. Minimal subarachnoid hemorrhage
   B. Subdural hematoma
   C. Retinal hemorrhage
   D. Normal

Match the following:

____ 6. Spondylolylis	A.	Degenerative changes of the vertebrae. Can include osteophyte formation at the disk spaces
____ 7. Spondylolisthesis	B.	Defect in the pars interarticulasis
____ 8. Spondylosis	C.	Slippage of the anterior portion of the superior vertebral body forward on the inferior vertebral body

Select the appropriate letter that correctly answers the question or completes the statement.

9. All of the following statements about low back pain are true, *except*:

   A. L_5-S_1 is the most frequent site of pain origination.
   B. Nerve root irritation pain rarely goes beyond the knee.
   C. New onset incontinence is a neurosurgical emergency.
   D. Spinal stenosis can be termed *pseudoclaudication*.

10. Which of the following is considered the diagnostic modality of choice for disk lesions, canal stenosis, and bony abnormalities?
   A. Radionuclide imaging
   B. Magnetic resonance imaging
   C. Myelogram
   D. Computed tomography

46
Pelvis and Thigh

Select the appropriate letter that correctly answers the question or completes the statement.

1. Avascular necrosis of the femoral head occurs most commonly after which of the following conditions?
   A. Acetabular fractures
   B. Femoral neck fractures
   C. Septic arthritis of the hip joint
   D. Congenital dislocation of the hip

2. The "Ortolani click test" is used in diagnosing:
   A. Slipped capital femoral epiphysis
   B. Avascular necrosis of the femoral head
   C. Congenital dilocation of the hip
   D. Acetabular fractures

3. The differential diagnosis of a mass lateral to the femoral vessels includes which of the following?
   A. Femoral hernia
   B. Iliopectineal bursitis
   C. Psoas abscess
   D. All of the above

4. A 24-year-old football player comes to the ED with a tender and swollen area over his anterolateral mid-thigh on the right. The patient states he was hit hard in that area 3 or 4 weeks ago, but he continued with his normal workouts. He is concerned because the injury doesn't seem to be improving. The most likely diagnosis is:
   A. Gluteus medius muscle strain
   B. Ilopectineal bursitis
   C. Traumatic periostitis of the iliac crest
   D. Myositis ossificans

5. All of the following statements are true *except*:
   A. Posterior hip dislocations are more common than anterior hip dislocations.
   B. The most common pelvic fractures are fractures of the pubic rami or the pubic bone.
   C. Anterior pelvic fractures are associated with more extensive hemorrhage than posterior pelvic fractures.
   D. The most common visceral injury seen with pelvic fractures is to the lower urinary tract.

Match the items on the right with their associated items on the left.

6. A 25-year-old with a history of a hip dislocation that occurred in an auto accident. The patient now has pain in the groin, and restriction of internal rotation and abduction of the previously dislocated hip.

7. This is often attributed to a mild traumatic episode or a low-grade febrile illness such as tonsillitis or otitis media.

8. *Staphylococcus aureus* is the most common organism.

9. A 10-year-old with a normal temperature and the insidious onset of pain in his left hip that radiates down into the left thigh and knee.

10. A 3-year-old with a temperature of 38.4°C, pain and swelling of his left hip joint, and no history of trauma to the hip.

a. Transient synovitis of the hip
b. Septic arthritis of the hip joint
c. Avascular necrosis of the femoral head

47
Proximal Femur and Femoral Shaft

Select the appropriate letter that correctly answers the question or completes the statement.

1. Which one of the following statements is true?
   A. Fractures of the superior aspect of the femoral head occur with posterior dislocations of the hip.

B. Impaction forces often cause comminuted fractures of the femoral head.

C. Fracture of the acetabulum rules out fracture of the femoral head.

D. Avascular necrosis is a rare complication following fracture of the femoral head.

2. All of the following statements regarding femoral neck fractures are true *except*:

A. A history of major trauma is nearly always obtained.

B. Adduction, external rotation, and shortening are pathognomic of displaced fractures.

C. Patients with such fractures are often ambulatory.

D. Hip dislocaton may be seen in association with the fracture.

3. All of the following statements are true *except*:

A. Solitary fractures of the greater or lesser trochanters results from an avulsion injury.

B. Subtrochanteric fractures occur in younger patients than intertrochanteric fractures.

C. A Thomas splint should be applied to disphyseal femur fractures, especially if bone is protruding.

D. Subtrochanteric fractures cause significant blood loss.

4. With which of the following can distal femoral fracture be associated?

A. Hip fracture or dislocation ipsilaterally

B. Vascular injury

C. Peroneal nerve injury

D. All of the above

Match the items on the right with their associated items on the left.

5. A 12-year-old with a history of strain to the right hip approximately 3 weeks ago. The patient is still limping and is complaining of right hip pain. Internal rotation of the hip is restricted.

a. Slipped capital femoral epiphysis

b. Tranient synovitis of the hip

c. Septic arthritis of the hip joint

d. Avascular necrosis of the femoral head

6. X-rays should include anterior views of both hips and lateral views taken in a "frog-leg" position (hip flexed 90° and abducted 45°).

48
Knee and Lower Leg

Select the appropriate letter that correctly answers the question or completes the statement.

1. Any disruption for the quadriceps mechanism requires:

A. Casting only for complete disruption

B. Casting for partial disruption

C. Surgical repair for partial or complete disruption

D. Nonweight-bearing only

2. A child with no history of trauma has an insidious onset of infrapatellar pain. Of the following, which is the most likely diagnosis?

A. Anserine bursitis

B. Baker's cyst

C. Osgood-Schlatter disease

D. Popliteal artery aneurysm

3. A patient complains of a painful swelling of his right knee. He states the swelling is sometimes very pronounced and painful, and other times he barely feels anything. You find a tense fluid-filled sac palpable in the popliteal fossa. This most likely represents:

A. Inflammation of the semimembranous or medial gastrocnemius bursa *Baker's cyst*

B. Anserine bursitis

C. Tibial artery aneurysm

D. Gouty arthritis

4. You diagnose a patient as having prepatelar bursitis following knee trauma. After several days of rest, immobilization, local heat, and antiinflammatory drugs the patient returns complaining of increasing swelling and pain. You would:

A. Aspirate fluid and send for appropriate studies

B. Reassure the patient that this is to be expected

C. Work-up for deep venous thrombosis

D. X-ray to check for ostomyelitis and if negative reassure the patient

5. A young female high school athlete complains of bilateral poorly localized knee pain. She states she just began training again after a period of inactivity and denies any trauma. The pain is worse when she climbs stairs. The patella compresion test is positive. This is consistent with:

A. Chondromalacia patella

B. Osgood-Schlatter disease

C. Baker's cyst

D. Anserine bursitis

6. All of the following statements are true _except_:
   A. Traumatic rupture of the gastrocnemius or soleus muscle requires surgical repair.
   B. Regarding tibial fractures, the presence of strong distal pulses excludes the possibility of a compartment syndrome.
   C. Patients with rupture of the plantaris tendon may be treated with splinting and immobilization.
   D. Stress fractures involve the fibula more often than the tibia.

49
Ankle and Foot

Select the appropriate letter that correctly answers the question or completes the statement.
1. A patient with a second-degree sprain would have all of the following _except_:
   A. Moderate flexion loss
   B. Swelling and local hemorrhage
   C. A partial ligamentous tear
   D. Initially no pain, then increasing pain
2. A patient complains of insidious onset of burning pain well measured on plantar surface of foot. The pain radiates superiorly along the medial side of the calf and rest decreases the pain. This suggests:
   A. Tarsal tunnel syndrome
   B. Tenosynovitis of extensor digitorum longus
   C. Cuboid ligament sprain
   D. Plantar fascitis
3. Nondisplaced third distal phalangeal fracture of the foot should be treated as follows:
   A. Cast to ankle
   B. Internal fixation
   C. Dynamic splinting
   D. Open toe orthopedic shoe

50
Osteomyelitis

Select the appropriate letter that correctly answers the question or completes the statement.
1. Which of the following patients are at risk for osteomyelitis caused by gram-negative organisms?
   A. Intravenous drug abusers
   B. Sickle cell anemia patients
   C. Patients with chronic osteomyelitis
   D. None of the above
   E. A and B
   F. A, B, and C

2. Which of the following patients are at risk for Pseudomonas osteomyelitis?
   A. A patient with osteomyelitis of the foot
   B. Osteomyelitis secondary to cat bites
   C. Osteomyelitis secondary to a wound with fresh water contamination
   D. A 3-year-old with acute hematogenous osteomyelitis
   E. A patient with diabetic foot osteomyelitis

51
Foreign Bodies

Select the appropriate letter that correctly answers the question or completes the statement.
1. A 25-year-old man comes to the ED complaining that he got something in his eye. After a thorough examination of his eye including fluorescein, you disgnose a corneal abrasion. Your treatment should be:
   A. Instillation of a topical antimicrobial and a prescription for antibiotic eye drops to be instilled every 4 hours, oral pain medication, and referral to an ophthalmologist the next day
   B. Instillation of a short-acting cycloplegic agent and a local anesthetic, a patch for 24 hours, and oral pain medication
   C. Instillation of a topical antimicrobial and a short-acting cycloplegic agent, and eye patch for 24 hours, and a referral to an ophthalmologist the next day
   D. Immediate ophthalmologic consultation
2. Which of the following methods should be used to remove a foreign body from the ear canal?
   A. Suction
   B. Removal with forceps
   C. Irrigation
   D. Any of the above
3. What symptoms are typical in patients who have aspirated a foreign body?
   A. Pneumonia, cough, and fever
   B. Wheezing, rhonchi, and stridor
   C. Absent breath sounds in one lung field and being short-of breath
   D. All of the above
4. A person with foreign body aspiration and complete airway obstruction is initially:
   A. Conscious and able to speak
   B. Unconscious and voiceless
   C. Conscious and voiceless
   D. Unconscious and stridorous

5. Regarding gastrointestinal foreign bodies, all of the following are true, *except*:
   A. Glucagon (0.5–2.0 mg) may be useful in the treatment of esophageal foreign bodies.
   B. Enzymatic degradation of impacted meat boluses in the esophagus should be the first treatment.
   C. Esophogeal disk batteries should be removed immediately.
   D. Chelation therapy may be required in patients who ingest disk batteries.

52
Animal Bites and Rabies

Select the appropriate letter that correctly answers the question or completes the statement.

1. Recommendations for tetanus prophylaxis include all of the following *except*:
   A. Tetanus-prone wounds require a booster dose of toxoid if more than 5 years has elapsed since the last dose.
   B. Tetanus prophylaxis is contraindicated during the first trimester of pregnancy.
   C. Tetanus immune globulin, 500 units, may be given for severe tetanus-prone wounds in persons not adequately immunized.
   D. If the patient has had 3 or more injections of tetanus toxoid, tetanus immune globulin is not necessary even if 10 years has elapsed since the last booster.

2. Which one of the following statements is true regarding the management of human bites?
   A. Lacerations should never be closed primarily, even if they involve the face.
   B. Penicillin is the drug of choice for human bite wound prophylaxis because of the preponderance of anaerobes in human mouth flora.
   C. Human bites of the hand that involve infection of deeper structures require parenteral antibiotics and intensive local surgical care.
   D. Judicious antibiotic prophylaxis may obviate the need for wound irrigation and debridement.

3. Bites of which of the following animals do not require antirabies prophylaxis?
   A. Bats   C. Rats
   B. Racoons   D. Skunks

4. All of the following statements are true regarding rabies *except*:
   A. Rabies has been reported in all states except Hawaii.
   B. The demonstration of Negri bodies is pathognomonic.
   C. Persons who work with farm animals are considered at risk for rabies and should be actively immunized.
   D. Postexposure treatment of rabies exposure requires both passive and active immunization.

53
Venomous Animal Injuries

Select the appropriate letter that correctly answers the question or completes the statement.

1. Appropriate treatment of venomous snakebites with envenomation includes all of the following *except*:
   A. Application of a loose tourniquet proximal to the bite
   B. Incision and suction if more than 1 hour from a medical facility
   C. Skin testing with antivenin prior to its administration only in patients with prior history of anaphylaxis
   D. Tetanus prophylaxis as indicated

2. All of the following statements regarding antivenin are true *except*:
   A. Antivenin injected around the bite area aids in venom neutralization and is thus indicated in most patients.
   B. Patients receiving more than 10 vials frequently develop serum sickness.
   C. The amount of antivenin required depends on the grade of envenomation.
   D. If no signs of envenomation develop within 4 hours, antivenin may be withheld and the patient discharged.

3. *Hymenoptera* stings and bites are common. Each of the following statements regarding them are true *except*:
   A. Subsequent fatalities are most commonly caused by toxic properties of the venom itself.
   B. Wasps and hornets can inflict multiple stings, while the *Hymenoptera* species is capable of a single sting only.
   C. Patients allergic to *Hymenoptera* stings should consider carrying bee sting kits.
   D. Evidence of a systemic reaction to *Hymenoptera* stings is an indication for skin testing and desensitization.

4. Which of the following statements is true regarding venomous marine animals?
   A. Bites occurring in the water do not require tetanus prophylaxis.
   B. Few deaths following marine animal envenomations are from drowning. Most are caused by toxic effects of the venom.
   C. Nematocysts may be fixed with formalin or alcohol before removal.
   D. Antivenin is available for most types of marine envenomations.

54
Soft-tissue Infections

Select the appropriate letter that correctly answers the question or completes the statement.

1. All of the following are characteristics of *Haemophilus influenzae* cellulitis *except*:
   A. Fever
   B. WBC count greater than 15,000
   C. Significant incidence of postive blood cultures
   D. A predilection for involving the extremities
   E. None of the above

2. Which of the following statements is true regarding impetigo?
   A. Impetigo may cause rheumatic fever.
   B. Poststreptococcal glomerulonephritis follows impetigo less frequently than streptococcal pharyngitis.
   C. Impetigo contagiosa may cause poststreptococcal glomerulonephritis.
   D. Bullous impetigo may cause poststreptococcal glomerulonephritis.

3. In which of the following cases may an abscess be sterile?
   A. Hidraderitis suppurativa
   B. Bartholin cyst
   C. Cutaneous abscess secondary to parenteral drug abuse
   D. Pilonidal abscess
   E. Perirectal abscess

55
Parasitology

Match the infective agent on the right with the disease on the left:

D	1. Swimmer's itch	A. *Anopheles* mosquito
F	2. Schistosomiasis	B. Tsetse fly
A	3. Malaria	C. Nematode microfilaira
B	4. Trypanosomiasis	
C	5. Elephantiasis	D. Ovarian schistosome
G	6. Chagas' disease	E. Flagellated protozoa
E	7. Giardiasis	F. Blood fluke
		G. Treatmid bug

Select the appropriate letter that correctly answers the question or completes the statement.

8. All of the following are consistent with the diagnosis of malaria, *except*:
   A. Drug of choice mebendazole
   B. History of shaking chills followed by fever
   C. Prior contact with *Anopheles* mosquito
   D. Life-threatening complication is cerebral involvement

Match the finding on the right to the disease on the left:

B	9. Cysticercosis	A. Pernicious anemia
D	10. Hookworm	B. New onset seizure
A	11. Fish tapeworm	
E	12. Onchocerciasis	C. Small bowel obstruction
F	13. Chagas' disease	D. Iron deficiency anemia
C	14. Roundworm	E. Blindness
		F. Acute myocarditis

Select the appropriate letter that correctly answers the question or completes the statement.

15. Which of the following best decribes giardiasis?
    A. Can result in ascending cholangitis
    B. Can be treated with suramin
    C. Can result in rectal prolapse in young children
    D. Can be associated with the "gay bowel syndrome"

16. Trichinosis is characterized by all of the following, *except*:
    A. Can be seen migrating through the subconjunctival tissue
    B. Caused from ingestion of undercooked pork
    C. Larval are found in striated skeletal and cardiac muscle
    D. Can be treated with thiabendazole and steroids

56
Common Ophthalmologic Problems

Select the appropriate letter that correctly answers the question or completes the statement.

1. Before dilating a patient's eye by pharmacologic means, one should routinely:
   A. Check pressures with tonometry
   B. Check pupillary reactivity
   C. Check anterior chamber depth
   D. Check for corneal abrasions
   E. Both *B* and *C*
2. True ophthalmologic emergencies require immediate initiation of therapy, often before even consulting with an ophthalmologist. Which one of the following is such an emergency?
   A. Central retinal vein occlusion
   B. Perforating globe injuries
   C. Temporal arteritis
   D. Central retinal artery occlusion   *Caustic burns*
3. Of the following, which can remain painless for 4 to 6 or more hours after the initial insult?
   A. A hot speck of metal penetrating the eye
   B. A contact lens worn improperly
   C. An arc welder who does not wear goggles and suffers ultraviolet damage to cornea
   D. All of the above
4. All patients should have visual acuity documented on the chart before detailed eye exam *except*:
   A. Alkali burns to eye
   B. Central retinal vein occlusion
   C. Patients who wear corrective lenses but did not bring them
   D. Acute angle closure glaucoma
5. Which conditions should topical steroids be used in the ED for?
   A. Herpes simplex infections
   B. Allergic conjunctivitis *+ zoster*
   C. Increased intraocular pressure
   D. Fungal infections
6. Which of the following statements about eye patches is true?
   A. They immobilize the lid preventing blinking.
   B. They cannot be worn for more than 4 hours. *≥ hrs*
   C. They should be periodically changed by the patient if infection is present.
   D. All of the above are true.
7. A 24-year-old woman without significant medical history complains of sudden bilateral visual loss. On examination you find no light perception or visual acuity and she has normal pupillary respon-

ses and normal funduscopic examination. The most likely diagnosis is:
   A. Temporal arteritis
   B. Vitreous hemorrhage
   C. Central retinal artery occlusion
   D. Hysteria
8. How are corneal ulcers best treated?
   A. Steroids and eye patching
   B. Culture drainage if any, then treat
   C. Ophthalmology consult at time of presentation
   D. All of the above
9. A rust ring will form in the cornea when metallic foreign bodies are present. How is this treated?
   A. It should be dissolved chemically.
   B. It requires immediate buffing before the rust infiltrates into deeper corneal layers.
   C. Appropriate management can be ophthalmologic follow-up in 24 to 48 hours.
   D. The rust ring will generally degenerate on its own and require only observation.
10. Of the following, which lid injury does not necessarily require ophthalmologic consultation?
    A. Lid lacerations associated with lid hematoma
    B. A laceration involving the lid margin
    C. Laceration of the medial one-sixth of the lid
    D. Protruding fat through laceration involving orbital septum
11. Of the following signs, which would suggest globe rupture?
    A. Hyphema
    B. Abnormally deep anterior chamber and soft eye to palpation
    C. Abnormally shallow anterior chamber and decreased visual acuity
    D. All of the above

57
Dental Emergencies

Select the appropriate letter that correctly answers the question or completes the statement.

1. A 28-year-old female underwent a third molar extraction for pericoronitis. She presents 3 days later with a sudden onset of excruciating pain over the mandibular extraction site accompanied by foul-smelling breath. The most likely diagnosis is:
   A. Alveolar osteitis   *dry socket*
   B. Recurrent pericoronitis
   C. Mandibular osteomyelitis
   D. Gingival abscess

2. Ludwig's angina is a bilateral board-like swelling involving the following space(s).
   A. Submental and submandibular
   B. Submental and sublingual
   C. Submental
   D. Sublingual
   E. Submandibular
   F. Submental, sublingual, and submandibular
3. For which of the following cases of dental trauma is treatment most urgently needed?
   A. Ellis Class I fracture
   B. Ellis Class II fracture
   C. Ellis Class III fracture
   D. Alveolar fracture
   E. Avulsion of a permanent tooth

58
Upper Respiratory Tract Infection

Select the appropriate letter that correctly answers the question or completes the statement.

1. All of the following are associated with peritonsillar abscesses *except*:
   A. Ipsilateral otalgia
   B. Odynophagia
   C. Trismus
   D. Submandibular indentation
   E. Uvular displacement
2. Which of the following is true about cellulitis of the floor of the mouth?
   A. It usually requires surgical intervention.
   B. Penicillin is the drug of choice.
   C. Diagnosis is often subtle and easily missed.
   D. Intubation may precipitate larynogospasm and respiratory arrest.
   E. All of the above
3. All of the following are advantages to treating presumed streptococcal pharyngitis with penicillin without awaiting culture results, *except*:
   A. Early treatment will shorten the duration of illness.
   B. Early treatment will decrease transmission of the illness.
   C. It will decrease the incidence of suppurative complications.
   D. Throat cultures are falsely negative in at least 10% of cases.
   E. All of the above
4. All of the following put the patient at increased risk for streptococcal pharyngitis, *except*:
   A. Age 5–20 years
   B. Crowded living conditions
   C. Late winter, early spring season
   D. Household contact with positive strep
   E. Prior history of strep pharyngitis
5. All of the following are true regarding the treatment of streptococcal pharyngitis, *except*:
   A. If treated on clinical grounds, a throat culture is not necessary.
   B. Treatment does not prevent subsequent acute glomerulonephritis.
   C. Any patient who has had a single attack of acute rheumatic fever should be on long-term prophylaxis with penicillin.
   D. Group B streptococcus has never been shown to be resistant to penicillin.
   E. Untreated carriers of streptococcus acquire a specific M-type immunity, which is prevented by treatment with penicillin.
6. All of the following increase the likelihood of streptococcal pharyngitis in a child, *except*:
   A. Temperature over 101°F
   B. Sore throat without other symptoms
   C. Tonsillar exudates
   D. Anterior cervical adenopathy
   E. All of the above
7. All of the following are possible complications of infectious mononucleosis, *except*:
   A. Upper airway obstruction
   B. Splenic rupture
   C. Hemolysis and thrombocytopenia
   D. Encephalitis
   E. All of the above
8. All of the following are true about *Corynebacterium diphtheriae*, *except*:
   A. It is often marked submandibular anterior neck adenopathy.
   B. Pharyngeal membrane is firmly fixed to underlying tissue.
   C. Temperatures are usually low grade.
   D. It can produce sudden airway obstruction.
   E. Treatment should await laboratory confirmation.
9. Which of the following would *not* be expected as a cause of pharyngitis?
   A. *Hemophilus influenzae*
   B. Epstein-Barr virus
   C. *Candida*
   D. *Neisseria gonorrhoeae*
   E. All of the above
10. A previously healthy 32-year-old construction worker presents with a 4-day history of the worst sore throat "I've had in my whole life." He was seen elsewhere 2 days ago and started on oral penicillin without effect. He is otherwise healthy and has no dental or ENT work done. Physical examination reveals a temperature of 101°F. His pharynx is

slightly red without tonsillar swelling or exudates. There is no adenopathy noted. He is not hoarse but his voice sounds muffled. The most appropriate next step for him would be:
A. Throat culture
B. Monospot
C. White blood cell count
D. Soft tissue neck film
E. Change penicillin to erythromycin

11. All of the following are true concerning Ludwig's angina, *except*:
A. Major cause of death is sudden and unpredictable airway occlusion.
B. Most patients require surgical decompression.
C. Attempted intubation may precipitate respiratory arrest.
D. Broad spectrum antibiotics including an aminoglycoside are usually required.
E. Most patients have an underlying chronic debilitating disease.

12. Which of the following statements is true regarding gonococcal pharyngitis?
A. It can be diagnosed by Gram's stain.
B. Spectinomycin is the treatment of choice.
C. It usually presents as a nonspecific sore throat.
D. It may progress to disseminated gonococcemia.
E. It is usually the only site of gonococcal infection.

13. A 22-year-old presents to the emergency department complaining of a rash. It started 2 days after being started on ampicillin for a sore throat. The rash is nonpuritic maculopapular and extends over the entire trunk. The most likely etiology of this rash is:
A. Scarlet fever
B. Allergic reaction to ampicillin
C. Infectious mononucleosis
D. Viral exanthem
E. Acute rheumatic fever

14. Tonsillar exudate, pharyngeal erythema, fever, and lymphadenopathy may all be seen in:
A. Streptococcal pharyngitis
B. Mononucleosis
C. Diphtheria
D. Gonococcal pharyngitis
E. All of the above

15. A 26-year-old factory worker complains of sore throat for 4 to 5 days, headache, difficulty swallowing, and fever to 101°F. He has had "strep throat" in the past and has had all of his immunizations. Physical examination reveals temperature 100°F, bilateral lymph nodes and adherent bluish tonsillar/palatal exudate that bleeds when removed. Proper management would be:
A. Throat culture, oral penicillin, discharge instructions to return if worse

B. Specify culture on Bordet-Gengou medium, ECG, discharge on penicillin
C. Hospitalization, IV penicilin, and proper throat culture
D. Hospitalization, penicillin, cardiac monitoring, diphtheria antitoxin

16. Which of the following is true regarding throat cultures in patients with pharyngitis?
A. A person with a negative throat culture does not have streptococcal pharyngitis.
B. A person with a positive culture has streptococcal pharyngitis.
C. *Streptococcus* can be cultured in at least 25% of asymptomatic children during winter months.
D. Any patient with a positive culture is at risk for developing acute rheumatic fever.
E. All of the above are true.

17. All of the following regarding prevertebral space infection are true *except*:
A. It is usually not associated with significant swelling of the neck.
B. It is often confused with a retropharyngeal abscess.
C. Fever is low grade and toxicity rare.
D. The usual source is hematogenous dissemination.
E. Lateral neck films usually show retropharyngeal swelling.

18. All of the following statements are true *except*:
A. Peritonsillar abscess is uncommon under 12 years of age.
B. Retropharyngeal abscess is most common under 3 years of age.
C. The key observation in peritonsillar abscess is medial displacement of the uvula and tonsil.
D. The patient preferring to lie prone suggests retropharyngeal abscess.
E. Virtually all cases of significant retropharyngeal abscess are associated with soft tissue swelling and forward displacement of the larynx.

19. You are evaluating a patient with acute pharyngitis. All of the following would make infectious mononucleosis more likely than streptococcal pharyngitis *except*:
A. Posterior cervical adenopathy
B. Splenomegaly
C. Age over 20
D. Fever less than 101°F
E. Conjunctivitis

20. What is the most important aspect of the treatment of *Corynebacterium diphtheriae*?
A. High dose penicillin
B. Antitoxin
C. Early intubation
D. Corticosteroids
E. All of the above

21. What is the most effective drug to treat streptococcal pharyngitis in a penicillin-allergic patient?
   A. Tetracycline
   B. Erythromycin
   C. Ampicillin
   D. Sulfonamides
   E. None of the above

22. All of the following statements about poststreptococcal rheumatic fever are true *except*:
   A. The incidence of rheumatic fever correlates directly with the amount of crowding and indirectly with comprehensive medical care.
   B. Because Group A *Streptococcus* is so sensitive to penicillin, acute rheumatic fever could be eliminated if all sore throats were appropriately treated.
   C. The attack rate for rheumatic fever after an epidemic of untreated streptococcal pharyngitis is 3%
   D. Treatment initiated within 5 days of the onset of symptoms will completely protect against rheumatic fever, although treatment as late as 10 days is of definite value.
   E. Acute rheumatic fever occurs 3 weeks after a streptococcal pharyngitis.

23. A previously healthy 22-year-old nonsmoker has a 3- to 4-day history of a nonproductive cough and a sore throat associated with a low-grade fever. He is noted to have bullous myringitis and a very few scattered rales on chest examination. The chest x-ray film shows patchy alveolar infiltrates of both lower lobes. The most likely pathogen is:
   A. *Haemophilus influenzae*
   B. Epstein-Barr virus
   C. *Mycoplasma pneumoniae*
   D. Rhinovirus
   E. *Actinomycosis*

24. Which of the following is true of acute epiglottitis in the adult?
   A. Patients rarely complain of dysphagia.
   B. There is prominent anterior cervical adenopathy.
   C. Pain in throat is disproportionate to objective signs of pharyngitis.
   D. Patients are usually hoarse.
   E. All of the above are true.

59
Sinusitis

Select the appropriate letter that correctly answers the question or completes the statement.

1. Which organisms are more commonly associated with chronic sinusitis than with acute sinusitis?
   A. *Hemophilus influenzae*
   B. *Streptococcus pneumoniae*
   C. *Streptococcus pyogenes*
   D. *Neisseria catarrhalis*
   E. Anaerobic streptococcus

2. The most accurate clinical indicator of acute sinusitis is:
   A. Appropriate history
   B. Tenderness to percussion over the sinus
   C. Purulent discharge from beneath the turbinates
   D. Opacification of sinus to transillumination
   E. Fever associated with facial pain radiating to the ear

3. Appropriate treatment of acute sinusitis should include all of the following, *except*:
   A. Ampicillin, 500 mg, 4 times daily
   B. Dexbrompheniramine (Drixoral) 3 times daily
   C. Oxymetazoline (Afrin) spray for 3 days only
   D. Nasal culture

4. A 55-year-old woman with a history of poorly controlled diabetes complains of right maxillary pain and facial tenderness. Physical examination reveals an oral temperature of 101°F, nasal mucosal congestion, and a dark nasal discharge. In addition to checking her blood sugar, the most appropriate treatment would be:
   A. Antibiotics and decongestants on an empiric basis with follow-up in 3 days
   B. Obtain sinus x-rays and if positive discharge on antibiotics and decongestants with follow-up in 3 days
   C. Obtain x-rays and if positive be admitted with urgent ENT referral
   D. Obtain x-rays and if positive to the OR for debridement

5. All of the following are true of cavernous sinus thrombosis *except*:
   A. It is characterized by third and sixth cranial nerve palsies.
   B. It usually occurs from extension of a sinusitis.
   C. The patients often have a low-grade temperature and may not appear toxic.
   D. Involvement is most often unilateral.
   E. Surgical intervention has not been shown to decrease morbidity or mortality.

6. The two most common pathogens in acute sinusitis are *Streptococcus pneumoniae* and:
   A. *Streptococcus pyogenes*
   B. *Staphylococcus aureus*
   C. *Hemophilus influenzae*
   D. *Neisseria catarrhalis*
   E. *Corynebacterium diphtheriae*

7. All of the following are true of sinusitis *except*:
   A. Obstruction to drainage is the etiology of both acute and chronic sinusitis.
   B. Culture of nasal swabs can be expected to yield pathogenic organism.

C. There is no correlation between antral leukocyte counts and chronic sinusitis.

D. An antral aspirate with a leukocyte count over 5,000 correlates well with acute sinusitis.

E. There is a lack of correlation of classic signs and symptoms with true infection.

8. Which of the following is true of Rhinocerebral phycomycosis?

A. Caused by anaerobic gram-negative organism

B. Characterized by a lack of intense inflammation

C. Seen most often in patients with underlying systemic disease

D. May cause cosmetic deformity but is rarely fatal

E. Is fairly common but usually unrecognized

60
Acute Bronchitis

Select the appropriate letter that correctly answers the question or completes the statement.

1. All of the following statements are true except:

A. Hemoptysis is uncommon in acute bronchitis.

B. Acute bronchitis is the leading cause of hemoptysis.

C. Coryza is commonly associated with both viral and bacterial bronchitis.

D. The development of purulent yellow or green sputum correlates with the presence of bacterial superinfection.

E. In most patients with tuberculosis, tuberculin positivity does not occur until 6 weeks after infection. 2 wks

2. All of the following are true about amantadine for influenza except:

A. It is only effective prophylactically.

B. It is comparable in efficacy to vaccination.

C. It is only effective against influenza A.

D. Its side effects include depression and congestive heart failure.

E. It is also used to treat Parkinsons' disease.

3. Influenza has a fairly typical course. Which of the following statements is incorrect?

A. The incubation period is 24–72 hours.

B. Acute illness lasts 24–36 hours. 2-6 days

C. Weakness and malaise may persist up to 3–4 weeks.

D. Viral pneumonia may be present.

4. Irritant bronchitis and allergic bronchitis have which component in common?

A. Both may develop chronic recurrent bronchitis.

B. Precipitating cough is the same.

C. Cortical steroid therapy is the standard mode of treatment.

D. None of the above

5. Which of the following is true of pneumomediastinum, a potential complication following vigorous coughing?

A. It may be associated with "crunching" heart sounds.

B. It is easy to recognize radiographically.

C. It is associated with pleuritic chest pain.

D. It is rarely associated with subcutaneous emphysema.

6. Physical examination of the patient with a cough should always include pulse, temperature, and respiratory rate. Which of the following statements is *not* true about the vital signs?

A. Absence of fever is a reliable indicator of the absence of pneumonia.

B. An increased respiratory rate may be a sign of early respiratory failure.

C. Increased respiratory rate may be benign.

D. An increased pulse merits investigation.

7. Indications for chest x-ray in a patient who presents with bronchitic symptoms include all of the following except:

A. Unexplained fever

B. Symptoms persisting for 3–5 days   >2 wks

C. Asymmetric breath sounds

D. Mediastinal crunch

8. Chest x-ray findings typical of bronchitic patients include:

A. Elevation of the diaphragm

B. Unilateral hilar adenopathy

C. Normal or slightly increased bronchopulmonary markings

D. Widened mediastinum

9. In regard to the treatment of bronchitis, which of the following is *not* true:

A. Oral hydration is the mainstay of nonpharmacologic therapy.

B. The most cost-effective expectorant is acetylcysteine.

C. It has been difficult to prove that antibiotics are useful in the treatment of bronchitis.

D. Bacterial species most commonly encountered in sputum are *S. pneumoniae*, and *H. influenza*.

10. Which of the following statements is true?

A. The pathologic hallmark of viral infection is mucorrhea.

B. Purulent secretions are commonly seen with a purely viral infection.

C. The most common pathogens found in purulent bronchitis are *S. pneumoniae* and *Klebsiella*. H flu

D. In the usual adult syndrome of adult bronchitis, high fever may be present.

61
Pneumonia

Select the appropriate letter that correctly answers the question or completes the statement.

1. A 50-year-old white woman with a 1-week history of upper respiratory infection symptoms has a sudden onset of fever, chills, and sweating, along with rusty-colored sputum. The most likely diagnosis is:
   A. *Streptococcus pneumoniae*
   B. *Hemophilus influenzae*
   C. *Mycoplasma*
   D. Influenza virus
   E. *Klebsiella pneumoniae*

2. A 25-year-old IV drug abuser with sudden onset of fever, chills, and sweating complains of shortness of breath for the last 24 hours. Chest x-ray film shows pneumatoceles. The most likely diagnosis is:
   A. *Streptococcus pneumoniae*
   B. *Hemophilus influenzae*
   C. *Klebsiella*
   D. Group B *Streptococcus*
   E. *Staphylococcus aureus*

3. A 30-year-old homosexual man with a known history of AIDS now with a 2-day history of nonproductive cough and fever. A chest x-ray reveals left lower lobe, fluffy infiltrates. What test would be most helpful in facilitating a diagnosis?
   A. Induced expectorated sputum for Gram's stain and C & S
   B. Induced expectorated sputum for acid fast stain and culture
   C. Blood cultures
   D. Transtracheal aspirate for specimen analysis
   E. Transthoracic needle aspiration

4. A previously healthy 40-year-old white man has a history of cough, sputum production, and one episode of severe shakes and sweats. Physical examination reveals a temperature of 101.5°F and a "non-toxic" looking apppearance. Chest x-ray film shows right middle lobe consolidation. Sputum Gram's stain shows gram-positive diplococci and white cells. The treatment of choice is:
   A. Start on IV penicillin 600,000 units every 6 hours and admit to hospital
   B. Oral penicillin VK 500 mg every 6 hours for 10 days and discharge
   C. IV pencillin 1.2 million units every 6 hours and admit to hospital
   D. Keflex 500 mg every 6 hours for 10 days and discharge
   E. IV aminoglycoside and ampicillin and admit to hospital

5. What is the most common cause of pneumonia in an immune compromised patient?
   A. *Hemophilus influenzae*
   B. *Klebsiella*
   C. *Pseudomonas*
   D. *Streptococcus pneumoniae*
   E. *Pneumocystis carinii*

6. All of the following are true about Legionnaires' disease *except*:
   A. It is caused by a gram-negative organism.
   B. Diarrhea is often a prominent part of the symptom complex.
   C. It usually occurs in winter months.
   D. The cough is usually nonproductive.
   E. Chest x-ray film shows a patchy alveolar infiltrate that may progress to cavitation.

7. Of the following, the laboratory test most likely to be positive in a patient with *Mycoplasma* pneumonia is:
   A. Sputum culture
   B. Sputum Gram's stain
   C. Cold agglutinins
   D. Blood culture
   E. Elevated white blood cell count

8. What is the most effective treatment for a suspected case of *Mycoplasma* pneumonia?
   A. Ampicillin 500 mg 4 times/day
   B. Cephalothin 500 mg 4 times/day
   C. Erythromycin 500 mg 4 times/day
   D. Tetracycline 500 mg 4 times/day
   E. Trimethoprim-sulfamethoxazole 160–800 mg 2 times/day

9. What is the best antimicrobial agent to treat Legionnaires' disease?
   A. Ampicillin
   B. Gentimycin
   C. Erythromycin
   D. Chloramphenicol
   E. Carbenicillin

10. A 45-year-old alcoholic has a sudden onset of fever with a single shaking chill. He is complaining of shortness of breath and producing purulent blood-tinged sputum. He has a temperature of 103°F, respiratory rate of 40, and pulse 140. Chest x-ray film shows lobar consolidation of the right lower lobe with an air bronchogram. WBC count is 19,000, and gram-positive lancet shaped diplococci are identified. He is allergic to penicillin. The most effective treatment for this patient would be:
    A. Erythromycin
    B. Cefoxitin
    C. Chloramphenicol
    D. Ampicillin
    E. Tetracycline

Match the items on the right with their associated items on the left. Each answer may be used once, more than once, or not at all.

_c_ 11. *Streptococcus pneumoniae*

_d_ 12. *Streptococcus aureus*

_b_ 13. *Hemophilus influenzae*

_e_ 14. *Legionella pneumoniae*

_e_ 15. *Mycoplasma pneumoniae*

a. Small bipolar gram-negative rods
b. Mixed gram-positive and gram-negative rods
c. Gram-positive diplococci
d. Gram-positive cocci in clumps
e. Negative Gram's stain

Select the appropriate letter that correctly answers the question or completes the statement.

16. Which of the following statements about pneumonia is _not_ true?
    A. Early pneumococcal pneumonia lacks physical or radiographic signs.
    B. Streptococcal pneumonia often shows abscess formation on chest x-ray at an early stage.
    C. Legionnaires' disease is an opportunistic disease process occurring in immunosuppressed patients.
    D. Most viral pneumonias are mild, self-limited, and without permanent sequellae.

17. Which one of the following patients with a pneumonia may need admission to the hospital for adequate therapy?
    A. Extensive pulmonary disease
    B. Sepsis
    C. Age greater than 60
    D. Lives alone
    E. Cavitating or necrotizing process
    F. All of the above

18. Which of the following statements is _not_ true regarding *pneumocystis carinii* pneumonia?
    A. The immunocompromised host with pneumocystis carinii is probably at greatest risk for a fatal outcome.
    B. Rapidly progressing pneumonia can occur in the face of a normal chest x-ray and physical examination.
    C. Early signs and symptoms correlate well with radiographic findings.
    D. The patients usually have fever, tachycardia, and a nonproductive cough.

19. Percutaneous transtracheal aspiration (PTTA) may be very helpful in identifying lower respiratory tract pathogens. In which of the following situations would this technique be recommended?

A. Infections of nonbacterial cause
B. Suspected superinfection in an established pulmonary infection
C. Fever of unclear cause when pulmonary infection is not suspected
D. Exacerbation of chronic lung disease without radiographically apparent pulmonary infiltrate

62
Acute Bronchial Asthma

Select the appropriate letter that correctly answers the question or completes the statement.

1. All of the following are effects of theophylline _except_:
   A. Increases cellular cyclic-AMP
   B. Increases diaphragmatic contractility
   C. Promotes diuresis
   D. Increases cardiac contractility
   E. Stimulates gastric acid secretion

2. All of the following statements about severe bronchospasm are true _except_:
   A. Patient may develop wheezing with appropriate treatment.
   B. Arterial blood gases may deteroriate with appropriate treatment.
   C. FEV_1 would be expected to less than 700.
   D. Chest x-ray film will show scattered infiltrates.
   E. EKG may show right ventricular hypertrophy with strain.

3. All of the following are useful for managing asthma in a young child _except_:
   A. Epinephrine 0.01 ml/kg
   B. Aminophylline 5.6 mg/kg
   C. Methylprednisolone 1 mg/kg
   D. Epinephrine in thioglycolate (Sus-Phrine) 0.005 ml/kg
   E. Mist tent

4. All of the following are true regarding sympathomimetic agents in acute asthma _except_:
   A. They are the most effective bronchodilators.
   B. Aerosolized agents cause fewer side effects.
   C. Terbutaline looses it $beta_2$ specificity when given subcutaneously.
   D. Aerosolized metaproterenol has the longest duration of action.
   E. They should never be used intravenously.

5. Which of the following statements about the use of corticosteroids is true?
   A. There is a general consensus that early administration of steroids makes little difference in the outcome of severe asthma.
   B. An initial PEFR of less than 100 liters per minute with improvement of less than 60 liters per minute suggests that aggressive therapy is indicated including steroids.
   C. Steroids should not be used in patients receiving long-term steroid treatment whose asthma is worsening.
   D. There is no place in the treatment of acute asthma for inhaled high potency steroids.

6. Which of the following statements regarding pharmacologic agents used in the treatment of acute adult asthma is *not* true?
   A. There is no place for the use of narcotics, sedatives, or tranquilizers in the treatment of acute asthma.
   B. Mucolitic agents can cause significant improvement in acute asthma.
   C. Routine use of antibiotics in acute exacerbations of asthma is unwarranted.
   D. Antihistamines are generally ineffective in acute asthma.

7. Which of the following are significant problems with the uses of isoproterenol?
   A. Dysrhythmias, hypoxemia, long duration of action
   B. Tachycardia, intrapulmonary shunting, long duration of action
   C. Ventricular fibrillation, hypoxemia, short duration
   D. Bradyarrhythmias, long duration of action, intrapulmonary shunting

8. Extrinsic asthma is characterized by which of the following?
   A. Sensitivity to specific inhaled allergens and increased levels of IGE
   B. A fall in forced expiratory volume in one second (FEV_1) after 6–10 minutes of exercise
   C. Psychological factors mediating changes in airway caliber
   D. None of the above

9. Organize the following sets of arterial blood gases as to their likely progression from normal to acute respiratory failure secondary to asthma.
   1. pH 7.5, Po_2 84, Pco_2 28
   2. pH 7.25, Po_2 65, Pco_2 55
   3. pH 7.52, Po_2 70, Pco_2 28
   4. pH 7.42, Po_2 84, Pco_2 38
   5. pH 7.42, Po_2 65, Pco_2 42
   A. 4, 1, 2, 3, 5
   B. 4, 3, 1, 5, 2
   C. 4, 1, 3, 2, 5
   D. 4, 1, 3, 5, 2

10. Which of the following statements is true regarding the presence of pulsus paradoxus in asthmatics?
    A. In initial pulsus paradoxus of greater than 10 Torr indicates immediate need for in-patient treatment.
    B. A significant pulsus paradoxus occurs in over half of acute asthmatic episodes.
    C. A significant pulsus paradoxus usually specifies severe airway obstruction.
    D. A significant pulsus paradoxus tends to persist in spite of clinical improvement.

11. Which of the following arterial blood gases would suggest the most serious sequella in a patient with acute asthma?
    A. pH 7.56, Pao_2 70, $Paco_2$ 28
    B. pH 7.44, Pao_2 84, $Paco_2$ 35
    C. pH 7.38, Pao_2 65, $Paco_2$ 46
    D. pH 7.37, Pao_2 80, $Paco_2$ 38

12. The symptoms of acute asthma consist of a triad of which of the following?
    A. Orthopnea, wheezing, sputum production
    B. Cough, dyspnea, wheezing
    C. Dyspnea, wheezing, sputum production
    D. Cough, wheezing, rales

13. A brief history needed in assessing an asthmatic patient should include all of the following, *except*:
    A. Duration and onset of current attack
    B. Identifying and precipitating cause
    C. Exercise tolerance
    D. Previous requirements for hospitalization
    E. Present or previous requirements for steroids

14. Recently an index that incorporates both objective and subjective factors has been used in the emergency department to measure asthma severity and predict the outcome. Which of the following symptom complexes would qualify for hospital admission using this index?
    A. Moderate dyspnea, pulse 125, moderate wheezing, respiratory rate 24
    B. Moderate dyspnea, pulse 110, pulsus paradoxus greater than 20, respiratory rate 28
    C. Moderate wheezing, pulse 125, moderate dyspnea, respiratory rate 30
    D. Pulse 110, mild wheezing, severe dyspnea, respiratory rate 30

15. Which of the following is not true regarding the use of calcium channel blockers in acute asthma?
    A. Calcium channel blockers may decrease airway smooth muscle sensitivity to contractile agonists.
    B. Some calcium channel blockers have been shown to inhibit exercise-induced bronchospasm.
    C. Calcium channel blockers may reduce chemical mediator release from Mast cells.
    D. Newer calcium channel antagonists are specific for airway smooth muscle.

16. A 60-kg male smoker comes to the emergency department with an acute asthmatic attack. He is on a theophylline preparation at home and has a serum theophylline level in the department of 6. The most appropriate loading dose of aminophylline for him would be:
    A. 100 mg   D. 600 mg
    B. 200 mg   E. 700 mg
    C. 400 mg
17. The physical finding that correlates best with the severity of an asthma attack is:
    A. Respiratory rate
    B. Pulse rate
    C. Pulsus paradoxus
    D. Extent of wheezing
    E. Adventitious breath sounds
18. All of the following will decrease the clearance of theophylline and thus require a lower dose except:
    A. Smoking
    B. COPD
    C. Congestive heart failure
    D. Liver dysfunction
    E. Old age
19. Which of the following is true concerning asthma in the pregnant patient?
    A. Most asthmatics will become worse.
    B. Terbutaline can inhibit uterine contractions.
    C. Theophylline can cause fetal abnormalities.
    D. Steroids can cause fetal respiratory distress.
    E. All of the above are true.

63

Chronic Obstructive Pulmonary Diseases

Select the appropriate letter that correctly answers the question or completes the statement.

1. A patient with known chronic bronchitis develops a cough, fever, and becomes acutely confused. The family calls an ambulance and during a transport time of 30 minutes, they give the patient 10 L of oxygen via a mask. On arrival in the ED the patient is comatose. The arterial blood gas measurements you would most expect to find would be:
    A. PO_2 65, PCO_2 100, pH 7.2
    B. PO_2 50, PCO_2 50, pH 7.3
    C. PO_2 70, PCO_2 45, pH 7.32
    D. PO_2 90, PCO_2 30, pH 7.25
    E. PO_2 90, PCO_2 80, pH 7.25
2. All of the following are true about advanced chronic bronchitis except:
    A. Cough is often the predominant symptom.
    B. Cardiac output would be expected to be increased.
    C. It is often associated with polycythemia.
    D. It is sometimes mistakenly diagnosed as biventricular failure.
    E. Total minute ventilation is usually increased.
3. All of the following regarding treatment of COPD are true except:
    A. Glyceryl guaiacolate is the best clinical expectorant.
    B. Phlebotomy should be considered if the hematocrit is over 60.
    C. Bronchitic patients have been shown to benefit from long-term low-dose broad-spectrum antibiotics.
    D. Digitalis should be avoided unless left-sided dysfunction coexists.
    E. MucoMyst (acetylcysteine), a mucus thinning agent, can precipitate bronchospasm.
4. A 65-year-old patient with known severe mixed obstructive pulmonary disease and decompensated cor pulmonale comes to the ED with increasing shortness of breath and a productive cough. He is alert and can speak in short sentences but has a respiratory rate of 40. The best initial treatment would be:
    A. 40% mist mask
    B. Terbutaline subcutaneously
    C. 24% Venturi mask
    D. Immediate intubation
    E. IV aminophylline
5. A patient with COPD has severe cor pulmonale. What is the most effective means to relieve the pulmonary vascular hypertension?
    A. Aminophylline   D. Furosemide
    B. Oxygen   E. Propranolol
    C. Nitroprusside
6. The most common cause of decompensation in a stable patient with COPD is:
    A. Noncompliance with medication
    B. Congestive heart failure
    C. Pulmonary embolus
    D. Infection
    E. Environmental stress
7. All of the following are true about primary emphysema except:
    A. It is associated with irreversible destruction of pulmonary architecture.
    B. It may be caused by a hereditary enzyme deficiency.
    C. Cardiac output would be expected to be high.
    D. Patients better tolerate chronic bronchitis than emphysema.
    E. Loss of elastic recoil is a major source of decreased airflow.

8. Which of the following statements about aminophylline is *not* true?
   A. Most COPD patients warrant at least a therapeutic trial even in the absence of bronchospasm.
   B. Serious toxic effects (ventricular tachycardia, seizures) are frequently seen when drug levels reach 25-30 UG/ML.
   C. Aminophylline has been shown experimentally to reduce the fibrillation threshold.
   D. In the severe COPD patient, one must be relatively sure subtherapeutic theophylline levels are present before aminophylline is given.

9. Which of the following statements regarding the use of antibiotics in COPD is *not* true?
   A. Stage B or C patients with acute nonallergic bronchitis should be treated.
   B. All bronchitic patients should be considered for long-term prophylactic treatment.
   C. Numerous antibiotic regimens have not been shown to shorten episodes of acute bronchitis.
   D. The choice of broad-spectrum antibiotics should be made on the basis of drug safety, patient acceptance, and cost.

10. Which of the following statements regarding management of COPD is *not* true?
    A. The most important therapeutic modality in the emergency department is oxygen administration.
    B. Adequate ventilation and oxygenation can reverse severe respiratory acidosis and correct severe hypoxemia in less than 1 minute.
    C. Following restored oxygenation, the patient may cease spontaneous respirations.
    D. If intubation cannot be accomplished in 15 seconds, the attempt must be halted.

11. All the following statements about COPD are true, *except*:
    A. Therapy that is useful in asthmatic patients is not necessarily useful in the reactive airway component of COPD.
    B. It is generally possible to determine to what degree a given patient has reactive airway disease.
    C. Bronchodilators may have beneficial effects in patients without any reactive airway disease.
    D. Some drugs provide subjective relief of dyspnea with little or no objective improvement.

12. A 55-year-old man comes to the emergency department in acute respiratory distress. You order blood gases to determine the extent of hypoxemia and acid base disturbance. His pH is 7.20; PO_2 65; PCO_2 55. Using ACLS golden rule #1, what is the expected pH?
    A. 7.35   C. 7.52
    B. 7.10   D. 7.28

13. The electrocardiogram may give useful information in COPD patients. Which of the following statements is true?

A. A vertical QRS axis of minus 90 or greater correlates with chronic pulmonary disease.
B. Low QRS voltage, clockwise rotation, and poor R-wave progression are sensitive and specific findings for COPD.
C. The absence of criteria for right ventricular hypertrophy effectively rules out cor pulmonale.
D. The presence of "p-pulmonale" may be present with acute increases in right atrial pressure.

Match the answers on the left with the correct diagnoses on the right.

_D_ 14. Hypoxemia, hypercarbia, polycythemia
_B_ 15. Blood pressure normal or slightly elevated
_B_ 16. Retrosternal heave
_A_ 17. Near-normal blood gases
_A_ 18. Dyspnea is the hallmark
_A_ 19. Pulmonary cachexia
_A_ 20. Normal tissue oxygenation with severe air hunger
_B_ 21. Profound hypoxemia, little ventilation
_D_ 22. Cor pulmonale
_B_ 23. Frequently misdiagnosed as left ventricular failure

A. Pink puffer
B. Blue bloater
C. Neither
D. Both

Select the appropriate letter that correctly answers the question or completes the statement.

24. The two principle mechanisms of airway obstruction in reactive airway disease are which of the following?
    A. Pulmonary edema and bronchoconstriction
    B. Air trapping and mucus plugging
    C. Bronchoconstriction and mucus plugging
    D. Air trapping and right-to-left shunt

25. Which of the following statements regarding COPD is *not* true?
    A. Clouding of consciousness should always suggest carbon dioxide narcosis.
    B. The number of words expressible at one time can be a crude measurement of FEV_1.
    C. A "silent chest" to auscultation generally indicates improvement.
    D. Many patients are able to assess their degree of airway restriction better than their physicians.

26. Which of the following would *not* be considered subacute aggravating factors in COPD?
    A. Lobar atelectasis
    B. Pneumonia
    C. Pleural effusion
    D. Small pulmonary emboli

27. Which of the following drugs may directly or indirectly produce bronchospasm?
    A. Reserpine
    B. Opiates
    C. Aspirin
    D. Cholinergics
    E. All of the above

64
Pulmonary Embolus

Select the appropriate letter that correctly answers the question or completes the statement.

1. A 35-year-old obese woman with a history of birth control use and varicose veins comes to the ED after a 6-hour plane flight. You suspect pulmonary embolism from her symptoms. Which symptom complex would be *most* compatible with pulmonary embolism?
    A. Dyspnea, cough, hemoptysis
    B. Chest pain, cough, hemoptysis
    C. Chest pain, dyspnea, apprehension
    D. Shoulder pain, hemoptysis, syncope
    E. Cough, abdominal pain, apprehension
2. What are the *most* likely physical findings you would expect in the above patient?
    A. Tachypnea, increased pulmonic valve closure, heart murmur
    B. Increased pulmonic valve closure, localized rales, tachycardia
    C. Tachycardia, S_3 or S_4 gallop, increased pulmonic closure
    D. I-II/VI systolic ejection murmur loudest over the pulmonic valve region, friction rub, tachycardia
    E. Tachypnea, tachycardia, fever
3. An ECG is next obtained. Which would support your diagnosis of pulmonary embolism?
    A. $S_1Q_3T_3$ pattern
    B. Normal ECG
    C. Left or right axis deviation
    D. Nonspecific ST-TW changes
    E. All of the above
4. Which of the following statements best describes pulmonary angiography versus ventilation/perfusion (V/Q) scans?
    A. A normal V/Q scan essentially rules out pulmonary embolism.
    B. V/Q scans are specific for pulmonary embolism.
    C. V/Q scans are not affected by asthma, CHF, or pleural effusions.
    D. Pulmonary angiograms are more sensitive than V/Q scans for pulmonary embolism.

5. Which of the following is the most common radiographic finding of a pulmonary emboli?
    A. Elevated hemidiaphragm
    B. Pleural-based wedge-shaped density
    C. Diminished peripheral vascularity
    D. Dilated pulmonary artery
    E. Segmental area of radiolucency
6. You are called to the floor to attend a patient admitted with a bleeding peptic ulcer who has just been given 10,000 units of heparin because of a medication error. The most effective treatment at this time would be:
    A. Observe the patient for any increased bleeding
    B. Administer 6 units of fresh-frozen plasma
    C. Administer 6 bags of platelets
    D. Administer 100 mg protamine/sulfate
    E. Administer 10 bags of cryoprecipitate
7. Which of the following is true concerning lung scans?
    A. It is the most sensitive test to detect pulmonary emboli.
    B. All normal people should have a normal lung scan.
    C. While pneumonia or congestive heart failure may produce an abnormal scan, acute reversible bronchospasm will not.
    D. It should not be done in patients allergic to iodine.
    E. All of the above are true.
8. Which of the following would *not* be considered a likely predisposing factor for pulmonary emboli?
    A. Malignancy
    B. Drug abuse
    C. Obesity
    D. Prolonged travel
    E. All of the above
9. The alveolar-arterial oxygen gradient may be a more sensitive index of an acute process than the PaO_2. The normal $P(A-a)O_2$ in a yound adult is:
    A. 4–8 mm Hg   C. 10–20 mm Hg
    B. 5–15 mm Hg   D. 25–30 mm Hg
10. The differential diagnosis for pulmonary emboli also includes pneumonia, viral pleurisy, acute pericarditis, muscular skeletal chest pain, hyperventilation syndrome, and many others. Which of the following symptom complexes helps most to rule out pulmonary emboli?
    A. Chest wall tenderness to palpation
    B. Pleuritic chest pain
    C. History of cough, fever, sputum production
    D. Acute onset of dyspnea

11. The major cause of decreased PaO_2 seen in acute pulmonary embolism is:
    A. Intrapulmonary left-to-right shunting
    B. A diffusion impairment in pulmonary vasculature
    C. The closing of pulmonary arteriovenous anastamosis from increased vascular pressure
    D. Pulmonary vasoconstriction
    E. Atelectasis
12. Which radiographic finding is most specific for a pulmonary emboli?
    A. Cardiomegaly
    B. Left-sided pleural effusion
    C. Elevation of the diaphragm
    D. Unilateral basilar atelectasis
    E. Pleural-based rounded density   *hampton's hump*
13. Which of the following hemodynamic consequences are found with a significant pulmonary emboli?
    A. Elevation of mean pulmonary arterial pressure
    B. Elevation of mean left atrial pressure
    C. Jugular venous distention with large V-waves
    D. Elevation of left ventricular end diastolic pressure
14. Deciding whether to institute antiocoagulant therapy when a pulmonary emboli is suspected can be a dilemma for the emergency physician. Which of the following would favor heparin therapy prior to definitive diagnostic studies?
    A. The unavailability of lung scan
    B. The presence of contraindications to anticoagulation
    C. Age of the patient
    D. The likelihood of recurrence of the embolus
15. Which of the following statements is true of patients with angiographically proven pulmonary emboli?
    A. Only 6% of patients have no predisposing factors.
    B. Tachypnea over 16 per minute was found in only 50%.
    C. Sinus tachycardia above 100 per minute occurred in 80% of cases.
    D. Less than 25% had a temperature over 38.5°F.
    E. All of the above are true.
16. All of the following are true of heparin in treating pulmonary emboli, *except*:
    A. It can cause thrombocytopenia.
    B. A PTT or thrombin time is the best test to monitor therapy.
    C. Heparin can reduce hypoxia by counteracting vasoactive substances released by the thrombus.
    D. Heparin will speed the resolution of pulmonary emboli.
    E. Heparin should be continued for at least 7 days.

65
Aspiration

Select the appropriate letter that correctly answers the question or completes the statement.

1. Which of the following might be useful immediately after a serious aspiration?
    A. Broad-spectrum antibiotics
    B. Corticosteroids
    C. Diuretics
    D. Intubation and mechanical ventilation
    E. All of the above
2. Which of the following is true about secondary bacterial infection after aspiration of gastric contents?
    A. It occurs in 50% of cases of acid aspiration.
    B. *Staphylococcus aureus* is the most common pathogen.
    C. Prophylactic antibiotics can prevent secondary infection.
    D. For aspiration in the hospital, an aminoglycoside and cephalosporin should be used.
    E. The use of positive end expiratory pressure has been shown to increase the incidence and severity of secondary infection.
3. Which are the most common organisms seen in pulmonary abscesses?
    A. *Staphylococcus aureus*
    B. Mixed anaerobes
    C. *Streptococcus pneumoniae*
    D. *Hemophilus influenzae*
    E. *Escherichia coli*
4. All of the following are true about radiographic features of aspiration, *except*:
    A. Alveolar infiltrates are present immediately.
    B. Infiltrates progress over the first 24–36 hours but no longer.
    C. Infiltrates are often unilateral.
    D. The extent of infiltrate does not correlate with the severity of hypoxia or mortality.
    E. All of the above.
5. An acute head injury patient is brought to the emergency department. Airway management is complicated by frequent seizures. Succinycholine is chosen to control the patient during intubation. Aspiration is a risk during this procedure because of which factor?
    A. Paralysis of the protective reflexes
    B. Paralysis of the esophageal sphincters
    C. Increased intraabdominal pressure during the vesiculation phase
    D. All of the above

6. Which of the following statements about aspiration is true?
   A. Massive aspiration of gastric contents is associated with an 85% mortality. *to 70%*
   B. 33% of presumed myocardial infarctions in patients who died in nursing homes were in fact aspiration.
   C. The diagnosis of patients with aspiration pneumonia is related to the volume of aspirate alone. *character + volume*
   D. Aspiration is rarely a silent event.

7. A 25-year-old male is brought to the emergency department by ambulance in a comatose state, apparently from a drug overdose. Among the interventions used to treat and stabilize the patient was the placement of a nasogastric tube. Which of the following statements is true?
   A. There is very little risk of aspiration once an N/G tube is placed.
   B. There may be an increased incidence of aspiration when an N/G tube is present.
   C. The risk of aspiration of patients with an N/G tube in place is related to the size of the tube.
   D. None of the above

8. Which of the following statements about aspiration is *not* true?
   A. In the initial phase of aspiration, infection does not appear to play a causative role.
   B. Aspiration of gastric contents is often silent.
   C. The major role of infection occurs during the convalescent period.
   D. The major factor determining progression of aspiration into pneumonitis is the content of the aspirate.

9. In reference to water and saline aspiration, which of the following is thought to occur immediately?
   1. Marked decreased compliance.
   2. Decreased O_2 saturation
   3. Increased O_2 saturation
   4. Marked increased compliance
   5. Increased shunt
   6. No change in shunt
   A. 1, 3, and 5   C. 2, 3, and 6
   B. 2 only   D. 1, 2, and 5

10. Which of the following are true regarding patients who have aspirated?
   1. Signs and symptoms occur within 1 hour of aspiration in 90% of patients.
   2. Apnea occurs in as many as one-third of patients.
   3. Chest x-ray done immediately often shows no changes.
   A. 1 and 2   C. 1, 2 and 3
   B. 2 only   D. 1 and 3

11. Which of the following hemodynamic changes are generally found following aspiration?
   A. High cardiac index, high CVP, high blood pressure
   B. High cardiac index, low CVP, pulmonary edema
   C. Low cardiac index, high CVP, pulmonary edema
   D. Low cardiac index, high CVP, low blood pressure

12. Which of the following is true about the use of antibiotics in acute aspiration?
   A. Prophylactic antibiotics are helpful in reducing pulmonary infection.
   B. Bacterial pneumonia occurs in as many as 90% of patients with acid aspiration.
   C. Indications for antibiotics include the presence of an infiltrate in the first 24 hours.
   D. None of the above

66
Thrombophlebitis

Select the appropriate letter that correctly answers the question or completes the statement.

1. It is currently thought that the necessary factors for the development of deep venous thrombosis (DVT) include:
   A. Vessel wall injury, hypercoagulable state, venous stasis
   B. Venous stasis, elevated antithrombin III, decreased factor X
   C. Decreased factor X, decreased fibrinogen, elevated antithrombin III
   D. Vessel wall injury, decreased factor X, elevated antithrombin III

2. When diagnosing DVT, the combination of signs that result in an acceptable level of sensitivity are:
   A. Leg edema, palpable thrombi, positive Homan's sign
   B. Leg tenderness, difference in calf circumference, leg hyperthermia
   C. Difference in calf circumference, positive Homan's sign, palpable thrombi
   D. Palpable thrombi, positive Homan's sign, positive Lowenberg's sign
   E. No combination of signs results in an acceptable level of sensitivity

3. A 45-year-old white woman arrives in the ED with signs, history, and risk factors suggestive of DVT. The single most helpful test to determine if DVT is the correct diagnosis is:
   A. Venogram
   B. Doppler ultrasound
   C. Electrical impedance plethysmography
   D. ^{125}I-fibrinogen scanning
   E. Radionuclide phlebography

4. The best therapy for a patient with thrombophlebitis involving only the deep veins of the calf is:
   A. Coumadin
   B. Elevation, heat, antiinflammatory drugs
   C. IV heparin
   D. Subcutaneous heparin with oral antiplatelet agents.
   E. Active leg exercises and antiembolic stockings

5. The mechanism by which estrogen-containing contraceptives promote thrombophlebitis is:
   A. Increased platelet count
   B. Increased platelet activity
   C. Increased thrombin activity
   D. Decreased levels of antithrombin III
   E. Activation of the intrinsic coagulation cascade

6. All of the following are true of the clinical diagnosis of deep venous thrombosis except:
   A. Fifty percent of patients with clinical signs and symptoms of DVT have normal venograms.
   B. Two-thirds of patients with DVT by ^{125}I-fibrinogen scans have no clinical signs or symptoms.
   C. Swelling is the most valid clinical sign.
   D. Most patients with DVT have some clinical risk factor.
   E. Bruits in the groin or popliteal fossa may be detected.

67
Aortic Aneurysms

Select the appropriate letter that correctly answers the question or completes the statement.

1. All of the following are associated with an increased incidence of dissecting aortic aneurysm except:
   A. Hypertension
   B. Coarctation
   C. Marfan's syndrome
   D. Cystic medial necrosis
   E. Patent ductus arteriosa

2. The most common problem requiring treatment in the emergency department with a dissecting thoracic aneurysm is:
   A. Hypovolemia
   B. Pericardial tamponade
   C. Hypertension
   D. Arrhythmias
   E. Respiratory failure

3. Which of the following is not a possible initial complaint in a patient with abdominal aortic aneurysm?
   A. Asymptomatic
   B. Hematuria
   C. Upper GI tract obstruction

D. Lower GI bleeding
E. All of the above

4. All of the following are possible complications of aortography to diagnose abdominal aortic aneurysm except:
   A. Iatrogenic dissection
   B. False-negative study
   C. Acute renal failure
   D. Dislodgement of mural thrombi
   E. All of the above

5. True statements about diagnosing abdominal aortic aneurysm include all of the following except:
   A. Physical examination is unreliable, missing up to 40% of abdominal aortic aneurysms.
   B. Ultrasound has a nearly 100% accuracy rate for detecting abdominal aortic aneurysms.
   C. Plain films of the abdomen, especially the lateral view, can detect 50-70% of abdominal aortic aneurysms.
   D. They are found on routine autopsies in 20% of the adult population.
   E. All of the above are true.

6. Most authorities feel that abdominal aortic aneurysms over _____ cm have a significantly greater risk of early rupture.
   A. 4 cm   D. 10 cm
   B. 6 cm   E. Size is of no
   C. 8 cm   predictive value

68
Arteriovascular Diseases

Select the appropriate letter that correctly answers the question or completes the statement.

1. The drug most frequently used to treat symptomatic Raynaud's syndrome is:
   A. Reserpine   D. Decadron
   B. Aldomet   E. Digoxin
   C. Nitroprusside

2. A 68-year-old man with a diagnosis of acute arterial occlusion of the left upper extremity has been transferred to your facility. On physical examination you may expect to find:
   A. A cool, painful hand with no flushing when an Allen's test is performed
   B. A paralyzed hand with painful ulcerations
   C. An erythematous-flushed hand with paresthesias
   D. Paresthesias and painless ulcerations of the hand, flushing of the hand when an Allen's test is performed

3. Statistically, the most common source of the occlusion found in the patient described in question 2 would be:
   A. Atherosclerotic disease of the left subclavian artery
   B. Oat cell cancer of the lung
   C. Atherosclerotic disease of the descending aorta
   D. Cardiac
4. A 45-year-old woman comes to the ED because her fingers occasionally turn very pale and tingle when exposed to cold air. Shortly thereafter her fingers become erythematous and throbbing. This has occurred 5 or 6 times. Evaluation of this patient should include all of the following *except*:
   A. ECG to rule out atrial fibrillation
   B. ANA and sedimentation rate to rule out connective tissue disease
   C. Exercising hyperabducted arms as well as Adson's maneuver to rule out thoracic outlet syndrome
   D. ABCs to rule out hypoxia
5. A patient seen earlier at a free-standing emergency clinic tells you he has been diagnosed as having thoracic outlet syndrome. This condition may be caused by all of the following *except*:
   A. Compression of the neurovascular bundle in the retroclavicular space anterior to the first rib when the arms are hyperabducted
   B. Compression of the neurovascular bundle when the shoulders are moved anterior and cephalad
   C. Compression of the neurovascular bundle as it passes through the interscalene triangle
   D. Compression of the subclavian artery by an anomalous cervical rib
6. Which of the following is the most common cause of the thoracic outlet syndrome?
   A. Scalenus anticus syndrome
   B. Cervical rib
   C. Costoclavicular syndrome
   D. Hyperabduction syndrome
7. The collagen vascular disease that is most often associated with Raynaud's syndrome is:
   A. Scleroderma
   B. Systemic lupus erythematosis
   C. Rheumatoid arthritis
   D. Sjögren's syndrome
   E. Ankylosing spondylitis
8. Which of the following statements is true about renal artery stenosis?
   A. Surgery for renal artery stenosis can improve blood pressure but not kidney function.
   B. With medical management of blood pressure, renal failure can progress.
   C. The renal vein renin index has little prognostic value about expected improvement with surgery.

D. Surgery for renovascular hypertension results in a cure in less than 50% of patients.
   E. Fibromuscular disease is usually seen in young men.
9. All of the following statements about cerebrovascular insufficiency are true *except*:
   A. Most strokes are due to atherosclerotic events.
   B. Most transient ischemic attacks are caused by embolic disease.
   C. A person with a stroke has a 60% chance of having another within 2 years.
   D. Blacks have a 4 times greater risk of TIA than whites.
   E. Anyone with a carotid bruit should have an arteriogram to rule out significant obstruction.
10. All of the following are true of Buerger's disease (thromboangiitis obliterans) *except*:
   A. It has a predilection for persons of Jewish descent.
   B. Most patients smoke cigarettes.
   C. It may present with intermittent claudication of the hand or foot.
   D. Pathology involves intimal proliferation and leukocyte infiltration of the small arteries.
   E. Main complication is acute myocardial infarction.

69

Infective Endocarditis and Acquired Valvular Heart Disease

Select the appropriate letter that correctly answers the question or completes the statement.
1. Prolapse of the mitral valve is a common, usually benign, disorder. All of the following are serious complications of this disorder, *except*:
   A. Bacterial endocarditis
   B. Paroxysmal supraventricular tachycardia
   C. Syncope
   D. Coronary artery spasm
   E. Third degree heart block
2. Which organism is the most common cause of subacute bacterial endocarditis?
   A. Alpha streptococcus   *S. viridans*
   B. *Staphylococcus epidemicus*
   C. Beta streptococcus
   D. Enterococci
   E. *Staphylococcus aureus*

3. All of the following are physical findings associated with mitral regurgitation, *except*:
   A. Loud S_1
   B. Holocystolic murmur
   C. S_3 gallop
   D. Left ventricular heave
   E. Radiation of murmur to the axilla

Match the valvular disorder on the left with the appropriate findings on the right.

_____ 4. Mitral stenosis
_____ 5. Mitral regurgitation
_____ 6. Aortic stenosis
_____ 7. Aortic regurgitation
_____ 8. Tricuspid stenosis
_____ 9. Tricuspid regurgitation
_____ 10. Pulmonic valvular disease

A. Hallmark of the disease is left atrial hypertension.
B. Atrial fibrillation is common.
C. Cardinal symptoms are dyspnea on exertion, angina, and exertional syncope.
D. Grade 3-6 holosystolic murmur radiating to the axilla
E. First symptoms are usually dyspnea and fatigue.
F. Systolic ejection murmur is the loudest in the left second intercostal space and increases with inspiration.
G. Prominent A-waves in the jugular venous pulse with diastolic murmur along the left sternal border

Select the appropriate letter that correctly answers the question or completes the statement.

11. The patient position or maneuver in which mitral stenosis is most easily heard is:
    A. Sitting up, leaning forward
    B. Left lateral decubitus position
    C. Squatting
    D. During Valsalva's maneuver
    E. After inhalation of amyl nitrate

12. The most common cause of infective endocarditis is:
    A. Gram-negative bacteria
    B. Streptococcus, gram-positive cocci
    C. *Staphylococcus aureus*
    D. None of the above

13. Which of the following statements about infective endocarditis is *not* true?

A. Any lesion that involves turbulent blood flow can predispose to endocarditis.
B. Echocardiography is especially helpful diagnostically.
C. Most commonly endocarditis affects the aortic valve.
D. Transient bacteremia is found in up to 60% of patients who develop endocarditis.

14. Complications of prosthetic valve such as thrombosis, infection, or valve deterioration is suggested by which of the following auscultatory characteristics?
    A. Sharp opening and closing sounds in aortic ball cage valves
    B. Apical diastolic rumble in mitral tissue valve
    C. Absence of high-pitched click in tilting disk valve
    D. Opening sound in central occluder disk valve

15. The most common valvular disorder in the United States is:
    A. Mitral stenosis secondary to rheumatic fever
    B. Mitral regurgitation associated with collagen vascular disorders
    C. Mitral valve prolapse
    D. Acute mitral regurgitation secondary to acute myocardial infarction

16. The greatest cause of morbidity and mortality in infectious endocarditis is related to which of the following?
    A. Lung abscess or infarction from septic emboli
    B. Dysrhythmias
    C. Neurologic event
    D. Congestive heart failure secondary to valvular destruction

17. A 10-year-old boy presents to the emergency department with a chief complaint of a sore throat. The current American Heart Association recommendations regarding a throat culture to prevent rheumatic fever is:
    A. Culture only if exudates are present
    B. No culture, treat prophylactically
    C. Culture only if the child is less than 4 years of age
    D. Culture in children ages 4–20

18. Which of the following symptom complexes is usually found in infective endocarditis?
    A. Chest pain, shortness of breath, malaise
    B. Fever, arthralgias, fatigue
    C. Malaise, fever, chest pain
    D. Headache, weight loss, shortness of breath

19. The cornerstone of the diagnosis of infectious endocarditis is:
    A. New heart murmur
    B. Leukocytosis
    C. Petechia
    D. Positive blood culture

20. Of the following Major Jones criteria for acute rheumatic fever, which is most commonly seen?
    A. Carditis
    B. Polyarthritis
    C. Chorea
    D. Erythema marginatum
    E. Subcutaneous nodules

21. The EKG finding most suggestive of prolapse of the mitral valve is:
    A. Left atrial enlargement
    B. Left bundle branch block
    C. First degree AV block
    D. Left ventricular hypertrophy
    E. Inferior wall ischemia

22. Which of the following correlates most closely with the severity of aortic stenosis?
    A. Intensity of S_2
    B. Length of the murmur
    C. Intensity of the murmur
    D. Quality of carotid pulses
    E. Ejection click

23. The most common organism causing right-sided endocarditis is:
    A. Alpha streptococcus
    B. *Staphylococcus epidemicus*
    C. *Candida albicans*
    D. Enterococci
    E. *Staphylococcus aureus*

24. The EKG finding that would be most suggestive of mitral stenosis is:
    A. Left ventricular enlargement
    B. Right bundle branch block
    C. First degree AV block
    D. Left atrial enlargement
    E. Prominent septal Q waves

25. Patients with mitral valve prolapse at greatest risk for malignant dysrhythmias have which of the following:
    A. Near syncope
    B. Inferior ST-T wave changes
    C. Prolonged Q-T interval
    D. Late systolic murmur preceded by a click
    E. All of the above

70

Hypertension

Select the appropriate letter that correctly answers the question or completes the statement.

1. What is the clinical hallmark of malignant hypertension?
    A. Papilledema
    B. Diastolic blood pressure over 130
    C. Signs of encephalopathy
    D. EKG evidence of left ventricular hypertrophy with strain
    E. All of the above

2. All of the following statements are true concerning hypertensive encephalopathy *except*:
    A. Nitroprusside is the agent of choice.
    B. It can be the initial manifestation of hypertension.
    C. CT scan is normal.
    D. Papilledema is usually present.
    E. Seizures are unusual.

3. Which is the most common cause of death in the preeclamptic woman?
    A. Cerebral hemorrhage
    B. Renal failure
    C. Intrauterine bleeding
    D. Septic pulmonary emboli
    E. Addisonian crisis

4. Aortic dissection is very difficult to distinguish clinically from myocardial ischemia. All of the following should suggest aortic dissection *except*:
    A. Radiation of pain to the back
    B. Tenderness along the course of a carotid artery
    C. Asymmetry of pulses
    D. Acute aortic insufficiency
    E. Systolic murmur radiating to both carotid arteries

5. All of the following about diazoxide are true *except*:
    A. It is a derivative of the thiazide class of antihypertensives.
    B. It causes a marked sodium and water retention.
    C. It can precipitate hyperglycemia.
    D. The duration of effect of a single IV bolus is 4 to 12 hours.
    E. It is especially useful if angina is present because its effect is rapid.

Match the antihypertensive on the left with the possible complications on the right.

___ 6. Minoxidil	A.	Coombs-positive hemolytic anemia
___ 7. Alpha-methyldopa	B.	Pericardial effusion
___ 8. Hydralazine	C.	Bronchospasm
___ 9. Propranolol	D.	Hypokalemia, hyperuricemia
___ 10. Furosemide	E.	Lupus-like syndrome with positive ANA

Select the appropriate letter that correctly answers the question or completes the statement.

11. A 50-year-old man presents with a sudden onset of extreme anxiety, tremor of both hands, palpitations, and headache. He reports that he lost his blood pressure medications 2 days ago. Physical examination reveals a diaphoretic, anxious white male with a fine tremor of both hands, blood pressure 170/120, and an S_4 gallop. Eye grounds reveal Grade 2 hypertensive changes. The most likely cause of this patient's symptoms are:
    A. Propranolol withdrawal
    B. Clonidine withdrawal
    C. Pheochromocytoma
    D. Hyperthyroidism
    E. Hydralazine withdrawal

12. A 54-year-old man comes to the emergency department with a sprained ankle. He is noted to have a sustained blood pressure of 200/120. He has no symptoms or history of hypertension. Physical examination shows AV nicking but no papilledema, hemorrhage, or exudates. There is an S_4 gallop but no other cardiac pathology noted. Laboratory workup includes a normal chest x-ray, and EKG shows left ventricular hypertrophy. Urinalysis is normal. Electrolytes and BUN are normal. The best step now is:
    A. Begin nitroprusside and admit to ICU
    B. Diazide IV
    C. Referral to Internist within 24 hours
    D. Admit for renal arteriograms and urinary metanephrines
    E. Begin hydrochlorothiazide and propanolol with prompt referral

13. All of the following are true about nitroprusside, *except*:
    A. It dilates both resistance vessls on the arterial side and capacitance vessels on the venous side.
    B. It can cause thiocyanate toxicity manifest as weakness, respiratory paralysis, nausea, and tinnitis.
    C. It should not be used during pregnancy because of the effect of thiocyanate on the fetus.
    D. Solution should be wrapped in aluminum foil to avoid precipitation and should be used before the solution is 4 hours old.
    E. It has been effective in reducing infarct size in acute myocardial infarction.

14. A healthy 26-year-old woman is found to have an elevated blood pressure. On a careful physical examination you find AV nicking of the fundi, an S_4 gallop, and a flank bruit. The most likely cause of her elevated blood pressure would be:
    A. Fibromuscular disease of the renal arteries
    B. Coarctation of the aorta
    C. Pheochromocytoma

D. Excessive ACTH production from an adrenal tumor
E. Chronic pyelonephritis

15. All of the following concerning labetalol in the treatment of acute hypertension are true, *except*:
    A. Its use requires admission to an intensive care unit.
    B. Because it is both an alpha and beta blocker, a reflex tachycardia is not seen.
    C. After intravenous administration, the patient should be kept in the supine position for several hours.
    D. It is contraindicated in the treatment of pheochromocytoma.
    E. Intravenous use is not associated with the profound decrease in blood pressure sometimes seen with diazoxide.

16. A 35-year-old immigrant who has never had medical care is sent to the emergency department because of an elevated blood pressure of 180/110. On a chest x-ray, you see left ventricular hypertrophy and bilateral notching of the posterior ribs. The physical finding you would expect in this patient is:
    A. Lower blood pressure in the lower extremities than the upper
    B. Bobbing of the head while at rest
    C. Blue sclera
    D. An opening snap with an end diastolic rumble
    E. Outstretched hands extend further than the patient's height

17. Which of the following are true statements about malignant hypertension?
    A. It is always associated with hypertensive encephalopathy.
    B. All patients with a sustained diastolic blood pressure greater than 130 will eventually develop malignant hypertension.
    C. The underlying pathology is fibrinoid necrosis of small arterioles.
    D. Immediate blood pressure reduction with nitroprusside is necessary.
    E. All of the above are true.

71
Dysrhythmias

Select the appropriate letter that correctly answers the question or completes the statement.

1. Which of the following is contraindicated as the sole agent to treat atrial fibrillation:
    A. Quinidine   D. Verapamil
    B. Digoxin   E. None of the above
    C. Propranolol

2. Which of the following is the drug of choice for uncomplicated supraventricular tachycardia?
   A. Verapamil
   B. Digoxin
   C. Edrophonium
   D. Propranolol
   E. Metaraminol

3. All of the following drugs will slow tachycardias (at least in part) because of their vagal influence *except*:
   A. Digitalis
   B. Edrophonium
   C. Metaraminol
   D. Carotid massage
   E. Verapamil

4. All of the following concerning Wolff-Parkinson-White syndrome are true *except*:
   A. Delta wave is caused by simultaneous conduction over the accessory bypass tract and the AV node.
   B. It can mimic ventricular hypertrophy, bundle branch block, or acute myocardial infarction.
   C. Cardioversion is particularly dangerous and can lead to ventricular fibrillation.
   D. Procainamide is the drug of choice for a patient with atrial fibrillation.
   E. In cases of atrial fibrillation, the R-R interval can be used to estimate the effective refractory period of the accessory pathway.

5. All of the following are contraindicated in a patient with atrial fibrillation who has Wolff-Parkinson-White syndrome *except*:
   A. Digitalis
   B. Propranolol
   C. Verapamil
   D. Procainamide
   E. Bretylium

6. A 45-year-old man has an ECG done in the ED that shows an atrial rate of approximately 300 bpm. The P waves have a sawtooth appearance. The QRS complexes have a rate of 150 bpm and are narrow and regular. The patient is asymptomatic. Initial therapy of this dysrhythmia is:
   A. Quinidine 200 mg IV
   B. Digitalis 0.5 mg IV then 0.25 mg every 30 minutes times 2
   C. Cardioversion at 10 joules
   D. Lidocaine 100 mg IV bolus

7. A 50-year-old man has an ECG done in the ED. The QRS complexes are 0.07 seconds and irregular with a rate of 160–170 bpm. There are no discernible P waves. The patient is asymptomatic. Initial therapy to slow the rate of this dysrhythmia includes all of the following *except*:
   A. Digitalization
   B. Cardioversion
   C. Verapamil
   D. Propranolol

8. A 58-year-old man has an ECG done in the ED. There are some beats that you think are PVCs. If present, factors that would support your diagnosis include all of the following *except*:
   A. The beat is premature.
   B. The T wave has a polarity that is opposite that of the QRS.

C. There is a compensatory pause following beat.
D. The QRS is 0.10 seconds in duration.
E. There is no P wave preceding the beat.

9. The patient in the previous question is now having 7 to 8 of these abnormal beats in a row. He is asymptomatic. Treatment of this dysrhythmia includes all of the following *except*:
   A. Procainamide up to 1 gm IV
   B. Lidocaine 1 mg/kg IV bolus, then 1 to 4 mg/minute drip
   C. Bretylium 5 mg/kg IV bolus, then 1 to 2 mg/min drip
   D. Digitalis 0.5 mg IV
   E. Cardioversion

10. A 54-year-old comes to the ED with a history of several hours of chest pain. After treatment with oxygen and nitroglycerin, he is free of pain but has a pulse of 50 and a blood pressure of 100/70. His ECG shows an anterior myocardial infarction with Mobitz type II second degree AV block. The best therapy at this point would be:
    A. Isoproterenol drip
    B. Atropine
    C. Transvenous pacemaker
    D. Careful observation
    E. Prophylactic lidocaine

11. Verapamil should not be given to a patient receiving which of the following medications?
    A. Lidocaine drip
    B. Bertylium drip
    C. IV propranolol
    D. Digitalis
    E. Procainamide

12. All of the following are true concerning the sick sinus syndrome *except*:
    A. The presenting complaint is usually syncope.
    B. The treatment is a pacemaker.
    C. It may be associated with tachyarrhythmias.
    D. It is usually associated with severe ischemic heart disease.
    E. It is often refractory to atropine.

13. Which of the following usually causes paroxysmal atrial tachycardia with block?
    A. Coronary artery disease
    B. Digitalis intoxication
    C. Conducting system disease
    D. Mitral valve disease
    E. No underlying cardiac disease

14. Which aberration on the ECG is the best way to differentiate a premature ventricular contraction from a premature atrial contraction?
    A. Inverted T waves with a PVC
    B. Compensatory pause with PVC
    C. PACs usually have a ibbb pattern
    D. PACs have a fixed coupling interval
    E. PACs have an initial vector different from normally conducted beats

15. Which clinical condition is most compatible with the ECG in Fig. 71-1?
    A. Right ventricular hypertrophy with strain
    B. Posterior myocardial infarction
    C. Wolff-Parkinson-White syndrome
    D. Idiopathic hypertrophic subaortic stenosis
    E. Nonspecific interventricular conduction delay

16. A 45-year-old man comes to the ED complaining of several hours of substernal chest pain. He has no cardiac history, but his ECG shows an inferior myocardial infarction. Shortly after arrival in the department he has the rhythm shown in Fig. 71-2. His chest pain has now resolved and his blood pressure is 110/70. This monitor strip shows:
    A. First degree A-V block
    B. Wenckebach block
    C. Mobitz type II block
    D. Intermittent sinus arrest
    E. Third degree A-V block

17. What arrhythmia is represented by the monitor strip shown in Fig. 71-3?
    A. Atrial fibrillation
    B. Multifocal atrial tachycardia
    C. PAT with block
    D. Sinus tachycardia with aberrant atrial conduction
    E. Second degree A-V block

18. A patient with an acute myocardial infarction is monitored in the Cardiac Care Unit. Which arrhythmia would suggest the worst prognosis?
    A. Over 6 PVCs in 24 hours
    B. Bigeminal pattern of PVCs
    C. Short interval between sinus beat and PVCs
    D. Runs of 3 or more PVCs in a row
    E. Multiform appearance of PVCs

19. When classifying patients with dysrhythmias as unstable, which of the following criteria apply?
    A. Blood pressure less than 90 mm Hg
    B. Change in the level of consciousness
    C. Chest pain unrelieved by nitroglycerin
    D. Pulmonary edema
    E. All of the above

20. A 55-year-old man presents to the emergency department with a history of 30 minutes of chest pain unrelieved with rest and associated with both shortness of breath and palpitations. His monitor shows a regular tachycardia with a rate of 150 per minute. No atrial activity is discernible. You should assume this rhythm to be which of the following?
    A. Sinus tachycardia
    B. Atrial flutter with 2-1 block
    C. Junctional tachycardia
    D. Regular atrial fibrillation
    E. Atrial tachycardia
    F. Superventricular tachycardia

21. The patient in the previous question now is asymptomatic yet the tachycardia persists. Which of the following maneuvers would be preferred at this point?
    A. Eyeball pressure   C. Pulling on the tongue
    B. Diver's reflex   D. None of the above

22. Which of the following statements about torsades de Pointes is *not* true?
    A. That dysrhythmia is frequently associated with Q-T prolongation.
    B. Pause-dependent type can be successfully treated with beta-adrenergic agonist.
    C. Pause-dependent type can be successfully treated with beta adrenergic blockers.
    D. Calcium antagonist may be effective.

23. What is the recommended treatment for accelerated idioventricular rhythm?
    A. Lidocaine, 1 mg/kg IV
    B. Atropine .5 mg IV
    C. No treatment is necessary.
    D. Pronestyl, 100 mg IV

24. That period of the action potential when a greater than normal stimulus is required to cause a new action potential is known as the:
    A. Threshold potential period
    B. Absolute refractory period
    C. Super normal period
    D. Relative refractory period

25. An impulse generated in the sinal atrial node is conducted through specialized intraatrial conduction tissue towards the A-V node. Which of the following are normal conduction pathways?
    1. Wenckebach's bundle
    2. Bundle of Kent
    3. Thorel's bundle
    4. Bachmann's bundle
    A. 1, 2, and 3   C. 2 and 4
    B. 4 only   D. 1, 3, and 4

26. The ectopic rhythm characterized by a changing coupling interval, a wide QRS, and frequent fusion beats is:
    A. Ventricular parasystole
    B. Multifocal PVCs
    C. PACs with aberrancy
    D. Interpolated PVCs

27. The sick sinus syndrome is associated with which of the following dysrhythmias?
    1. Atrial tachycardia
    2. Sinus block
    3. A-V block
    4. Sinus bradycardia
    A. 1, 2, and 4
    B. 1 and 2
    C. 2 and 3
    D. 1, 2, 3, and 4

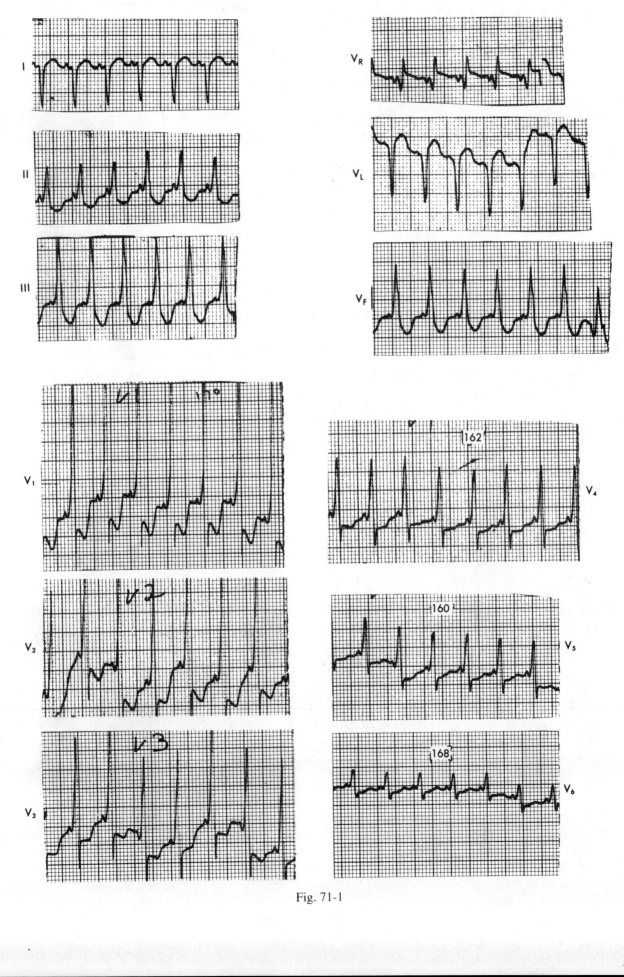

Fig. 71-1

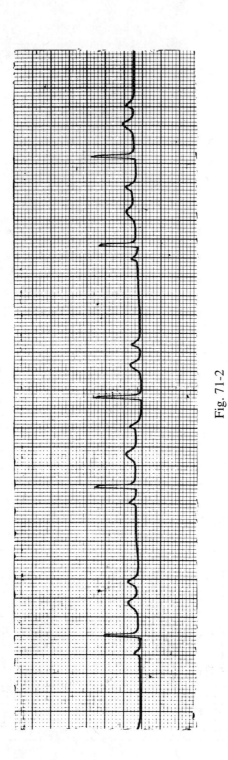

Fig. 71-2

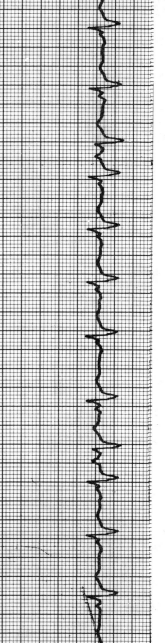

Fig. 71-3

68

28. The underlying disease causing multifocal atrial tachycardia usually is:
A. Chronic obstructive pulmonary disease
B. Coronary artery disease
C. Mitral stenosis
D. Viral myocarditis
E. No underlying cardiac pathology

29. The repolarization phase (3) of the ventricular myocardial cell is reflected by which portion of the electrocardiogram?
A. P wave   D. P-R interval
B. R wave   E. Q-T interval
C. T wave

30. A 65-year-old man presents to the emergency department with a history of acute onset of chest pain unrelieved by nitroglycerin. His electrocardiogram shows ST-segment elevation in leads 2-3 and AVF. His blood pressure was 100/60 and the chest pain has now been relieved with 4 mg of morphine. His monitor shows arrythmia in Fig. 71-4.
A. Second degree A-V block
B. A-V dissociation
C. Wandering atrial pacemaker
D. None of the above

31. Which of the following statements pertaining to electrophysiology is true?
1. In myocardial working cells, slow channels allow the influx of sodium ions.
2. The energy-dependent (ATP) pump mechanism maintains resting potential.
3. In pacemaker cells there is a spontaneous increase in negativity called diastolic depolarization.
4. The steeper the slope of phase 4, the greater the automaticity.
A. 1, 2, and 3   C. 2, 3, and 4
B. 1 and 3   D. 2 and 4

32. The two major theories as to the mechanism of cardiac dysrhythmias are:
1. Enhanced automaticity
2. Reentry phenomena
3. Triggered automaticity
4. Increased excitability
A. 1 and 3
B. 2 and 4
C. 2 and 3
D. 1 and 2

72
Congestive Heart Failure

Select the appropriate letter that correctly answers the question or completes the statement.
1. What is the earliest radiographic finding of left-sided congestive heart failure?
A. Cardiomegaly
B. Redistribution of blood flow to upper zones
C. Interstitial edema
D. Pleural effusion
E. Dilatation of the azygos vein

2. Management of congestive heart failure in the infant differs from that of an adult in all of the following ways *except*:
A. You must be careful to keep a warm environmental temperature.
B. Bicrbonate is used earlier and more often to correct acidosis.
C. Digitalis toxicity is less likely to occur.
D. Morphine is contraindicated because of increased respiratory depression.
E. Definitive treatment is usually surgical

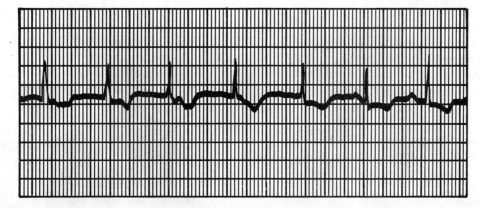

Fig. 71-4

3. All of the following are true about calcium channel blockers *except*:
   A. Verapamil has little effect on ventricular ectopy.
   B. Diltiazem is associated with the fewest side effects.
   C. Nifedipine is the most likely to induce hypotension.
   D. Verapamil can induce an increase in the serum level of digoxin.
   E. Nifedipine induces a marked depression of atrioventricular conduction.

4. A 55-year-old woman with known coronary artery disease comes to the ED with a 2-hour history of substernal chest pain, diaphoresis, and shortness of breath. She has a history of hypertension as well as chronic bronchitis. Her medications at home include hydrochlorothiazide, isosorbide dinitrate, and theophylline. She is mildly cyanotic with a respiratory rate of 30 and a blood pressure of 100/70. Chest examination reveals bibasilar rales and scattered ronchi. Cardiac examination shows an S_4 gallop. Her electrocardiogram is shown in Fig. 72-1. All of the following are appropriate in the management of this patient *except*:
   A. Intravenous lidocaine
   B. O_2 via nasal cannula
   C. Isosorbide dinitrate
   D. Morphine sulfate
   E. Digitalis

5. A previously healthy 47-year-old is seen in the ED with a sudden onset of shortness of breath without chest pain after jogging 5 miles. He has a history of an unknown type of heart murmur, but no other cardiac problems. Physical examination reveals rales one-half way up all lung fields, and S_4 gallop, and a grade 4/6 sea-gull type murmur radiating to the base and axilla. The most likely cause of this acute condition is:
   A. Silent myocardial infarction
   B. Ruptured chordae tendineae
   C. Aortic valve obstruction from IHSS
   D. Reversal of shunt through ASD
   E. Thrombus obstructing the mitral valve

6. All the following are true of furosemide *except*:
   A. Causes both potassium and magnesium wasting
   B. Causes a significant venodilatation before any effect on diuresis
   C. Decreases calcium exertion   excretion (↑)
   D. Causes ototoxicity in large doses
   E. May cause an allergic reaction in a person sensitive to sulfonamides

7. All of the following can precipitate acute pulmonary edema in a patient with underlying congestive heart failure *except*:
   A. Pulmonary emboli
   B. Pneumonia
   C. Bronchospasm

D. Myocardial infarction
E. All the above

8. The most common cause of congestive heart failure in an adult is:
   A. Coronary artery disease
   B. Valvular heart disease
   C. Cardiomyopathy
   D. Hypertension
   E. Congenital cardiac disease

9. The most common arrhythmia seen in the Digitalis-toxic patient is:
   A. PAT with block
   B. Nodal tachycardia
   C. Premature ventricular contractions
   D. Atrial fibrillation/flutter
   E. Wenckebach type II heart block

10. Which of the following electrolyte disturbances would predispose a patient to Digitalis toxicity?
    A. Hypermagnesemia
    B. Hypocalcemia
    C. Hyponatremia
    D. Hypokalemia

11. Which of the following best describes the effect of nitroglycerin on MVO_2 (myocardial oxygen demand)?
    A. Acceleration of heart rate from VENO dialation increases MVO_2.
    B. Dilatation of capacitance veins decreases left ventricular wall stress and decreases MVO_2.
    C. Both of the above
    D. None of the above

12. A 60-year-old patient in CCU, recently admitted for refractory congestive heart failure, is decompensating. The patient has previously received morphine, oxygen, and Lasix, 40 mg IV. You are called at 2 A.M. because the patient has now become significantly hypotensive. The best approach right now would be:
    A. Lasix 100 mg IV
    B. Nitroglycerin drip
    C. Fluid challenge of 300 cc, normal saline over 15 minutes
    D. Start dopamine infusion at 5 μg/Kg/min
    E. Swan-Ganz catheter insertion

13. The presence of acute pulmonary edema with normal heart size on x-ray may indicate all of the following *except*:
    A. Constrictive pericarditis
    B. Massive myocardial infarction
    C. Mitral regurgitation   (stenosis)
    D. Noncardiogenic pulmonary edema

14. On a short-term basis, which of the following is *not* a method the heart uses to cope with increasing demand?
    A. Hypertrophy of cardiac chambers
    B. Frank-Starling mechanism
    C. Maximizing the ionotropic state
    D. Variation of heart rate

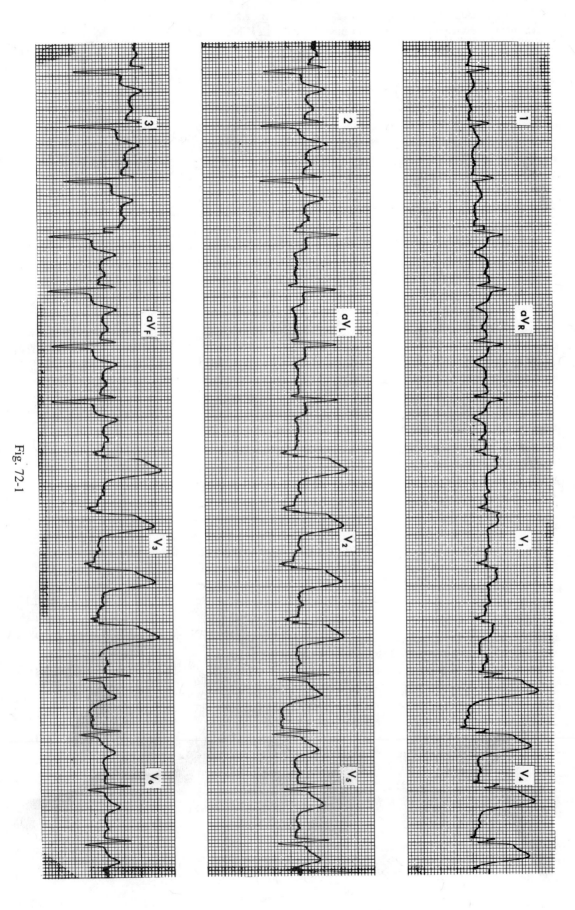

Fig. 72-1

71

15. Which of the following drugs used for vasodilatory effect in the treatment of congestive heart failure has the most balanced preload and afterload reducing properties?
    A. Hydralazine
    B. Captopril
    C. Nifedipine
    D. Prazosin

16. Which of the following statements regarding ionotropic agents is true?
    A. Dobutamine is different from dopamine in that it decreases afterload without tachycardia.
    B. The best indication for Digitalis is congestive heart failure and a large left ventricle.
    C. Dopamine is preferred to dobutamine because of a decreased frequency of dysrhythmias.
    D. Amrinone is the newest catecholamine ionotropic agent to increase cardiac output.

17. Chest x-ray interpretation can be essential in assessing congestive heart failure. The presence of non-branching short lines in a reticular or honeycomb pattern in the lower lung fields are known as:
    A. Kerley a lines
    B. Kerley b lines
    C. Kerley c lines
    D. None of the above

18. Morphine is felt by many to be the drug of choice for management of acute congestive heart failure. Its actions include all the following except:
    A. Alleviates anxiety
    B. Decreases arterial resistance
    C. Increases venous capacitance
    D. May dilate coronary arteries
    E. Decreases stroke-work index

19. The last few years have seen a major shift in the treatment of congestive heart failures toward vasodilator therapy. Which of the following statements regarding vasodilator therapy is true?
    A. Venodilators reduce filling pressure and afterload.
    B. Arterial dilators increase systemic vascular resistance but do not affect preload.
    C. Vasodilators primarily affect preload.
    D. Some vasodilators primarily affect afterload.

20. Which of the following statements is most true?
    A. Dyspnea is a sensitive specific symptom in congestive heart failure.
    B. Proxysmal nocturnal dyspnea is specific for congestive heart failure.
    C. The patient's general appearance and neck vein examination are helpful indicators of congestive heart failure.
    D. The S_4 gallop is a very specific indicator of a failing ventricle in the adult patient.
    E. None of the above are true.

21. The most valuable ancillary test for congestive heart failure is:
    A. EKG
    B. Arterial blood gases
    C. Chest x-ray
    D. Blood chemistry

73
Cardiogenic Shock

Select the appropriate letter that correctly answers the question or completes the statement.

1. Complications of a Swan-Ganz catheter include all of the following except:
   A. Pulmonary infarction
   B. Pulmonary artery rupture
   C. Thrombosis of catheter tip
   D. Ventricular arrhythmias
   E. Ventilation-perfusion mismatching

2. You are called to the Cardiac Care Unit to attend a 54-year-old man admitted 2 days ago with an anterior myocardial infarction. Initially his blood pressure was 145/90 with a pulse of 100 and no signs of congestive heart failure. Now he has suddenly developed severe shortness of breath with a blood pressure of 90/70, pulse of 125, and a respiratory rate of 30. There are bilateral rales up 3/4 of the chest wall and a new grade 3 over 6 systolic murmur at left sternal border radiating across to the right side of the chest. The most likely diagnosis is:
   A. Extension of the infarction to involve the inferior wall
   B. Papillary muscle rupture
   C. Acute pulmonary embolus
   D. Rupture of the ventricular septum
   E. Pericardial effusion with tamponade

3. A patient is seen in the ED complaining of severe chest pain of several hours duration. He has had one infarction in the past. Medications include digoxin, Lasix, Nitro paste, and propranolol. He is pale, diaphoretic with a blood pressure of 70/40. His lungs are clear. There is an S_3 gallop. The electrocardiogram shows an acute anterior wall myocardial infarction. A Swan-Ganz catheter reveals a pulmonary artery wedge pressure of 8. The most effective therapy now would be:
   A. Begin dopamine drip
   B. IV digoxin
   C. Normal saline fluid challenge
   D. Intraaortic balloon pump
   E. Dobutamine drip

4. A 40-year-old man is seen in the ED after a syncopal episode. He now denies any symptoms but remains hypotensive with a blood pressure of 80/50. His neck veins are flat, his chest is clear but there is an S_3 gal-

lop at the apex with an apical lift. His EKG is shown in Fig. 73-1. The best way to initiate treatment of this patient is:

A. Dopamine infusion
B. Temporary transvenous pacemaker
C. Swan-Ganz catheter
D. IV heparin pending pulmonary angiography
E. Rapid digitalization

5. All of the following are true about cardiogenic shock *except*:

A. Left ventricular end diastolic pressure should be elevated.
B. Central venous pressures accurately reflect the hemodynamic derangement.
C. Cardiac index would be expected to be less than 2 $l/min/m^2$.
D. It occurs in 15–20% of patients with myocardial infarction.
E. All of the above are false.

6. A 65-year-old man comes to the emergency department following 3 days of chest pain. He now has a blood pressure of 60/0; heart rate 120; respiratory rate 24. The skin is pale, cool, and clammy. A fluid challenge of 250 cc of Ringer's lactate did not improve his vital signs. A Swan-Ganz catheter is placed. The pulmonary capillary wedge is 8 Torr. What would be the next step in this patient's management?

A. Ringer's lactate wide open until systolic blood pressure is greater than 90.
B. 100 cc Ringer's lactate wide open until pulmonary capillary wedge pressure is up to 18 Torr.
C. Ringer's lactate at 200 cc per hour and Lasix 40 mg IV.
D. 200 cc Ringer's lactate bolus until pulmonary capillary wedge pressure is up to 12 Torr.

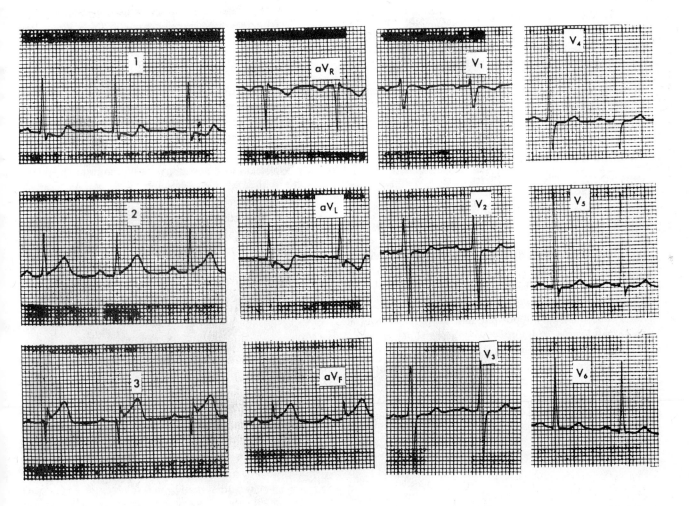

Fig. 73-1

7. Which of the following statements about pharmacologic agents used in the treatment of cardiogenic shock is *not* true?
   A. In severely hypotensive patients treated with doputamine, another agent may be required to increase systemic vascular resistance.
   B. A primary benefit of norepinephrine infusion is redistribution of blood flow to the heart and brain.
   C. Dopamine has been shown to be the most effective agent in decreasing mortality of cardiogenic shock.
   D. Substantial increase in cardiac output has been shown in patients with severe congestive heart failure caused by cardiomyopathy when treated with amrinone.

8. In cardiogenic shock which of the following carries the worst prognosis?
   A. Evidence of both right and left ventricular damage
   B. LVEDP greater than 29 Torr.
   C. Cardiac index less than 2 l/min/m², LVEDP less than 15
   D. Myocardial infarction in which 40% of the left ventricular mass has been damaged

9. Which of the following extra cardiac influences is most important in cardiogenic shock?
   A. Volume loss
   B. Sinus tachycardia
   C. Acidosis
   D. Vasodilators
   E. All of the above

10. Which of the following are not indicators for placement of pulmonary artery lines?
    A. Hypotension responsive to volume challenge
    B. Hypotension and congestive heart failure
    C. Unstable angina requiring intravenous nitroglycerin
    D. Distinguishing cardiogenic from noncardiogenic pulmonary edema

11. Cardiogenic shock is best defined by which of the following?
    A. Persistent low blood pressure after correcting hypovolemia, pulmonary wedge pressure greater than 16, urine output less than 20 cc per hour
    B. Altered mental status, peak systolic blood pressure less than 90
    C. Cool clammy skin, decreased level of consciousness, low blood pressure, urine output less than 20 cc per hour
    D. None of the above

Ischemic Heart Disease

Select the appropriate letter that correctly answers the question or completes the statement.

1. All of the following are true concerning sudden cardiac death *except*:
   A. Most patients have prodromal symptoms of chest pain.
   B. Ventricular fibrillation is the initial arrhythmia in 62% of cases.
   C. It is the initial manifestation of ischemic heart disease in 25% of patients.
   D. Prognosis for survivors of sudden cardiac death is better when not associated with an acute infarction.

2. All of the following are true regarding the difference between anterior and inferior myocardial infarctions *except*:
   A. An inferior myocardial infarction is associated with increased parasympathetic tone, which can contribute to nausea, vomiting, and diarrhea.
   B. An anterior myocardial infarction is likely to involve a larger area of the ventricle.
   C. An anterior infarction is more likely to be associated with ventricular wall thrombi.
   D. Right ventricular infarction is likely to complicate an inferior wall infarction.
   E. Sudden death is more likely as the initial manifestation of an anterior myocardial infarction.

3. In which of the following does coronary artery spasm play some role?
   A. Classic angina pectoris
   B. Prinzmetal's variant angina
   C. Acute myocardial infarction
   D. Sudden cardiac death
   E. All of the above

4. All of the following may cause ST segment elevation *except*:
   A. Pericarditis
   B. Digitalis toxicity
   C. Left bundle branch block
   D. Hyperkalemia
   E. Ventricular aneurysm

5. All of the following are true about the difference between subendomyocardial infarction and transmural myocardial infarction *except*:
   A. The presence or absence of Q waves does not differentiate a transmural myocardial infarction from an endocardial infarction.
   B. The incidence of hypotension is the same in each.
   C. Subendocardial infarction is more likely to be associated with pericarditis.

D. Both have the same incidence of ventricular arrhythmias.
   E. All of the above.
6. All of the following happen during Valsalva's maneuver *except*:
   A. Murmur of mitral valve prolapse increases in intensity.
   B. Murmur of aortic stenosis increases in intensity.
   C. Murmur of mitral regurgitation decreases in intensity.
   D. Coronary blood flow decreases by 45%.
   E. There is a reflex increase in parasympathetic tone.
7. All of the following are capable of causing Q waves, which can mimic an acute myocardial infarction, *except*:
   A. Left ventricular hypertrophy
   B. Idiopathic hypertrophic subaortic stenosis
   C. Wolff-Parkinson-White syndrome
   D. Pneumothorax
   E. Pericarditis
8. All of the following are true concerning left bundle branch block *except*:
   A. It can mask an acute myocardial infarction
   B. It can mimic an acute myocardial infarction.
   C. A right ventricular pacemaker will produce a left bundle branch block pattern.
   D. It can be confused with left ventricular hypertrophy.
   E. It is often associated with congenital heart disease.
9. Which of the following statements concerning cardiac enzymes in the emergency department is true?
   A. Rise in serum enzymes does not occur until 4 hours after an acute myocardial infarction.
   B. With special isoenzymes such as CPK-MB false positives do not occur.
   C. False negatives for all practical purposes do not occur.
   D. With increasing speed and availability, cardiac enzymes are becoming an important part of the ED evaluation of a patient with chest pain.
   E. All of the above are true.
10. The physical finding that would be the most helpful in differentiating a ventricular tachycardia from a supraventricular tachycardia with aberrancy would be:
    A. Intermittant cannon A waves
    B. Difference in blood pressure between two arms
    C. Reverse split of S_2
    D. Hepatojugular reflux
    E. Waterhammer pulses
11. The earliest EKG manifestation of acute myocardial ischemia is:
    A. Increase in R-wave voltage of precordial leads
    B. Elevated "hyper-acute" T waves

C. ST segment depression
    D. Inverted T waves
    E. ST segment elevation
12. Prinzmetal's variant angina is associated with all of the following *except*:
    A. EKG changes indistinguishable from an acute myocardial infarction
    B. Infrequently associated with serious arrhythmias
    C. Pain typically occurs at rest
    D. Pain frequently occurs at night
    E. May include normal coronary arteries or those with major occlusive disease
13. All of the following are true of postinfarction angina *except*:
    A. It may occur in up to 85% of patients.
    B. Treatment is essentially the same as noninfarction-associated angina.
    C. Ischemia at a distance from the infarct zone has a better prognosis.
    D. Ischemia involving the infarct zone most likely represents an incomplete infarct zone with a severely narrowed coronary artery supplying a hypokinetic ventricular wall segment.
    E. All of the above are true.
14. With which classic transmural infarction is a right ventricular infarction most likely to be found?
    A. Anterior
    B. Inferior
    C. Lateral
    D. Apical
    E. Any of the above
15. The single best way to differentiate acute pericarditis from acute myocardial infarction on the electrocardiogram is:
    A. ST segment clevation is diffuse with an upward concavity.
    B. Deviation of the P-R segment
    C. ST segments are elevated more diffusely.
    D. Lack of reciprocal changes
    E. Lack of acute T-wave inversion
16. Which of the following patients with an acute myocardial infarction needs a pacemaker?
    A. Right bundle branch block with left anterior hemiblock
    B. Alternating right bundle branch block and left bundle branch block
    C. Mobitz type 2, second degree AV block
    D. Right bundle branch block with first degree AV block
    E. All of the above

17. All of the following are true concerning conduction delay due to bundle branch block *except*:
    A. Complete heart block develops in 40% of patients with an acute myocardial infarction and EKG findings of right bundle branch block with left anterior hemiblock.
    B. Left anterior hemiblock is 10 times as common as left posterior hemiblock.
    C. Lidocaine can induce complete heart block in patients with an acute myocardial infarction and bilateral bundle branch block.
    D. An asymptomatic patient with a new left bundle branch block should be admitted and monitored.
    E. All of the above are true.

18. Right ventricular infarction is being recognized as a more important clinical entity than in years past. Which of the following statements is *not* true regarding right ventricular infarction?
    A. In general aggressive fluid resuscitation distinguishes its treatment from other types of infarction.
    B. Right ventricular infarction should be suspected with any inferior wall myocardial infarction.
    C. Jugular venous distention with the absence of congestive heart failure should suggest right ventricular infarction.
    D. Invasive hemodynamic monitoring is essential.
    E. None of the above.

19. It is well documented that a normal EKG does not exclude an acute myocardial infarction and that many "ischemic" or injury patterns may be related to causes other than ischemia. Which of the following is *always* related to an acute myocardial infarction?
    A. ST segment elevation and pathologic Q waves
    B. ST segment depression
    C. T-wave inversion
    D. None of the above

20. The earliest EKG manifestation of acute myocardial ischemia is which of the following?
    A. A marked increase in R-wave voltage
    B. Peaked T waves
    C. Hyperacute ST elevation
    D. Pathologic Q waves

21. Which of the following statements reflects lessons learned from the institution of Coronary Care Units?
    A. Ischemic heart disease patients have the highest risk in developing ventricular fibrillation after the onset of symptoms. *before*
    B. The aggressive containment of lethal rhythm disturbances is feasible.
    C. All of the above
    D. None of the above

22. Myocardial ischemia is defined as myocardial oxygen deficit resulting from reduced coronary profusion. This decrease in perfusion involves which of the following?

A. Delivery of oxygen to the heart
B. Delivery of metabolic substances to the heart
C. Removal of deleterious metabolic end products from the heart
D. All of the above

23. The relationship between hypoxemia and myocardial ischemia can best be described by which of the following?
    A. Hypoxemia always results in ischemic hypoxia of the myocardium.
    B. Both syndromes have reduced oxygen delivery to the heart.
    C. Both are associated with coronary perfusion deficits.
    D. None of the above.

24. The past 10 years have shown a decline in mortality related to ischemic heart disease. This is best attributed to:
    A. Lifestyle changes that would reduce coronary risk factors
    B. Impact of emergency medical services
    C. Impact of coronary artery bypass surgery
    D. The reason for the decline is unknown.

25. A 60-year-old man presents to the emergency department with a sudden onset of chest pain while mowing his lawn. The vital signs include a blood pressure of 130/90; heart rate 120; respiratory rate 20. Current medications include Lopressor hydrochlorathiazide and nitroglycerin PRN. Which of the following most likely precipitated his acute myocardial ischemia?
    A. A sudden decrease in coronary perfusion in the face of normal demand
    B. A sudden acceleration of myocardial demand in the face of normal coronary perfusion
    C. A mix of stable restriction of coronary perfusion exceeded by a sudden acceleration of myocardial demand
    D. A sudden increase in coronary perfusion in the face of increased demand

26. Myocardial oxygen demand (MVO_2) is a key factor that determines whether ischemia is present in a given situation. Much of our therapy is aimed at decreasing MVO_2. Which of the following are primary determinates of MVO_2?
    1. Systolic wall tension
    2. Ventricular size
    3. Duration of systolic wall stress
    4. Contractile state of the heart
    A. 1, 2, and 3   C. 1, 3, and 4
    B. 1 and 3   D. 1, 2, 3, and 4

27. Current indications for the use of thrombolytics include all but which of the following?
    A. The patient should present to the emergency

department within a few hours of the onset of symptoms.

B. ST segment elevation should be without Q waves on EKG

C. Capacity to do emergency follow-up cardiac catheterization should exist.

D. None of the above.

28. A 65-year-old man presents to the emergency department with an apparent acute inferior wall myocardial infarction confirmed by ST segment elevation in leads 2, 3 and AVF with reciprocal changes in the 1 through V-3. An initial CPK is elevated with positive MB isoenzymes. Chest pain has been relieved with 30 mg of IV morphine. He now has a blood pressure of 88/60, heart rate of 110, and urine output of 10 cc for the past hour and is beginning to exhibit signs of mental confusion. The lungs remain clear to auscultation. The chest x-ray is within normal limits. How would you proceed at this juncture?

A. 40 mg of Lasix to increase urine output

B. 500 cc of normal saline over 30 minutes

C. Dopamine infusion at 5-10 µg/kg/min.

D. Place a Swan-Ganz catheter before proceeding

29. Which of the following are characteristic of EKG findings in hypothermia?

1. Delta waves
2. Bradycardia
3. Q-T shortening
4. Osborn waves

A. 2, 3, and 4   C. 3 and 4
B. 1 and 3   D. 2 and 4

30. Which of the following statements regarding the significance of Q waves is *not* true?

A. The failure to find a new Q wave in the presence of an old one excludes the presence of acute myocardial infarction.

B. Abnormal and normal Q waves look alike.

C. The presence of Q waves does not alone establish the age of acute myocardial infarction.

D. The resolution of Q waves after acute myocardial infarction to an apparently innocent Q wave renders the EKG nondiagnostic.

31. Which of the following is *not* a cause of prominent T waves resembling those of acute myocardial ischemia?

A. Benign early repolarization
B. Idiopathic hypertropic subaortic stenosis
C. Subarachnoid hemorrhage
D. Hypokalemia

32. Which of the following statements regarding benign early repolarization (BER) is true?

A. BER is more often found in the mid- and left precordial leads than the right precordial leads.

B. ST segment elevation of BER is not associated

with reciprocal ST segment depression.

C. A distinctly notched J point is considered pathognomonic of BER.

D. BER can be confirmed when the ST segment contour is convexed upward and the ST segment elevation exceeds 5 mi.

33. A pseudoinfarction pattern can be represented by all of the following *except*:

A. Capacity to obscure the EKG changes of myocardial ischemia

B. Tendency to mimic the initial QRS force and ST-T abnormalities of myocardial infarction

C. Clinically associated with the chest pain, dyspnea, or syncope

D. All of the above

34. Bifascicular blocks, other than left bundle branch block, have clinical importance because adequate conduction depends entirely upon the integrity of the remaining third fascicle. Which of the following statements is *not* true about bifascicular block?

A. Bifascicular blocks have a well recognized risk for the development of sudden death.

B. Right bundle branch block and left posterior fascicular block (LPFB) are the most common type of bifascicular block.

C. The distal complete heart block caused by a sudden trifascicular block is generally unresponsive to atropine.

D. The acute myocardial infarction patient with bifascicular block merits consideration for a pacemaker.

35. You are called by the paramedics regarding a 55-year-old patient who has just experienced a syncopal episode. She denies chest pain and her monitor shows complete heart block with a wide QRS pattern and a ventricular rate of 40. Atropine 1 mg IV twice and an isoprel drip have been ineffective in restoring A-V conduction or accelerating ventricular rate. Her blood pressure is now 70/0 and she is having some ventricular ectopy. Which of the following would you now recommend?

A. Increase the Isoprel infusion
B. No change in therapy, rapid transport
C. Decrease the Isoprel infusion
D. Start a lidocaine infusion

36. Which of the following is *not* one of the actions of nitroglycerin?

A. Venous and arterial vasodilatation
B. Decreased heart rate and blood pressure
C. Decreased preload and afterload
D. Coronary artery vasodilatation
E. Direct relief of coronary vasospasm

75
Acute Abdominal Pain

Select the appropriate letter that correctly answers the question or completes the statement.

1. All of the following patients may complain of pain on the top of the shoulder *except*:
   A. Ruptured spleen
   B. Ectopic pregnancy
   C. Cholecystitis
   D. Perforated ulcer
   E. All of the above
2. What is the most common diagnosis of a patient with abdominal pain seen in the ED?
   A. Gastroenteritis
   B. Pelvic inflammatory disease
   C. Appendicitis
   D. Intestinal obstruction
   E. Abdominal pain of unknown etiology
3. Which of the following can have initial symptoms of abdominal pain as the chief complaint?
   A. Myocardial infarction
   B. Pneumonia
   C. Diabetic ketoacidosis
   D. Sickle cell crisis
   E. All of the above
4. A 5-year-old boy with a 2-day history of fever, anorexia, 2 episodes of vomiting, and diffuse abdominal pain is seen in the ED. He is a fussy uncooperative child who complains "everything hurts," but bowel sounds are positive and there is no definite guarding or rebound. His temperature is 103.5°F and urinalysis is normal. WBC is 16,000 with 82 segs and 10 bands. The next step would be:
   A. Exploratory laparotomy
   B. Flat plate of the abdomen
   C. Barium enema
   D. Serum and urine amylase
   E. Chest x-ray
5. Ultrasound is useful in evaluation of all of the following *except*:
   A. Cholelithiasis
   B. Abdominal aortic aneurysm
   C. Detection of ascitic fluid
   D. Ectopic pregnancy
   E. Acute pancreatitis
6. All of the following statements about appendicitis are true *except*:
   A. Diarrhea is more likely than constipation.
   B. Eighteen percent of patients will report prior episodes of similar pain.
   C. Abdominal pain usually occurs before the onset of nausea or vomiting.

D. Over 50% of the patients will not have a significant fever.
E. Ninety-six percent of patients with appendicitis will have either a WBC count over 10,000 or a shift to the left.
7. The most important cause of abdominal pain in a patient over age 70 is:
   A. Nonspecific abdominal pain
   B. Acute cholecystitis
   C. Diverticular disease
   D. Peptic ulcer disease
   E. Incarcerated hernia
8. The finding that is most predictive of an abnormality on abdominal radiography is:
   A. Distention
   B. Increased high-pitched bowel sounds
   C. Blood in the urine
   D. History of abdominal surgery
   E. Flank pain, tenderness

76
Upper Gastrointestinal Tract Disorders

Select the appropriate letter that correctly answers the question or completes the statement.

1. True statements about laboratory tests in patients with acute upper gastrointestinal bleeding include all of the following *except*:
   A. It may take 36 hours before the hematocrit drops to reflect the full extent of blood loss.
   B. Reticulocytosis can be expected within 24 hours.
   C. A PT, PTT, and platelet count will detect over 90% of bleeding disorders.
   D. BUN and creatinine can be expected to be elevated even without renal failure.
   E. A significant leukocytosis can be expected even without infection.
2. All of the following are useful in the treatment of esophageal reflux *except*:
   A. Elevation of the head of the bed
   B. Anticholinergic drugs
   C. Antacids
   D. Elimination of smoking, alcohol, and caffeine
   E. Cimetadine
3. What is the most common cause of massive upper gastrointestinal hemorrhage?
   A. Duodenal ulcer   D. Mallory-Weiss tear
   B. Gastric ulcer   E. Esophageal varices
   C. Erosive gastritis

78

4. Which of the following is most suggestive of a penetrating ulcer?
   A. Diminished response to antacids
   B. Radiation of pain to the back
   C. Onset of pain at night
   D. Signs of peritoneal irritation
   E. Diminished bowel sounds

5. Which of the following is true of diffuse esophageal spasm?
   A. May be relieved by nitroglycerin
   B. Usually requires surgical therapy
   C. Rarely is associated with dysphagia
   D. Pain is usually precipitated by activity
   E. Diagnosis is by endoscopy

6. Which procedure will most accurately diagnose Borehaave's syndrome?
   A. Gastrograffin swallow
   B. Chest radiograph
   C. Mediastinoscopy
   D. Acid perfusion (Berstein's test)
   E. Endoscopy

7. All of the following are helpful in distinguishing chest pain due to esophageal reflux from that of coronary artery disease except:
   A. Exacerbation of symptoms on bending forward
   B. Dysphagia
   C. Regurgitation into the back of the throat
   D. Relief of pain by antacids
   E. Pain waking the patient from sleep

8. All of the following are true about upper GI bleeding, except:
   A. Fifty percent of patients actively bleeding with known esophageal varices will be bleeding from some other source.
   B. Twenty-five percent of patients bleeding from a duodenal ulcer will have no history of ulcer symptoms.
   C. Twenty percent of patients complaining of intestinal bleeding are in fact not bleeding.
   D. Bleeding from Mallory-Weiss tears and esophageal varices is almost always painless.
   E. All of the above are true.

9. All of the following are true about the superior mesenteric artery syndrome except:
   A. Precipitating factors include weight loss, prolonged bed rest, body cast, and increased lordosis.
   B. Predominant symptom is midabdominal crampy pain.
   C. Eating a meal usually provides relief of pain.
   D. Usually diagnosed by an upper GI series.
   E. All of the above are true.

10. The classic electrolyte abnormality seen with protracted vomiting is:
    A. Metabolic acidosis with increased potassium
    B. Metabolic acidosis with decreased potassium
    C. Metabolic alkalosis with increased potassium
    D. Metabolic alkalosis with decreased potassium

11. All of the following are true about the Mallory-Weiss syndrome except:
    A. Often associated with alcohol
    B. Rarely requires surgical management
    C. Best diagnosed by endoscopy
    D. Associated with hiatal hernia
    E. Laceration occurs most often in the esophagus

12. All of the following can cause apparent melena except:
    A. Iron
    B. Charcoal
    C. Bismuth
    D. Aluminum hydroxide
    E. All of the above

13. Frequent complications seen with penetration of a duodenal ulcer include all of the following except:
    A. Hemorrhage
    B. Pancreatitis
    C. Weight loss
    D. Intractable pain
    E. Abscess formation

Match the items on the left with the correct items on the right.

D 14. Can be expected to have a low gastric PH.

C 15. Pain relieved by food.

D 16. Rapid gastric emptying.

A 17. May have a palpable supraclavicular lymph node (Virchow's node).

D 18. Surgery is the therapy of choice.

A. Gastric ulcer
B. Peptic ulcer
C. Both
D. Neither

Select the appropriate letter that correctly answers the question or completes the statement.

19. All of the following are associated with perforation of a peptic ulcer except:
    A. Vomiting
    B. Severe abdominal pain
    C. Hyperperistalsis
    D. Guaiac positive stools
    E. Diffuse abdominal guarding

20. All the following are true about bleeding esophageal varices except:
    A. Emergency portacaval shunt should be used only as a last ditch effort.
    B. Vasopressin, if infused directly into the superior mesenteric artery, is more effective than peripheral IV infusion.
    C. A major complication of a Sengstaken-Blackemore tube is aspiration.
    D. A major complication of vasopressin is coronary ischemia.
    E. All of the above.

21. All of the following concerning treatment of peptic ulcer disease are true *except*:
    A. Most antacids tend to be constipating.
    B. Antiacids should be given 1 hour and 3 hours after each meal and at bedtime.
    C. Bland diets are no more effective than a regular diet.
    D. Cimetadine is a histamine antagonist and a potent inhibitor of gastric acid excretion.
    E. Anticholinergic agents can decrease gastric secretion by 50%.

22. All of the following are true regarding gastric outlet obstruction due to peptic ulcer disease *except*:
    A. Most patients have had typical ulcer symptoms for years.
    B. Vomiting typically occurs 30–60 minutes after a meal.
    C. Most patients will require surgery.
    D. Anticholenergic medication often produces symptomatic relief.
    E. An N/G tube will drain 400 cc of fluid in 30 minutes.

23. Ranitidine is superior to cimetidine in all of the following areas *except*:
    A. Fewer side effects
    B. Fewer drug interactions
    C. More potent acid suppression
    D. More convenient dosage

77

Disorders of the Liver, Biliary Tract, and Pancreas

Select the appropriate letter that correctly answers the question or completes the statement.

1. A 44-year-old alcoholic with known cirrhosis is seen in the ED. He has had increasing confusion and lethargy for several days. On physical examination he is somnolent but arousable, oriented once with positive asterixis. Vital signs are: temperature 100°F, blood pressure 110/70, and pulse 100. The liver edge is palpable 5 cm below the right costal margin and there is a large accumulation of fluid. White blood cell count is 9,700 and hemoglobin is 12. The most appropriate therapy would be:
    A. Paracentesis of the abdomen
    B. Nasogastric tube drainage
    C. IV neomycin
    D. Rectal neomycin
    E. IV Lasix

2. Which of the following serologic markers indicate immunity to hepatitis B?

A. HBsAg   D. Anti-HBcAg
B. Anti-HBsAg   E. None of the above
C. HBcAg

3. A 70-year-old man with long-standing diabetes comes to the emergency department with a 2-week history of abdominal pain, fever, and vomiting. He appears acutely ill with a temperature of 102°F. His abdomen is diffusely tender, greater in the right upper quadrant, but no guarding or rebound is apparent. His white blood cell count is 18,000 and glucose is 250. His abdominal flat plate is shown in Fig. 77-1. The best management of this patient now would be:
    A. Schedule ultrasound of gallbladder
    B. Immediate laparotomy
    C. Order liver enzymes and a serum amylase
    D. Admit for high-dose antibiotics
    E. Immediate endoscopy

4. A 50-year-old alcoholic comes to the emergency department. He has a 3-month history of mid-epigastric abdominal pain without nausea, vomiting, or diarrhea and a 20-pound weight loss. You suspect a pancreatic carcinoma. The best test for this patient's initial evaluation would be:
    A. Pancreatic ultrasound
    B. Serum carcinoembryonic antigen levels
    C. Fasting blood sugar
    D. Upper GI series
    E. Paracentesis

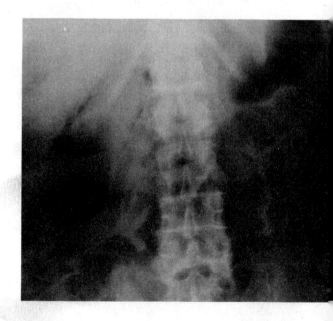

Fig. 77-1

Match the items on the right with their associated items on the left.

_A_ 5. Jaundice, anorexia, nausea, tender liver, increased ALT and SGOT, normal alkaline phosphatase

_D_ 6. Jaundice, anorexia, nausea, tender enlarged liver, SGOT elevated above ALT

_B_ 7. Jaundice, right upper quadrant tenderness with mild rebound, and leukocytosis with elevated SGOT, ALT, and alkaline phosphatase

_C_ 8. Jaundice, hepatosplenomegaly, moderately increased ALT, hypergammaglobulinemia

A. Viral hepatitis
B. Acute cholecystitis
C. Chronic active hepatitis
D. Alcoholic hepatitis

Select the appropriate letter that correctly answers the question or completes the statement.

9. A 16-year-old presents with a history of intermittent asymptomatic jaundice. He has a brother with similar symptoms. Physical examination is normal. The liver function tests show a bilirubin of 4 with .9 direct; SGOT and alkaline phosphatase are normal. CBC and reticulocyte count are also normal. The most appropriate therapy would be:
A. Cholecystectomy
B. Bone marrow biopsy
C. Splenectomy
D. Corticosteroids
E. None of the above

10. The best diagnostic test for a patient with suspected acalculus cholecystitis is:
A. Ultrasound
B. CT scan
C. ERCP
D. Hida scan
E. None of the above

11. All of the following conditions involve risk for developing gallstones except:
A. Pancreatitis
B. Obesity
C. Estrogen use
D. Hemolytic anemia
E. Ileal resection

12. All of the following reflect a poor prognosis in pancreatitis except:

A. Glucose over 200
B. White cells greater than 16,000
C. Calcium less than 8
D. LDH over 700 IU/dl
E. Amylase over 1,500 IU/dl

13. All of the following can precipitate hepatic encephalopathy except:
A. Gastrointestinal bleeding
B. Bacterial peritonitis
C. Phenothiazines
D. Hypokalemia
E. Hypertension

14. All of the following would be expected with a liver abscess except:
A. Hepatic tenderness radiating to the shoulder
B. Elevated alkaline phosphatase
C. Decreased breath sounds at the right lung base
D. Jaundice
E. Palpable liver edge

15. All of the following are causes of pancreatitis except:
A. Thiazide diuretics
B. Hypothyroidism
C. Hyperlipidemia
D. Trauma
E. Hypercalcemia

16. All of the following are causes of an elevated amylase except:
A. Perforated ulcer
B. Strangulated bowel
C. Acute cholecystitis
D. Ectopic pregnancy
E. All of the above

17. An icteric patient with presumed hepatitis B has a negative HBsAg with a negative anti-HBsAg. Which of the following conclusions is most valid?
A. The patient does not have hepatitis B.
B. The patient may have hepatitis B, but it would be too early in the course to detect serologic markers.
C. The patient may have hepatitis B, but may be in a state between serologic markers.
D. If the patient does have hepatitis B, he is prone to acute hepatic necrosis.
E. None of the above.

18. Non-A, Non-B hepatitis shares all these traits with hepatitis B except:
A. Carrier state does not develop
B. Fulminant hepatic necrosis does not develop
C. Postnecrotic cirrhosis does not develop
D. Non-A, Non-B is transmitted only via blood products.
E. All of the above.

19. Which of the following patients with acute hepatitis should be treated with immune serum globulin?
A. Hepatitis A
B. Hepatitis B
C. Non-A, Non-B
D. All of the above
E. None of the above

20. All of the following have been implicated as causing hepatic injury in therapeutic doses *except*:
   A. Isoniazid
   B. Erythromycin estolate
   C. Chloropromazine
   D. Alpha-methyl dopa
   E. All of the above

21. All of the following statements about alcoholic hepatitis are true *except*:
   A. There is a progression to cirrhosis after alcoholic hepatitis despite abstinence in some people.
   B. The risk of alcoholic hepatitis is unrelated to the amount of alcohol consumed.
   C. It can occur even in well-nourished alcoholics.
   D. It can lead to death in the acute episode.
   E. Definitive diagnosis is made by liver biopsy.

Match the items on the left with the correct item on the right.

22. Usually do not see jaundice	A. Hepatitis A
23. Can cause acute fulminant hepatic necrosis and death	B. Hepatitis B
24. Can lead to chronic active hepatitis	C. Both
25. Evidence of disease in 50% of the population over age 50	D. Neither
26. May develop Laennec's cirrhosis	

Select the appropriate letter that correctly answers the question or completes the statement.

27. Elevated transaminase levels may be caused by all of the following *except*:
   A. Congestive heart failure
   B. Shock
   C. Inflammatory bowel disease
   D. Respiratory failure
   E. Constrictive pericarditis

28. The delta agent is:
   A. Serologic marker for pancreatic cancer
   B. Elevated in cases of hepatic obstruction
   C. A virus that can complicate hepatitis B
   D. Detected in the blood after any cause of hepatic damage
   E. Thought to confer immunity from hepatitis B

78

Disorders of the Small Intestine

Select the appropriate letter that correctly answers the question or completes the statement.

1. All of the following are true regarding mesenteric vascular occlusion *except*:
   A. Diarrhea with occult blood is an expected finding.
   B. Many people will have intermittent preliminary symptoms.
   C. Required therapy is immediate surgical intervention.
   D. Large volumes of plasma pool in the bowel raising the hematocrit.
   E. Lactic acidosis with adequate peripheral perfusion is a common finding.

2. All of the following are true of intussusception *except*:
   A. Bowel sounds are usually normal.
   B. It typically involves the terminal ileum.
   C. It usually occurs in an older child.
   D. Meckel's diverticulum is the most common intrinsic bowel lesion.
   E. Adults are more likely to have a tumor as the initiating event.

3. Differentiation of pelvic inflammatory disease from appendicitis includes all of the following *except*:
   A. Bilateral adnexal tenderness with tenderness on cervical motion suggests pelvic inflammatory disease.
   B. There are equal degrees of leukocytosis, but the sedimentation rate tends to be higher in PID.
   C. Patients with PID will typically have had pain longer than with appendicitis.
   D. Pain of PID usually starts just after menstrual flow.

4. The radiographic finding most suggestive of appendicitis is:
   A. Right lower quadrant ileus
   B. Separation of right colon from flank stripe
   C. Blurring of right flank stripe
   D. Soft tissue mass in the right lower quadrant
   E. Fecalith

5. What is the "historic triad" that should suggest small bowel obstruction?
   A. Pain, vomiting, and prior surgery
   B. Pain, vomiting, and alcohol use
   C. Vomiting, lack of stool, and peritoneal irritation
   D. Pain, absent bowel sounds, and abdominal distention
   E. Absent bowel sounds, abdominal mass, and peritoneal irritation

6. All of the following are true regarding regional enteritis *except*:
   A. It can involve the colon, small bowel, or more frequently both.
   B. Inflammatory process affects all layers of the bowel wall and mesentery.
   C. Fistulas are a common complication.
   D. Extra intestinal complications are few.
   E. All of the above are true.
7. All of the following can be associated with regional enteritis *except*:
   A. Hydronephrosis
   B. Ankylosing spondylitis
   C. Conjunctivitis
   D. Megaloblastic anemia
   E. All of the above
8. The best way to differentiate an ileus from a small bowel obstruction is:
   A. Plain film of the abdomen
   B. Lack of pain with ileus
   C. Absence of bowel sounds with ileus
   D. Lack of abdominal distention with ileus
   E. Peritoneal irritation with obstruction
9. All of the following are recognized as causes of ileus *except*:
   A. Appendicitis
   B. Fracture of the lumbar spine
   C. Anticholinergic drugs
   D. Hyperkalemia
   E. Diabetic ketoacidosis
10. The most common cause of small bowel obstruction is:
    A. Adhesions   D. Tumor
    B. Hernia   E. Volvulus
    C. Intussusception
11. True statements about appendicitis in children include all of the following *except*:
    A. Perforation rate exceeds 50%.
    B. Forty to fifty percent of children with ruptured appendics have seen a physician earlier in their course.
    C. It is less likely to lead to generalized peritonitis.
    D. Diarrhea with other associated symptoms is more likely.
    E. All of the above.
12. Regional enteritis includes all of the following features *except*:
    A. Involves all layers of the bowel wall and mesentery
    B. Typified by skip areas of involved bowel with normal areas
    C. Incidence is increasing yearly
    D. Usually limited to the small bowel
    E. Fistula formation is a common complication
13. All of the following are true of a nonocclusive mesenteric infarction *except*:

   A. It accounts for 10% of cases of mesenteric vascular disease.
   B. It may be precipitated by arrythmias or transient episodes of hypotension.
   C. Digitalis has been implicated as a causative agent.
   D. It usually involves the superior mesenteric artery.
   E. It may begin insidiously and progress over several days or even weeks.

79
General Disorders of the Large Intestine

Select the appropriate letter that correctly answers the question or completes the statement.

1. Which of the following is the most common source of bright red rectal bleeding?
   A. Hemorrhoids
   B. Diverticular disease
   C. Intestinal polyps
   D. Meckel's diverticulum
   E. Carcinoma
2. Common causes of colonic obstruction include all of the following *except*:
   A. Carcinoma   D. Adhesions
   B. Volvulus   E. All of the above
   C. Diverticulitis
3. All of the following treatments of acute diarrhea are correct *except*:
   A. Oral fluids with glucose content will stimulate gastrointestinal absorption.
   B. Milk should be avoided because there is a transient lactase deficiency.
   C. Kaolin-pectin increases the incidence of formed stools and decreases total stool salt loss.
   D. The use of antimotility agents has been shown to increase the duration of fever, diarrhea, and excretion of organisms in patients with invasive diarrhea.
   E. Bismuth-subsalicylate (Pepto-Bismol) can improve fluid and electrolyte losses in toxigenic diarrhea.
4. What is the most common cause of rectal bleeding in a child?
   A. Anal fissure   D. Diverticulae
   B. Polyps   E. Infectious colitis
   C. Angiodysplasia
5. All of the following are metabolic causes of constipation *except*:
   A. Hypokalemia   D. Diabetes
   B. Hypercalcemia   E. Uremia
   C. Hypothryoidism

83

6. The best way to distinguish a toxin-mediated gastroenteritis from one due to an invasive organism is:
   A. Lack of true abdominal tenderness
   B. Lack of fever
   C. Absence of fecal leukocytes
   D. Diarrhea greater than nausea and vomiting
   E. Peripheral leukocytosis

7. The most common cause of massive lower GI bleeding is:
   A. Carcinoma
   B. Angiodysplasia
   C. Inflammatory bowel disease
   D. Polyps
   E. Diverticulosis

Match the descriptions on the left with the most appropriate lesion causing rectal bleeding listed on the right.

_____ 8. A small amount of blood mixed with the stool in an elderly patient with right lower quadrant pain and recent weight loss of 10 pounds.

_____ 9. Bloody diarrhea with diffuse cramps, generalized arthralgias, and fever in a 25-year-old.

_____ 10. Painless bright red blood per rectum occurring on 3 separate occasions in a 33-year-old.

_____ 11. Small amount of blood noticed coating the stool associated with rectal irritation in a 27-year-old.

   A. Colonic carcinoma
   B. Diverticular disease
   C. Ulcerative colitis
   D. Adenomatous polyps
   E. Internal hemorrhoids

80
Acute Gastroenteritis and Colon Disorders

Select the appropriate letter that correctly answers the question or completes the statement.

1. A 90-year-old resident of a local nursing home has a history of progressive abdominal distention and no stool for 2 weeks. He has a long history of senile dementia and chronic constipation. His blood pressure is 110/85, pulse is 90, and temperature is 98°F. He is in mild distress from pain, and the abdomen is distended and typmanitic with diffuse tenderness. A flat plate of the abdomen shows a single dilated loop of colon on the left side with both ends in the pelvis. The best initial therapy would be:
   A. Decompression with a Levine tube
   B. Immediate laparotomy
   C. Sigmoidoscopy with rectal tube
   D. Peritoneal lavage
   E. Broad-spectrum antibiotics and nasogastric tube

2. In a patient with inflammatory bowel disease how is ulcerative colitis clinically most likely to be differentiated from granulomatous colitis?
   A. Grossly bloody stools
   B. Elevated erythrocyte sedimentation rate
   C. Peripheral arthritis
   D. Colonic ulcerations
   E. Weight loss

3. Which of the following is true regarding treatment of salmonellosis?
   A. Antibiotics have not been shown to shorten the clinical course and may prolong the carrier state.
   B. Amoxicillin is the drug of choice.
   C. Erythromycin is the drug of choice.
   D. Trimethoprim-sulfamethoxazole is the drug of choice.
   E. Chloramphenicol is the drug of choice.

4. Which of the following is true regarding treatment of *Shigella*?
   A. Antibiotics have not been shown to shorten the clinical course.
   B. Amoxicillin is the drug of choice.
   C. Erythromycin is the drug of choice.
   D. Trimethoprim-sulfamethoxazole is the drug of choice.
   E. Chloramphenicol is the drug of choice.

5. Toxic megacolon is a serious complication seen in:
   A. Ischemic colitis
   B. Radiation colitis
   C. Shigellosis
   D. Ulcerative colitis
   E. Diverticulitis

6. All of the following are true of enterobius vermicularis *except*:
   A. Pruritis ani is the most common complaint.
   B. It can cause vaginitis, endometritis, or salpingitis.
   C. All children of the same family should be treated even if not infected.
   D. Treatment should be repeated 2 weeks after the initial dose.
   E. Diagnosis is by microscopic exam of the stool.

7. All the following are true about diarrhea caused by ecoli *except*:
   A. It can produce diarrhea either by mucosal invasion or production of an enterotoxin.
   B. The most common cause of "Tourista" in visitors to Mexico.
   C. Antibiotic prophylaxis is effective, but antibiotics are ineffective once symptoms have begun.
   D. Bismuth subsalicylate has been found to decrease enteric cyclic AMP and thus decrease diarrhea.
   E. It cannot be diagnosed on stool culture.

8. All of the following are true about amebic dysentery (entamoeba histolytica) *except*:
   A. It is usually associated with peripheral esophinilia.
   B. Serologic tests are the most common mode of diagnosis.
   C. The most common complication is liver abscess.
   D. Attacks are often precipitated by the use of steroids.
   E. Barium, antimotility agents, and antacids all interfere with recovery and identification of trophozoites.

9. A 30-year-old man presents with severe abdominal cramps and bloody diarrhea. He has been on high doses of ampicillin for 3 weeks due to a severe sinusitis. He has been otherwise healthy. His vital signs are blood pressure 110/70, pulse 120, and temperature 101°F. Physical examination is negative except for mild diffuse abdominal pain and increased bowel sounds. The most effective therapy would be:
   A. Supportive therapy with IV fluid replacement only
   B. Begin IV gentamycin and cephalothin
   C. Oral vancomycin
   D. Oral tetracycline
   E. Exploratory laporatomy

10. All the following are true regarding pin worms (*Enterobius vermicularis*) *except*:
    A. The best diagnosis by the scotch tape test.
    B. Mebendazole (Vermox), a single dose of 100 mg, is the drug of choice.
    C. Asymptomatic children in the family should be tested as well.
    D. Nocturnal puritis ani is the most common symptom.
    E. The human body is the only natural host.

11. A 33-year-old presents with intermittent abdominal cramps, occasional diarrhea, and foul-smelling stools since returning from a camping trip in Colorado 4 weeks ago. He has previously been in good health. Physical examination is normal and stool culture and ova and parasites are all negative. The best diagnostic test now is:

A. Sigmoidoscopy
B. Serologic titer for *Entamoeba histolytica*.
C. Duodenal aspirate.
D. Barium enema

12. Antibiotic-associated enterocolitis can be seen after all of the following *except*:
    A. Clindamycin
    B. Ampicillin
    C. Tetracycline
    D. Trimethoprim-sulfamethoxazole
    E. All of the above

13. The enteric pathogen most likely to mimic appendicitis is:
    A. *Yersinia enterocolitica*
    B. *Vibrio parahaemolyticus*
    C. *Campylobacter fetus*
    D. *Bacillus cereus*
    E. *Entamoeba histolytica*

14. The single best diagnostic test for suspected ulcerative colitis is:
    A. Barium enema
    B. Sigmoidoscopy
    C. Microscopic examination of diarrheal stool
    D. Gallium scan
    E. Serology

15. Scombroid fish poisoning should be treated with:
    A. Tetracycline
    B. Fluid replacement alone
    C. Antihistamines
    D. Vancomycin
    E. Nasogastric suction

16. Which of the following is the most common source of acute food poisoning in the United States?
    A. Staphylococcal
    B. Clostridium perfringens
    C. Bacillus cereus
    D. Toxigenic ecoli

17. All of the following are true regarding gastroenteritis due to *vibrio parahaemolyticus*, *except*:
    A. It is the most common cause of bacterial enteritis in Japan.
    B. It is limited to warmer months.
    C. It is only pathogenic for humans.
    D. A preformed enterotoxin is responsible for symptoms.
    E. It is a self-limited illness lasting 1–2 days.

18. Which of the following infections can be confused with acute ulcerative colitis?
    A. Entamoeba histolytica
    B. Shigella
    C. Campylobacter fetus
    D. All of the above

19. All of the following are true of diverticular disease *except*:
    (A) Most people present with pain.
    B. Diverticuli are due to chronic increased intra-luminal pressure.
    C. Morphine and codeine are contraindicated because of their effect on intraluminal pressure.
    D. Barium enema may cause perforation of an acutely inflamed diverticula.
    E. Vasopressin is often effective in stopping large amounts of bleeding.
20. Which of the following is true regarding treatment of *Campylobacter fetus*?
    A. Antibiotics have not been shown to shorten the clinical course and may prolong the carrier state.
    B. Amoxicillin is the drug of choice.
    (C) Erythromycin is the drug of choice.
    D. Trimethoprim-sulfamethoxazole is the drug of choice.
    E. Chloramphenicol is the drug of choice.

81
Disorders of the Anorectum

Select the appropriate letter that correctly answers the question or completes the statement.
1. True statements about hemorrhoids include all of the following *except*:
    (A) Thrombosed external hemorrhoids require evacuation of the clot.
    B. Of people over age 40, 70% have hemorrhoids.
    C. Internal hemorrhoids are always covered by mucous membrane.
    D. Intraabdominal tumors are frequently associated with hemorrhoids.
    E. Straining at stool is a major etiologic factor.
2. Which type of anal rectal abscess can be safely drained in the emergency department?
    A. Perianal abscess   D. Supralevator abscess
    B. Ischiorectal abscess (E) *A* and *C*
    C. Submucosal abscess
3. All of the following are true about proctalgia fugax *except*:
    A. Anal spasm lasts 5–10 minutes.
    B. It is relieved by nitroglycerin
    C. There is a high incidence of psychiatric disorders
    (D) It can be triggered by digital exam.
4. The most common initial presentation of internal hemorrhoids is:
    A. Painful bright red rectal bleeding
    (B) Painless bright red rectal bleeding

C. Prolapse
D. Thrombosis
E. Spasm of the anal sphincter

82
Genitourinary Disease

Select the appropriate letter that correctly answers the question or completes the statement.
1. Which of the following statements is true concerning acute prostatitis?
    A. Trimethoprim-sulfamethoxazole is bacteriostatic and should not be used.
    B. Vigorous massage of the prostate prevents localization of pus and decreases the need for surgery.
    C. If urinary retention occurs, a Foley catheter is indicated.
    (D) Culture of voided urine will usually reveal the responsible organism.
    E. None of the above is true.
2. A 38-year-old man has a sudden onset of left flank pain radiating to his groin. He is afebrile and appears normal on physical examination. Urinalysis shows a pH of 6 with many red blood cells. An IVP shows a 4-mm stone at the ureterovesicular junction. Correct management of this patient would be:
    A. Admit for vigorous hydration and analgesia
    B. Admit for IV and antibiotics
    C. Discharge with urine strainer, antibiotics, and analgesia
    (D) Discharge with urine strainer and analgesia
    E. Immediate urologic consultation
3. Urgent urologic consultation should be orderd for a patient with a kidney stone and which of the following?
    A. Solitary kidney
    B. Stone diameter greater than 6 mm
    C. High degree of obstruction
    D. Intractible vomiting
    (E) Evidence of infection
4. All of the following are true anout kidney stones *except*:
    A. Of stones 4 mm or less 90% will pass spontaneously.
    (B) The narrowest point along the ureter is the ureteropelvic junction.
    C. About 90% of stones are radiopaque.
    D. Most stones are composed of calcium oxalate.
    E. Most people with one kidney stone will have another.

5. A 13-year-old boy reports pain and swelling of his right testicle that has awakened him from sleep. All of the following make torsion of the testicle more likely than epididymitis *except*:
   A. The patient's age
   B. Sudden onset of symptoms
   C. History of similar pain that has resolved spontaneously
   D. Absence of urinary symptoms
   E. Relief of pain on elevation of the testicle

6. All of the following are true about urinary tract infection during pregnancy *except*:
   A. All asymptomatic bacteriuria should be treated.
   B. All patients with evidence of pyelonephritis should be admitted for parenteral antibiotics.
   C. Asymptomatic bacteriuria has little effect on the developing fetus.
   D. Cephradine is the antibiotic of choice for a penicillin-allergic patient.
   E. All of the following are true

7. All the following conditions involve risk for post-IVP renal failure *except*:
   A. Preexisting renal disease
   B. Diabetes
   C. Multiple myeloma
   D. Sepsis
   E. All of the above

8. All of the following are true about hematuria *except*:
   A. The degree of hematuria is related to the seriousness of the etiology.
   B. Red blood cell casts indicate a source of bleeding from the kidney.
   C. Myoglobinuria should be suspected when the dip stick is positive but no red blood cells are seen.
   D. Hemorrhage from benign prostatic hypertrophy is the most common cause of hematuria in a man over age 60.
   E. Terminal hematuria is caused by disease of the bladder neck or prostate.

9. The most common cause of painless gross hematuria in a middle-aged man is:
   A. Kidney stone
   B. Hemorrhage cystitis
   C. Bladder tumor
   D. Renal carcinoma
   E. Prostatic hypertrophy

10. All of the following are true of acute urinary retention *except*:
   A. An emergency IVP should be done on the initial presentation.
   B. An increase in BUN to creatinine ratio may be expected.
   C. The patient is at risk for postobstructive diuresis and possible dehydration.
   D. If a coudé catheter cannot be passed, a suprapubic tap can be used for temporary symptomatic relief.
   E. Antihistamine, anticholinergic agents and tricyclic antidepressants have all been implicated as etiologic agents.

11. For which of the following women with a urinary tract infection would single-dose therapy be appropriate?
   A. The patient with hemorrhagic cystitis
   B. The patient with symptoms longer than 48 hours
   C. Recurrence of bacteriuria 3 days after treatment
   D. Symptomatic patient with pyuria but not bacteriuria
   E. None of the above

12. All of the following concerning urinary tract infection in a child are true *except*:
   A. Suprapubic aspiration is the preferred method for obtaining a urine sample in a child under 1 year.
   B. Bacturemia is present in 50% of neonates with urinary tract infections.
   C. Boys have an increased risk of infection with *Proteus*.
   D. All demand an urgent referral to a urologist.
   E. All of the above

13. The only age group in which urinary tract infection is more common in a male than a female is:
   A. Neonates
   B. Preschool-age
   C. School-age
   D. Reproductive age
   E. Geriatrics

14. Which antibiotic is the drug of choice for urinary tract infection due to *Proteus mirabilis*?
   A. Ampicillin
   B. Tetracycline
   C. Gentamicin
   D. Trimethoprim-sulfamethoxazole
   E. Cephalexin

15. All the following are true about epididymitis *except*:
   A. It is a sexually transmitted disease in a young patient.
   B. It usually requires operative intervention.
   C. Most cases of orchitis are secondary to extension of epididymitis.
   D. It may result in sterility.
   E. Forty percent of patients will have pyuria.

16. The most common organism causing epididymitis in a 20-year-old is:
   A. *Chlamydia trachomatis*
   B. *Neisseria gonorrhoea*
   C. *Escherichia coli*
   D. *Staphylococcus aureus*
   E. *Herpes genetalis*

17. All of the following are true of testicular torsion *except*:
   A. It can occasionally be managed nonsurgically.
   B. It involves an underlying bilateral anatomic abnormality.
   C. Doppler studies and isotopic scans are equally effective in their ability to confirm lack of blood flow.
   D. A reactive hydrocele may be present.
   E. With vascular compromise for 6 hours, there may be irreversible loss of spermatogenesis.

18. A previously healthy 26-year-old presents with the sudden onset of right lower quadrant abdominal pain radiating to the testicle associated with nausea and vomiting. He is afebrile and has a normal physical exam. Urinalysis shows a specific gravity of 1.010 and pH of 5.0 with many erythrocytes. A flat plate of the abdomen reveals an opaque stone. The most likely etiology of this patient's stone is:
   A. Primary hyperoxaluria
   B. Uric acid stone
   C. Renal tubular acidosis
   D. Magnesium-amonium-phosphate stone
   E. Idiopathic hypercalcuria

83
Pelvic Pain

Select the appropriate letter that correctly answers the question or completes the statement.

1. A 24-year-old gravida 1 para 0 in her sixth month of pregnancy complains of a 2-day history of pain just below the right costal margin. She has persistent nausea and vomiting. She is afebrile with a WBC of 12,7000, and a urinalysis shows 3 to 4 WBC/hpf. The most likely diagnosis is:
   A. Round ligament strain
   B. Uterine contractions
   C. Acute pyelonephritis
   D. Penetrating ulcer
   E. Appendicitis
2. All of the following concerning pyelonephritis in pregnancy are true except:
   A. All should be admitted to the hospital.
   B. Tetracycline should be avoided.
   C. Progesterone causes decreased peristaltic activity and dilatation of the ureter.
   D. Relapse rate is high and patients should be treated for 4 to 6 weeks.
   E. Classic signs and symptoms are usually absent.
3. All of the following are true concerning appendicitis in pregnancy except:
   A. Appendicitis may initiate premature labor.
   B. Pregnant woman are at increased risk for appendicitis.
   C. Leukocytosis up to 15,000 is normal in pregnancy.
   D. Fever is uncommon.
   E. There is greater risk of generalized peritonitis during pregnancy.
4. All of the following are true concerning the potential risk of birth control pills except:
   A. The risk of pregnancy and its complications is greater than with any birth control pill.
   B. The use of birth control pills in early pregnancy doubles the risk of congenital abnormalities.
   C. The most common serious risk is from thromboembolic events.
   D. Increased blood pressure is seen in 5% of women on birth control pills.
   E. All of the above are true.
5. All of the following are true concerning intrauterine devices except:
   A. They are equally effective as birth control pills in preventing pregnancy.
   B. IUDs are associated with an increased risk of ectopic pregnancy.
   C. Asymptomatic uterine infection is a common early complication.
   D. They can be safely removed with ring forceps without local anesthesia.
   E. If a patient gets pregnant with an IUD in place, it should be removed.
6. The drug of first choice to treat premenstrual tension is:
   A. Naprosyn
   B. Spironolactone
   C. Medroxyprogesterone
   D. Pyridoxine (vitamin B-6)
   E. None of the above
7. All of the following are causes of secondary dysmenorrhea except:
   A. Endometriosis   D. Follicular cyst
   B. Adenomyosis   E. Intrauterine device
   C. Uterine leiomyomata
8. Which of the following is true concerning mittelschmerz syndrome:
   A. Withdrawal spotting may occur.
   B. A major complication is endometritis.
   C. It can be prevented with a D & C.
   D. It is often associated with pelvic trauma.
   E. Oral contraceptives have no effect.

84
Complications of Pregnancy

Select the appropriate letter that correctly answers the question or completes the statement.

1. A 19-year-old gravida 1, para 0,36 weeks gestation has a 2-day history of headaches associated with nausea and vomiting. She has had an uneventful pregnancy until now. Blood pressure is 150/100, pulse is 108, and temperature is 97°F. The fundi are benign, neck is supple, and chest and abdomen are normal. The uterus is at an ap-

propriate height with fetal heart tones of 160, she has 2+ pedal edema, and reflexes are 3+ with unsustained clonus. Laboratory data include: CBC 13,500, II & II 13/36, and urinalysis with 3+ protein, 1 to 2 WBC, and 0 RBC. The agent of choice for this patient is:
A. Hydralazine
B. Nitroprusside
C. Diazoxide
D. Propranolol
E. Reserpine

2. All of the following statements concerning magnesium sulfate in eclampsia are true *except*:
A. It has a significant antihypertensive effect.
B. It causes depression of deep tendon reflexes.
C. The effects are reversed with calcium gluconate infusion.
D. Initial dose should be 4 gm IV.
E. All of the above are true.

Match the item on the left with the appropriate item on the right.

_A_ 3. Associated with painless bright red vaginal bleeding
_B_ 4. Associated with abdominal pain and dark vaginal bleeding
_B_ 5. High incidence of clotting abnormalities
_D_ 6. Diagnosis by careful manual examination

A. Placenta previa
B. Abrupto placenta
C. Both
D. Neither

Select the appropriate letter that correctly answers the question or completes the statement.

7. All of the following are suggestive of a hydatidiform mole *except*:
A. Uterus is larger than expected by gestational age.
B. Nausea and vomiting begin earlier and are more severe.
C. There is a low level of serum HCG.
D. It is frequently associated with increased blood pressure.
E. All of the above.

8. Delayed postpartum hemorrhage is usually due to:
A. Retained portions of the placenta
B. Inadequate oxytocin production
C. Clotting abnormalities
D. Trauma from delivery
E. Uterine infection

9. All of the following are important components of therapy for postpartum hemorrhage due to uterine atony *except*:

A. Intravenous oxytocin
B. Manual uterine massage
C. Replacement of blood loss
D. Uterine curettage
E. All of the above

10. All of the following are associated with normal pregnancies *except*:
A. Carpal tunnel syndrome
B. Acute cholecystitis
C. Pituitary infarction
D. Amniotic fluid embolism
E. Hyperemesis gravidarum

11. All of the following statements about pregnancy are true *except*:
A. Rupture of membranes can be confirmed with nitrazine paper showing a pH of 7.0.
B. Current treatment of hyperemesis gravidarum is with pyridoxine.
C. Amniotic fluid embolus is a frequent, often unrecognized complication of normal delivery.
D. A temporizing maneuver for a breech presentation is to place the patient in Trendelenburg position.

12. All of the following are true of toxemia of pregnancy *except*:
A. It complicates 10% of all pregnancies.
B. It is more common in multiparous women.
C. Seizures should be controlled with magnesium sulfate.
D. Definitive treatment is delivery of the infant and placenta.
E. The primary pathophysiologic event is vasospasm due to an unknown toxin.

13. The most common complication of a missed abortion is:
A. Clotting abnormalities
B. Sepsis
C. Hemorrhage
D. Pulmonary emboli
E. Infertility

14. Uterine rupture is associated with all of the following *except*:
A. Previous uterine surgery
B. Cessation of contraction
C. Clinical hypovolemia out of proportion to vaginal bleeding
D. Peritoneal irritation
E. 100% fetal mortality

85

Ectopic Pregnancy

Select the appropriate letter that correctly answers the question or completes the statement.

1. Features that suggest a threatened intrauterine abortion as opposed to an ectopic pregnancy include all of the following *except*:
   A. Bleeding is heavier
   B. Soft, nontender cervix
   C. Anemia greater than expected from the amount of bleeding
   D. Longer period of amenorrhea
   E. Pain localized more in the midline

2. All of the following are true concerning culdocentesis to diagnose ectopic pregnancy *except*:
   A. A dry tap effectively excludes ectopic pregnancy.
   B. Obtaining straw-colored fluid effectively excludes an ectopic pregnancy.
   C. It is impossible to differentiate a true positive tap from a false positive secondary to vascular aspiration.
   D. Aspirate with a hematocrit of less than 10% favors the diagnosis of ectopic pregnancy.
   E. None of the above are true.

3. Which of the following presentations is compatible with an ectopic pregnancy?
   A. 21-year-old posttubal ligation with a 2-day history of lower abdominal pain, last period 6 weeks ago
   B. 28-year-old with an IUD in place complaining of low back pain, urinary frequency, and low-grade fever, last period 4 weeks ago.
   C. 18-year-old with 2-day history of lower abdominal pain, vaginal discharge, fever, nausea, and vomiting, just started her period
   D. 25-year-old who passed out while shopping, blood pressure 100/70 lying down, 80/40 sitting, hematocrit 28%
   E. All of the above

4. Which of the physical findings listed is most suggestive of an ectopic pregnancy?
   A. Fullness of cul-de sac
   B. Normal sized uterus with a positive pregnancy test
   C. Rebound tenderness
   D. Adnexal mass
   E. Abdominal pain referred to shoulder

5. Features that suggest a threatened intrauterine abortion as opposed to an ectopic pregnancy include all of the following *except*:
   A. Bleeding is heavier
   B. Soft, nontender cervix
   C. Anemia greater than expected from the amount of bleeding
   D. Longer period of amenorrhea
   E. Pain localized more in the midline

6. Which is the *least* frequent sign of ectopic pregnancy?
   A. Abdominal pain D. Vaginal bleeding
   B. Amenorrhea   E. Adnexal mass
   C. Cervical tenderness

7. All of the following are associated with an increased incidence of ectopic pregnancy *except*:
   History of
   A. Salpingitis
   B. Therapeutic abortion
   C. Tubal ligation
   D. IUD
   E. Pelvic adhesions

8. All of the following are true about birth control methods and ectopic pregnancy *except*:
   A. Birth control pills have the lowest incidence of both intrauterine and ectopic pregnancy.
   B. Tubal ligation is a very effective form of contraception, but if pregnancy occurs there is a 50% chance it will be ectopic.
   C. IUD users have a greater risk of ectopic pregnancy especially during the first 2 years.
   D. Patients with an IUD are at increased risk for ectopics for up to 6 months after the IUD is removed.

9. Which of the following statements concerning pregnancy tests is the *most* true?
   A. Whole molecule radial receptor assay for HCG is the most specific test.
   B. A gestational sac should be identified by ultrasound when the quantitative HCG is over 3,000.
   C. A quantitative level of HCG, which does not increase by 66% in 48 hours, should suggest an ectopic pregnancy.
   D. The more specific the pregnancy test, the fewer the number of false negatives.
   E. The rapid receptor assay can detect HCG levels as low as 40 m/v.

10. Which of the following is true concerning an ectopic pregnancy?
    A. The ratio of ectopic to intrauterine pregnancies has more than doubled in the past 10 years.
    B. The incidence of ectopic pregnancies has decreased but more are being recognized.
    C. Ectopic pregnancy is relatively more common in a younger age group.
    D. The most common predisposing factor is an IUD.
    E. None of the above.

86
Vaginal Bleeding

Select the appropriate letter that correctly answers the question or completes the statement.

1. All of the following are true of uterine leiomyomas *except*:
   A. They frequently undergo malignant degeneration.
   B. They are usually asymptomatic.
   C. They are seen in 20% of women over age 35.
   D. Estrogenic stimulation is an important etiologic factor.
   E. They frequently regress after menopause.

2. Which is not associated with uterine myomata (fibroids)?
   A. Palpable mass
   B. Heavy periods
   C. Urinary frequency
   D. Pressure sensation on the rectum
   E. Midcycle bleeding

3. Which of the following is true regarding cervical polyps?
   A. They usually cause heavy cyclic bleeding.
   B. They often degenerate to cervical carcinoma.
   C. Diagnosis is by colposcopy.
   D. They are the cause of postcoital bleeding.

4. All of the following are true about normal menstrual bleeding *except*:
   A. Cycles from 18–40 days are considered normal.
   B. Variation within the cycle of as many as 5 days is normal.
   C. Duration of menses is from 3–7 days.
   D. Normal blood loss is 25–60 cc.
   E. Some women normally pass clots.

5. All of the following are true of anovulatory cycles *except*:
   A. It is the most common cause of dysfunctional uterine bleeding.
   B. It often presents like a threatened abortion.
   C. Treatment is a "Medical curettage" with IM progesterone.
   D. The underlying pathology is an inadequate endometrial phase.

6. The most common cause of abnormal vaginal bleeding not related to pregnancy is:
   A. Birth control pills
   B. Uterine myomata
   C. Cervical cancer
   D. Corpus luteum cyst
   E. Pelvic inflammatory disease

87
Genital Infections

Select the appropriate letter that correctly answers the question or completes the statement.

1. Which of the following types of venereal disease is caused by a *Chlamydial* organism?
   A. Chancroid
   B. Lymphogranuloma venereum
   C. Granuloma inguinale
   D. Condylomata accuminata

Match the items on the right with their associated items on the left.

   2. Thick cheesy vaginal discharge with plaques adherent to vaginal mucosa
   3. Punctate red foci on the cervix associated with a copious, foul smelling, frothy discharge
   4. Grey homogeneous vaginal discharge with clue cells
   5. Liquid filled vesicles and ulcers on the cervix and vagina with a clear discharge

   a. Tetracycline, 500 mg qid
   b. Metronidazole, 250 mg tid
   c. Local Acyclovir cream, 1%
   d. Local clotrimazole cream

Match the items on the right with their associated items on the left.

   6. It can cause an acute urethral syndrome in both men and women.
   7. It can exist as an asymptomatic infection in both men and women.
   8. Tetracycline is effective therapy.
   9. Ampicillin, 3.5, plus 1 g Probenecid orally is curative.
   10. It frequently coexists with other sexually transmitted diseases.

   a. *Neisseria gonorrhea*
   b. *Chlamydia*
   c. Both
   d. Neither

Select the appropriate letter that correctly answers the question or completes the statement.

11. A 25-year-old man presents to the emergency department "to be checked for VD." A sexual partner told him she had it, but he doesn't know what type. He has been completely asymptomatic. The best management of this patient would be:
    A. Urethral culture and await results prior to treatment
    B. Urethral Gram's stain and treat if any gram-negative intracellular organisms are seen
    C. Urethral Gram's stain and treat if any leukocytes are seen
    D. One gram Probenecid with 4.8 million units of penicillin
    E. Tetracycline, 500 mg qid

12. All of the following concerning herpes genitalis are true except:
    A. Acyclovir ointment is as effective as oral acyclovir for initial infection.
    B. Mothers with herpes genitalis should be delivered by cesarean section.
    C. Diagnosis is by a Tzanck smear showing multinucleated giant cells.
    D. There is an increased risk of cervical cancer.
    E. It can cause fever blisters on lips and gums.

13. All of the following are true about the toxic shock syndrome except:
    A. Vigorous fluid resuscitation is the most important aspect of therapy.
    B. Antistaphylococcal antibiotics shorten the duration of symptoms.
    C. An erythematous macular rash with desquamation during recovery is expected.
    D. Any form of contraception decreases the risk.
    E. Blood cultures are negative.

14. All the following antibiotics are contraindicated in pregnancy except:
    A. Erythromycin   D. Metronidazole
    B. Tetracycline   E. Trimethroprim
    C. Sulfonamides

15. The most common cause of vaginitis among premenarch girls is:
    A. Foreign body vaginitis
    B. Monilial vulva vaginitis
    C. Trichomoniasis
    D. Herpes genitalis
    E. Chemical irritant vaginitis

16. The treatment for condyloma acuminatum (veneral warts) is:
    A. IM procaine penicillin
    B. Acyclovir cream
    C. Oral tetracycline
    D. Podofhyllin locally
    E. IM benzathene penicillin

17. The most commonly seen vaginal infection among adult women is:
    A. Monilial vaginitis   D. Herpes genitalis
    B. Trichomoniasis   E. Atropic vaginitis
    C. Hemophyilis vaginalis

18. All of the following are effective treatments for incubating syphilis (zero-negative without clinical signs) except:
    A. 1 g probenecid followed by 4.8 million units procaine penicillin IM
    B. Tetracycline, 500 mg qid, for 7 days
    C. Ampicillin, 3.5 g by mouth after 1 g probenecid
    D. Amoxicillin, 3 g by mouth after 1 g of probenecid
    E. Spectinomycin, 2 g IM

19. True statements concerning gonorrhea include all of the following except:
    A. It is responsible for 20–40% of cases of pelvic inflammatory disease.
    B. Forty percent of women with gonorrhea may be asymptomatic.
    C. The incubation period is 3-10 days.
    D. Men are almost never asymptomatic.
    E. The only natural reservoir is man.

20. All of the following statements are true about syphilis except:
    A. Serologic tests are often negative during the primary stage of chancre formation.
    B. The rash of secondary syphilis is one of few that typically involves the palms and soles.
    C. Penicillin, tetracycline, and erythromycin in appropriate doses are all curative.
    D. All patients require follow-up for 1 year.
    E. The hallmark of primary syphilis is a painful and endurated genital ulcer.

21. All of the following statements are true about pelvic inflammatory disease except:
    A. Less than 65% of patients clinically diagnosed have laparoscopic evidence of PID.
    B. PID was found at laparoscopy in 15% of patients believed not to have the disease.
    C. Most patients will have an elevated white blood cell count but a relatively normal erythrocyte sedimentation rate.
    D. Neisseria gonorrohea and Chlamydia together account for 80% of cases of PID.
    E. PID represents a leading cause of ectopic pregnancy, infertility, and chronic pelvic pain.

22. Persistent monilial vulvovaginitis is often associated with which systemic disease?
    A. Lupus erythematosus
    B. Diabetes mellitus
    C. Renal failure
    D. Epilepsy
    E. Regional enteritis

88
Anemia and White Blood Cell Disorders

Select the appropriate letter that correctly answers the question or completes the statement.

1. The reticulocyte count should be elevated in all of the following *except*:
   A. Sickle cell disease
   B. Polycythemia vera
   C. Aplastic anemia
   D. Coombs' positive hemolytic anemia
   E. Occult gastrointestinal bleeding

2. All of the following are expected to have elevated mean corpuscular volume and mean corpuscular hemoglobin (macrocytic picture) *except*:
   A. Thalassemia   D. Liver disease
   B. B_{12} deficiency   E. Hypothyroidism
   C. Folate deficiency

3. All of the following are decreased in iron deficiency anemia *except*:
   A. Serum iron level
   B. Serum iron binding capacity
   C. Serum ferritin
   D. Bone marrow stainable iron
   E. Hemoglobin

4. All of the following are important in the treatment of sickle cell vasoocclusive crisis *except*:
   A. Fluid restriction
   B. Oxygen
   C. Analgesics
   D. Folic acid

5. Which of the following is true of chronic myelogenous leukemia?
   A. It is the most common leukemia of adults.
   B. Splenomegaly is rare.
   C. It has elevated leukocyte alkaline phosphatase.
   D. While the total white blood cell count is elevated, the differential is normal.
   E. It is associated with increased platelets and red blood cells.

6. You see a patient whom you suspect has a leukomoid reaction. The best way to differentiate this from chronic myelogenous leukemia would be:
   A. Bone marrow biopsy
   B. Leukocyte alkaline phosphatase
   C. Immune electrophoresis
   D. Cold agglutinins
   E. Examination of the peripheral smear

7. All the following are true about white blood cells *except*:
   A. One-half of the total circulating neutrophils are adherent to vessel walls and not measured on a blood sample.
   B. Only 5% of the total body lymphocytes are in the circulation at any one time.
   C. Normally one can expect one band form for each 10 neutrophils.
   D. An increase in total white blood cell count without an increased number of bands can be seen as the result of exercise, stress, or epinephrine.
   E. Lymphocytes can be divided morphologically into T cells, B cells, and null cells.

8. The disorder most likely to be found in a patient with sickle cell trait is:
   A. Osteomyelitis   D. Vasoocclusive crisis
   B. Retinal hemorrhages   E. Hematuria
   C. Splenic autoinfarction

9. The most common cause of death in a patient with sickle cell anemia is:
   A. Aplastic crisis
   B. Cerebrovascular accident
   C. Renal failure
   D. Infection
   E. Hemorrhage

10. A 4-year-old child with a history of sickle cell anemia presents with osteomyelitis. Which of the following is the *most* likely pathogen?
    A. *Hemophilis influenzae*
    B. *Salmonella*
    C. *Staphylococcus*
    D. *Streptococcus*
    E. *Pseudomonas*

11. Which of the following is the specific test for paroxysmal nocturnal hemoglobinuria?
    A. Osmotic fragility
    B. Hemoglobin electrophoresis
    C. Sucrose and acid hemolysis
    D. Bone marrow biopsy
    E. Direct Coombs' test

12. Neutrophilic leukocytes with greater than 5 lobes are seen in which disease?
    A. Folate deficiency
    B. Hereditary spherocytosis
    C. Autoimmune hemolytic anemia
    D. Thalassemia
    E. Aplastic anemia

13. A child who presents with a microcytic anemia associated with basophylic stippling of red blood cells on the peripheral smear should have which disease excluded?
    A. Sickle cell disease
    B. Folate deficiency
    C. Lead poisoning
    D. B_{12} Deficiency
    E. Aplastic anemia

14. A patient with sideroblastic anemia should have a trial of which type of therapy?
    A. Iron   C. Pyridoxine (B$_6$)
    B. Folate   D. Serum electrophoresis
15. The site of erythropoietin production is:
    A. Liver   D. Hypothalamus
    B. Kidney   E. Adrenal gland
    C. Bone marrow
16. Decreased serum haptoglobin would be expected in which of the following disorders?
    A. Iron deficiency anemia
    B. Thalassemia
    C. B$_{12}$ deficiency
    D. Hemolytic anemia
    E. Sideroblastic anemia
17. All the following are true of chronic lymphocytic leukemia *except*:
    A. Most patients will have lymphocytosis.
    B. It is often associated with autoimmune disorders.
    C. It often terminates in a blastic crisis.
    D. It is the most common leukemia in patients over age 50.
    E. It may require no therapy.

89

Disorders of Hemostasis and Polycythemia

Select the appropriate letter that correctly answers the question or completes the statement.

1. All of the following can be expected in a patient with thrombotic thrombocytopenic purpura *except*:
   A. Microangiopathic anemia
   B. Elevated PT and PTT
   C. Renal disease
   D. Fever
   E. Fluctuating neurologic symptoms
2. What is the single best test to confirm your suspicion that a patient has disseminated intravascular coagulation?
   A. Increased fibrinogen degradation products
   B. Prolonged PTT
   C. Prolonged PT
   D. Decreased platelet count
   E. Prolonged bleeding time
3. Which of the following statements are true about thrombocytopenia?
   A. An elevated PTT and normal PT is usually seen.
   B. Aspirin is a leading cause.
   C. Spontaneous bleeding is unlikely to occur at platelet counts above 20,000.
   D. The most common initial clinical manifestation is

   hemarthrosis.
   E. It is usually caused by a genetically transmitted defect.
4. A 50-year-old man develops gastrointestinal bleeding after ingestion of 25 Coumadin tablets as a suicide attempt. His blood pressure is 90/40, pulse 125. His PT is 80, and PTT is 35 with a hematocrit of 32%. The best initial therapy for the clotting defect is:
   A. Antihemophilic factor
   B. Whole blood
   C. Fresh-frozen plasma
   D. Vitamin K
   E. Protamine sulfate
5. All of the following cause a prolonged bleeding time *except*:
   A. Normal patient taking aspirin
   B. Patient with idiopathic thrombocytopenic purpura
   C. Patient with scurvy
   D. Patient being treated with heparin for pulmonary emboli
   E. Patient on large doses of steroids for rheumatoid arthritis
6. All of the following are associated with a secondary or reactive thrombocytosis (platelet count over 1,000,000) *except*:
   A. Iron deficiency   D. Autoimmune disorders
   B. Postsplenectomy   E. Malignancy
   C. Infection
7. Classic hemophilia and von Willebrand's disease have all of the following in common *except*:
   A. Both have low levels of factor VII activity.
   B. Both are genetically transmitted disorders.
   C. Both have a prolonged PTT.
   D. Both have a prolonged bleeding time.
   E. Cryoprecipitate is effective treatment for both.
8. What is the most common cause of death in the hemophiliac?
   A. Gastrointestinal bleeding
   B. Intracranial hemorrhage
   C. Exsanguination after trauma
   D. Myocardial infarction
   E. Transfusion reaction
9. All of the following are true regarding treatment of hemophilia, *except*:
   A. 1 unit of factor VIII activity is equal to that found in 1 cc of normal plasma.
   B. After cryoprecipitate has been thawed it must be transfused within 4 hours.
   C. Desmopressin (DDAVP) can increase factor VIII activity in mild disease.
   D. Heat-treated factor VIII concentrate will result in a lower titer of AIDS-associated virus.
   E. A patient should wait for symptomatic bleeding before treatment is begun.

10. The emergency treatment for symptomatic polycythemia is:
    A. Rapid saline infusion
    B. Diuresis with Lasix
    C. Phlebotomy
    D. Splenectomy
    E. Hydroxyurea
11. All of the following help to differentiate polycythemia vera from secondary polycythemia except:
    A. Arterial blood gases
    B. Platelet count
    C. Leukocyte alkaline phosphatase
    D. Serum B_{12}
    E. Bone marrow biopsy
12. Which of the following is true of von Willebrand's disease?
    A. It is transmitted as an autosomal recessive trait.
    B. Both the PT and the PTT are elevated.
    C. It is associated with thrombocytopenia.
    D. Single treatment with cryoprecipitate will last up to 40 hours.
    E. Because of multiple clotting defects, it is more severe than hemophilia A.
13. All of the following are true regarding idiopathic thrombocytopenic purpura except:
    A. Posttransfusion thrombocytopenia is associated with bleeding 1 week after transfusion.
    B. Acute ITP of childhood is usually secondary to a viral illness.
    C. Chronic ITP is associated with splenomegaly.
    D. Corticosteroids do not help acute ITP but are useful for chronic ITP.
    E. Platelet transfusions are used only for life-threatening bleeding.

90
Oncologic Emergencies

Select the appropriate letter that correctly answers the question or completes the statement.

1. All of the following are true regarding epidural spinal cord compression except:
    A. Most are located in the thoracic spine.
    B. Pain is the initial symptom in 95% of cases.
    C. The most common treatment is radiation therapy.
    D. Plain films seldom show any abnormalities.
    E. It is most commonly caused by lymphoma and lung, breast, or prostatic carcinoma.
2. The most commonly recommended combination of antibiotics for a granulocytopenic febrile patient includes:

    A. Clindamycin and gentamycin
    B. Ampicillin and gentamycin
    C. Carbenicillin and gentamycin
    D. Kefzol alone
    E. Nafcillin and tobramycin
3. Which is the most common electrolyte abnormality in the oncology patient?
    A. Increased sodium
    B. Decreased sodium
    C. Increased potassium
    D. Increased calcium
    E. Decreased calcium
4. Which of the following metabolic abnormalities is not part of the acute tumor lysis syndrome?
    A. Hyperuricemia
    B. Hypokalemia
    C. Hyperphosphatemia
    D. Hypocalcemia
    E. All of the above
5. Which of the following is true of the superior vena cava syndrome?
    A. The patient should be kept in a recumbent position.
    B. All IVs should be in the lower extremities.
    C. Early chemotherapy is the most important therapeutic modality.
    D. With certain tumors steroids are an important part of therapy.
    E. Diuretics are of no benefit.
6. Emergency department therapy of the hyperviscosity syndrome should include:
    A. Vigorous diuresis
    B. Phlebotomy with saline replacement
    C. Allopurinol
    D. Dilantin
    E. Hydroxyura
7. All of the following are useful in the treatment of the acute tumor lysis syndrome except:
    A. Hydration
    B. Alkalinization
    C. Allopurinol
    D. Hemodialysis
    E. Calcium chloride
8. All of the following regarding infection in a cancer patient are true except:
    A. Hodgkin's disease can present with a significant fever due to the tumor mass itself.
    B. Any patient with a fever over 38.5°C and less than 500 polymorphonuclear leukocytes should be admitted and started on antibiotics.
    C. Infection is the number one cause of cancer death.
    D. Untreated infection in a cancer patient has a 25–50% chance of 48-hour mortality.
    E. A careful history and physical examination will usually reveal the site of infection in a granulocytopenic patient.

9. A febrile patient with granulocytopenia should have all of the following done before starting antibiotics *except*:
   A. Chest x-ray
   B. Urinalysis and culture
   C. Lumbar puncture
   D. Blood cultures
   E. Sputum culture

10. Which of the following is true regarding CNS infection in the oncology patient?
   A. Meningismus is often absent.
   B. White blood cells may be absent from the CSF.
   C. Lumbar puncture is not helpful in diagnosing a brain abscess.
   D. Neutropenic patients are usually infected with a gram-negative organism.
   E. All of the above are true.

91
Arthritis

Select the appropriate letter that correctly answers the question or completes the statement.

1. True statements about Reiter's syndrome include all of the following *except*:
   A. It occurs more frequently in men than women.
   B. Conjunctivitis is the least likely of the characteristic triad to be present.
   C. Late complications include iritis, ankoylosing spondylitis, and aortic insufficiency.
   D. Cultures for gonorrhea should be performed.
   E. Most acute attacks require treatment with corticosteroids.

2. A 22-year-old woman comes to the ED with a 4-day history of fever, tenderness and swelling of the right knee, and tenderness without swelling of both wrists. Physical examination shows an effusion with heat and erythema of the knee and tenderness over both wrists. There are no skin lesions or other joints involved. The most correct answer concerning this patient is:
   A. A Grams stain of the knee aspirate will show the offending organism.
   B. The most likely organism is staphylococcus.
   C. A response within 12 hours to appropriate antibiotics can be expected.
   D. Repeated joint aspirations are contraindicated because of the possibility of secondary infection.
   E. Antibiotics should be withheld pending culture results.

3. Each of the following patients needs to be admitted to the hospital *except*:

   A. A 30-year-old woman with newly diagnosed systemic lupus erythematosus.
   B. A 21-year-old man with gonococcal arthritis of the wrists.
   C. A 10-year-old girl with acute rheumatic fever.
   D. A 40-year-old man with staphylococcal arthritis.
   E. A 5-year-old with osteomyelitis of the tibia.

4. Which of the following is true of synovial fluid anaylsis?
   A. Normal synovial fluid has a white blood cell count of 5–10,000 mostly mononuclear cells.
   B. Normal synovial fluid will form a string 3 cm long.
   C. Both uric acid and calcium pyrophosphate crystals are negatively birefringent under a polarizing microscope.
   D. Normal synovial fluid will not form a mucin clot with ascetic acid.
   E. High levels of lactic acid should suggest gonoccal arthritis.

5. The complication of rheumatoid arthritis most likely to require emergency treatment in the emergency department is:
   A. Vasculitis
   B. Felty's syndrome
   C. Sjögren's syndrome
   D. Subcutaneous nodules

6. Which of the following is true about Felty's syndrome?
   A. It may be initial manifestation of rheumatoid arthritis.
   B. Leukocystosis with predominantly lymphocytes is expected.
   C. Splenomegaly is an expected finding.
   D. Associated with dry eyes and dry mouth.
   E. It often complicates seronegative rheumatoid arthritis.

7. All of the following drugs are known to induce a lupus reaction *except*:
   A. Isoniazid   D. Hydrochlorothiazide
   B. Procainamide   E. Dilantin
   C. Hydralazine

8. Of the following Jones criteria for acute rheumatic fever, which is most commonly seen?
   A. Carditis
   B. Polyarthritis
   C. Chorea
   D. Erythema Marginatum
   E. Subcutaneous nodules

9. All of the following are useful to treat acute gouty arthritis *except*:
   A. Allopurinol   D. Phenylbutazone
   B. Indomethacin   E. ACTH
   C. Colchicine

10. All of the following statements about pseudogout are true *except*:
   A. X-rays reveal calcification of articular cartilage.
   B. The great toe is the most frequently involved joint.
   C. It is associated with hyperparathyroidism.
   D. Treatment is joint aspiration and antiinflammatory drugs.
   E. The etiologic agent is calcium pyrophosphate crystals.

11. Pitting of the nail beds is seen in over 90% of patients with:
   A. Gout
   B. Pseudogout
   C. Psoriatic arthritis
   D. Systemic lupus erythematosis
   E. Rheumatoid arthritis

92
Dermatologic Problems

Select the appropriate letter that correctly answers the question or completes the statement.

1. All of the following are true statements about impetigo *except*:
   A. It requires systemic antibiotic treatment.
   B. Bullous impetigo is caused by staphylococci.
   C. It can cause both glomerulonephritis and acute rheumatic fever.
   D. It is very contagious among infants and children.
   E. Late complications are not prevented by antibiotics.

2. All of the following are true concerning the relationship between chickenpox and shingles (herpes zoster) *except*:
   A. Chickenpox can be acquired from exposure to shingles.
   B. Shingles can be acquired by direct exposure to chickenpox.
   C. Shingles can be acquired by exposure to shingles.
   D. Shingles is caused by a reactivation of latent virus present since the initial infection of chickenpox.
   E. Both chickenpox and shingles can result in central venous system involvement.

3. All of the following are true of measles *except*:
   A. It is considered contagious as long as the rash is present.
   B. It can be modified or prevented by human immune serum globulin.
   C. Koplick's spots on the buccal mucosa are characteristic.
   D. Otitis media is the most common complication.

E. The predominant life-threatening complication is encephalitis or pneumonia.

4. Your are called to the x-ray department to attend a 50-year-old man with known coronary artery disease who is having a severe anaphylactoid reaction to an IVP. He is diaphoretic and wheezing, with a blood pressure of 55/0. Although all of these agents have a place in therapy, the best initial treatment is:
   A. Rapid fluid infusion with Ringer's lactate
   B. 300 mg hydrocortisone IV
   C. 50 mg diphenhydramine IV
   D. 0.3 ml epinephrine 1:1000 subcutaneously
   E. 3 ml epinephrine 1:10,000 IV

5. Roseola infantum is characterized by all of the following *except*:
   A. High fever for 3 to 4 days
   B. Toxic-appearing child
   C. Possibility of febrile seizures
   D. Rash that appears as the fever defervesces
   E. Affects children from 6 months to 3 years of age

6. After a week-end camping trip, a 13-year-old Boy Scout comes to the ED with localized vesicular eruptions that are now crusting and oozing over both forearms and hands. The lesions itch but he has no fever or other symptoms. The best initial therapy is:
   A. Oral prednisone 20 mg qid
   B. Dicloxacillin 250 mg qid
   C. Wet compresses of Burow's solution qid
   D. Calamine lotion qid
   E. Hydrocortisone cream 1% qid

7. All of the following are true about erythema nodosum *except*:
   A. Birth control pills are the leading cause of drug-induced cases.
   B. Potassium iodine may provide pain relief.
   C. They usually occur over the anterior tibia.
   D. A thorough systematic search for the underlying cause is mandatory.

8. The most common cause of erythema nodosum is:
   A. Sarcoidosis
   B. Ulcerative colitis
   C. Idiopathic
   D. Birth control pills
   E. Tuberculosis

9. The staphylococcal scalded skin syndrome:
   A. Is a benign form of toxic epidermal necrolysis.
   B. Is indistinguishable from other causes of toxic epidermal necrolysis.
   C. Can lead to large fluid losses.
   D. Include steroids as an important part of therapy.
   E. Affects all age groups equally.

10. A 6-year-old girl presents with a 2-week history of puritis of the scalp. She has a 4-cm area of scaling associated with broken hair strands, 1-2 mm above the scalp. She is in good general health, has no fever or other complaints. True statements concerning her disorder include all of the following *except*:
    A. Lesion will fluoresce under an ultraviolet (Woods) light.
    B. Treatment is with topical clotrimazole (Lotrimin).
    C. Permanent hair loss can result.
    D. It may be transmitted by child-to-child contact.
    E. Shaving or cutting the hair is not necessary.
11. Which of the following is true concerning corticosteroids in patients with herpes zoster?
    A. They should be given to everyone except the immune-compromised.
    B. They should be avoided if there is ocular involvement.
    C. They should be used routinely in those over age 60.
    D. They will lessen the severity of pain in postherpetic neuralgia.
    E. They are equally effective topically or systemically.
12. All of the following statements concerning scabies are true *except*:
    A. All family members and sexual contacts should be treated.
    B. Gamma benzene hexachloride (Quell) has been associated with neurotoxicity in small children.
    C. The most common area of involvement is the interdigital web spaces and flexor surfaces of the wrist.
    D. In addition to topical therapy, bed linens and underwear should be washed in very hot water.
    E. It is not necessary to treat the face and scalp, especially in small children.
13. Which of the following is true regarding pediculosis:
    A. With generally improved sanitation there has been a decrease in infestations in recent years.
    B. Nits appear as black dots cemented to the hair shaft while adults are white grains.
    C. A second treatment with lindane is usually necessary after 1 week.
    D. All persons in the household should be treated.
    E. None of the above are true.
14. Which of the following is true regarding serologic tests for syphilis?
    A. Patients with tertiary syphilis may retain a positive serology even though adequately treated.
    B. The most sensitive specific serologic test is the RPR.
    C. A biological false positive is defined as a negative VDRL but a positive fluorescent treponemal antibody absorption (FTA-ABS).

D. The VDRL is positive in nearly 100% of cases of primary syphilis but only 75% of secondary syphilis.
    E. A dark field microscopic examination is preferred to serology to diagnose secondary syphilis.
15. All of the following statements concerning urticaria are true *except*:
    A. It affects 15–20% of the population.
    B. Penicillin and aspirin are the most commonly implicated drugs.
    C. Cholinergic urticaria can be induced by exercise.
    D. Antihistamines alone usually provide symptomatic relief.
    E. A thorough search for the etiology must be initiated.
16. Generalized lymphadenopathy, particularly including the suboccipital and postauricular nodes with a pinkish maculopapular rash that first appears on the face, is most typical of which illness?
    A. Measles
    B. Rubella
    C. Rocky Mountain spotted fever
    D. Scarlet fever
    E. Roseola infantum
17. Which of the following is true about meningococcemia?
    A. Typical rash develops in over 90% of cases.
    B. Cefazolin is the drug of choice in the penicillin-allergic patient.
    C. Rifampin is recommended only for immediate household contacts and those directly involved in the resuscitation.
    D. Waterhouse-friderichsen occurs in about 50% of cases.
    E. The rash is pathognomonic for meningococcemia.
18. The disorder shown in Fig. 92-1 is best treated with:
    A. 5% hydrocortisone cream
    B. Oral griseofulvin, 5 mg/kg per day
    C. Lindane (Quell lotion).
    D. Pencillin V, 25–50 mg/kg per day
    E. Clotrimazole (Lotrimin) ointment

93
Stroke

Select the appropriate letter that correctly answers the question or completes the statement.
1. Which of the following is the most important predisposing factor for stroke?
    A. Hypertension   D. Hyperlipidemia
    B. Heart disease   E. Oral contraceptives
    C. Diabetes mellitus

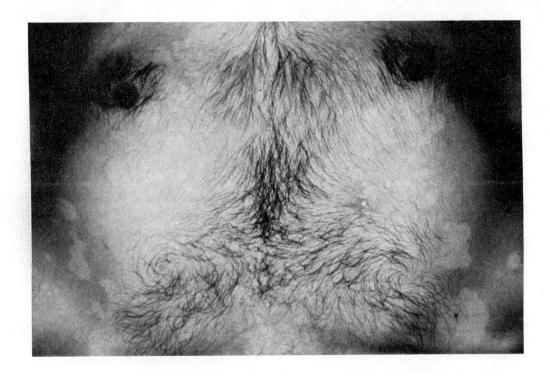

Fig. 92–1.

2. A 72-year-old woman with adult-onset diabetes controlled by diet alone was placed on oral coumadin therapy 4 months ago for transient ischemic attacks. She comes to the ED with a history of headache, drowsiness, and confusion that has increased in severity over the last 7 days. There is no history of fall or other trauma. She has a normal temperature, pulse, and respiratory rate, and her blood pressure is 160/100. Other findings are an incomplete right hemiplegia, aphasia, and a questionable left hemianopsia. Lab studies reveal a normal partial thromboplastin time and clotting time and a therapeutic prothrombin time. The most likely cause of this patient's condition is:
   A. Recurrent TIA
   B. Evolving thrombotic stroke
   C. Hypoglycemic episode
   D. Pontine hemorrhagic stroke
   E. Subdural hematoma
3. A 68-year-old hypertensive man comes to the ED with acute onset of dysarthria, loss of usual dexterity of his dominant hand, and weakness with clumsiness of the arm on the same side. Careful attention to his speech reveals mild slurring. These symptoms are all new since yesterday, according to the patient's wife. The patient has no other complaints. The most likely cause of this patient's problem is:

   A. A lacunar infarction of the pons
   B. Cerebellar infarction
   C. Subarachnoid rupture of a berry aneurysm
   D. Migraine
   E. Acute myocardial infarction
4. In which of the following disorders are embolic infarctions more common?
   A. Patients with rheumatic heart disease with atrial fibrillation
   B. Patients with coronary artery disease with a recent myocardial infarction
   C. Patients with deep vein thrombophlebitis in the lower extremities without congenital heart disease
   D. Patients on anticoagulant therapy
   E. A and B
5. A 75-year-old hypertensive woman with a unilateral transient loss of vision in her left eye is seen. The most likely area of her lesion causing this problem is:
   A. Vertebral basilar artery
   B. Middle cerebral artery
   C. Posterior cerebral artery
   D. Circle of Willis
   E. Carotid artery

6. A 73-year-old hypertensive man comes to the ED with acute onset of dizziness, nausea, vomiting, and ataxia. He is unable to ambulate without steadying from his wife. The remaining examination reveals no other areas of involvement, but the patient's blood pressure is 160/105. This type of infarction varies from others primarily because:
   A. Symptoms tend to resolve on their own.
   B. There are usually the result of remote trauma.
   C. Completely irreversible bilateral blindness is a frequent concomitant finding.
   D. Surgical decompression may remedy developing postacute symptoms.
   E. CT scan is of no value in identifying this lesion.

7. A 45-year-old previously healthy man comes to your ED with acute onset of an excruciating headache that began while running to catch a plane. He had a transient loss of consciousness, then a period of confusion, nausea, and vomiting. He admits to upper back pain and photophobia, which are both new. Vital signs are normal except for a temperature of 100°F. There is some questionable nuchal rigidity on physical examination, but no focal neurologic deficits. Laboratory tests yield only a mild leukocytosis with a normal differential. The only true statement about this patient's probable pathology is:
   A. Lumbar puncture is the procedure of choice for making the diagnosis.
   B. A bruit over the eyeball is strongly suggestive of this patient's pathologic problem.
   C. This patient is unusually young to be experiencing this event.
   D. Ergotamine alkaloids are the treatment of choice for this problem.
   E. CT scan will detect all acute cases of this problem.

8. A 75-year-old woman comes to your ED via ambulance. She arouses to painful stimulus by movement of her left arm and leg. Babinski reflex is positive on the right, but other right-sided reflexes are markedly depressed. Her vital signs are stable except for a blood pressure of 190/120. She exhibits anisocoria with the right pupil at 8 cm and poorly reactive, and with the left pupil at 4 cm and normally reactive. Funduscopic examination reveals no papilledema. What would be contraindicated in this patient?
   A. Lumbar puncture
   B. Intravenous steroids
   C. Intravenous mannitol or glycerol
   D. CT scan
   E. Hyperventilation on a respirator

94
Seizure

Select the appropriate letter that correctly answers the question or completes the statement.

1. All of the following are thought to exert an inhibitory role over seizures or contribute to ictal cessation *except*:
   A. GABA (gamma-aminobutyric acid)
   B. A failure of oxidative metabolism
   C. Acetylcholine
   D. The cerebellum

2. All of the following statements are true *except*:
   A. Tumors tend to be an uncommon cause of epilepsy in children.
   B. Infratentorial tumors more commonly cause seizures than do supratentorial tumors.
   C. Slowly growing, more benign tumors are most commonly epileptogenic.
   D. Arteriosclerotic cerebrovascular insufficiency and cerebral infarctions are much more commonly the cause of seizures from vascular disorders than is a subarachnoid hemorrhage.

3. Which of the following is a characteristic that distinguishes complex febrile convulsions from simple febrile convulsions?
   A. Duration
   B. Focal vs. generalized
   C. Single episode vs. occurring in a series
   D. All of the above

4. Which of the following seizure types has little or no alteration of consciousness?
   A. Simple partial
   B. Complex partial
   C. Psychomotor (temporal lobe)
   D. Absence (petit mal)

5. True statements about status epilepticus include all of the following *except*:
   A. The definition generally accepted for status epilepticus is a seizure that persists for over 1 hour or repeated seizures that produce a fixed and enduring epileptic condition for more than 1 hour.
   B. Convulsive status occurs approximately 6 times more commonly in patients with a primary epilepsy as opposed to secondary epilepsy.
   C. Absence (petit mal) status is more common in adults than in children.
   D. Status epilepticus has an acute mortality lower than 10%.

6. Which of the following true statements distinguish a true seizure from a simple syncopal episode?
   A. Headache may occur after a synocopal episode, whereas after a seizure it doesn't.
   B. Seizures usually have a more gradual onset with a prodrome of visual blurring and nausea, whereas syncope does not.
   C. Syncope almost always occurs when the patient is upright.
   D. Syncope is often associated with injuries from falling or with incontinence.

7. A mother brings her 3-year-old son to the emergency room and states that she was scolding him and he was crying. During this he started hyperventilating for a period of time and then suddenly stopped breathing. This was followed by the child turning blue, passing out, and she thinks she saw some muscle jerks. He is now awake and looks well. Which of the following characteristics of the above scenario would be consistent with a breath-holding spell?
   A. The hyperventilation
   B. The cyanosis
   C. The muscle jerks
   D. All of the above

8. All of the following statements are true *except*:
   A. The closed tonic jaw should be opened and a "bite block" inserted in the seizing patient's mouth to prevent intraoral injury.
   B. The vast majority of seizure episodes are relatively benign in nature and short in duration, with spontaneous termination and prompt recovery.
   C. The first priority of therapy is to correct the underlying cause if possible, and the second is to control the seizures, if necessary.
   D. The seizing patient should be placed in a lateral decubitus position to avoid aspiration.

9. In which of the following patients is phenytoin (Dilantin) the drug of first choice?
   A. A 3-year-old child who had a febrile seizure and is not presently seizing.
   B. A 25-year-old otherwise healthy man in status epilepticus who has been given a maximum dose of diazepam (Valium) and is still seizing.
   C. A patient who has been on phenobarbital for seizures, had one seizure today, his compliance with his medications is suspect.
   D. A 59-year-old with a heart rate of 50 and a left bundle branch block who is in status epilepticus and did not respond to maximum diazepam.

10. Phenobarbital should be used with caution in which of the following patients?
    A. Patients with severe cardiac conduction disturbances
    B. Children under the age of six
    C. Patients allergic to phenytoin (Dilantin)
    D. Patients with myasthenia gravis

95
Vertigo and Syncope

Select the appropriate letter that correctly answers the question or completes the statement.

1. The presence of true vertigo implies disturbance in which of the following?
   A. Semicircular canals, utricle, eighth cranial nerves
   B. Semicircular canals, posterior columns, and eye muscles
   C. Tendons, muscles, joints, posterior columns
   D. Visual system

2. How would rhythmic eye movements in which the eyes move quickly to the right and return slowly to the left best be termed?
   A. Right vertical nystagmus
   B. Left vertical nystagmus
   C. Right horizontal nystagmus
   D. Left horizontal nystagmus

3. A 23-year-old patient complains of sudden onset of *true* vertigo and tinnitus. The most likely cause is:
   A. VIII nerve tumor
   B. Otosclerosis
   C. Labyrinthitis (viral)
   D. Foreign body in the ear canal

4. A patient relates a history of progressive hearing loss, which he states "runs in his family." He recently experienced episodes of imbalance, but no true vertigo. The ear appears normal except for a slight orange hue of the tympanic membrane, as well as a negative Rinne test. Most likely diagnosis in this patient is:
   A. VIII nerve tumor
   B. Acute otitis media superimposed with chronic serous otitis media
   C. Otosclerosis
   D. Acute labyrinthitis

5. What is the most likely valvular lesion that would cause syncope?
   A. Aortic regurgitation
   B. Mitral insufficiency
   C. Aortic stenosis
   D. Mitral stenosis

6. Which of these statements is true concerning vasovagal syncope?
   A. It may result from a period of asystole caused by stimulation of vasovagal pathways.
   B. It may be associated lesions of the larynx or mediastinum.
   C. Tincture of belladonna may be used to prevent episodes.
   D. All of the above are true.
7. A patient comes to the ED with a history of severe pain in the oropharynx and ear associated with coughing and swallowing. He has fainted several times with this pain after coughing. He most likely is experiencing:
   A. Episodes of vasovagal syncope
   B. Glossopharyngeal neuralgia-realated syncope
   C. Orthostatic hypotension
   D. VIII cranial nerve syncope
8. How does drug ingestion produce syncope?
   A. Dysrhythmias
   B. Orthostatic hypotension
   C. Intoxication
   D. All of the above
9. A patient who is feigning syncope may be very convincing. Cold caloric testing may be necessary. In the patient who is *truly* unconscious the response to cold water instillation would be:
   A. Horizontal nystagmus away from the lavaged ear
   B. Tonic eye deviation toward the lavaged ear
   C. No eye movement
   D. Vertical upbeat nystagmus

96
Weakness

Select the appropriate letter that correctly answers the question or completes the statement.
1. Guillain-Barré syndrome may be differentiated from myasthenia gravis and botulism on the basis of all of the following *except*:
   A. Eye involvement is common with botulism and myasthenia gravis and rare with Guillain-Barré.
   B. Fever is common with botulism but rare with myasthenia gravis and Guillain-Barré.
   C. Reflexes are decreased with Guillain-Barré but intact with myasthenia gravis.
   D. Paralysis is ascendling in Guillain-Barré and descending in botulism.
2. Which one of the following are characteristic of the Guillain-Barré Syndrome?
   A. Asymmetric leg weakness
   B. Asymmetric facial weakness

C. A CSF protein count of less than 400 mg/L
D. A CSF cell count of greater than 10 per ml (mostly granulocytes)
3. All of the following statements are true regarding myasthenia gravis *except*:
   A. In 20% of patients, manifestations will be confined to the eye muscles.
   B. A previously untreated patient presents with muscle weakness, sweating, salivation, miosis, and tachycardia.
   C. Antibodies against acetylcholine receptors cause myasthenia gravis.
   D. Edrophoniun can transiently reverse weakness caused by myasthenia gravis.
4. Which one of the following statements is true?
   A. Botulism is caused by a toxin that destroys acetylcholine receptors.
   B. Infantile botulism is caused by growth of *C. botulinum* spores in the gut. Boiling formula before giving will not destroy the spore.
   C. Eaton-Lambert syndrome is associated with lymphoma.
   D. Tick paralysis is an ascending paralysis that develops over 1 to 2 weeks. (days)

97
Adult Meningitis

Select the appropriate letter that correctly answers the question or completes the statement.
1. All of the following factors are predisposing host factors to the development of meningitis *except*:
   A. Age less than 5 years
   B. Household contact with case
   C. Female sex
   D. Thalassemia major
   E. Bacterial endocarditis
2. Which one of the following physical findings is inconsistent with meningitis?
   A. Nuchol rigidity
   B. Laterol rectus ophthalmoplegia
   C. Seizures
   D. Papilledema
3. Which one of the following is *not* an indication for CT Scan before lumbar puncture in patients with suspected bacterial meningitis?
   A. Ophthalmoplegia
   B. Papilledema
   C. Altered mental status
   D. History or evidence of head trauma

4. Xanthochromia with a low CSF protein (less than 150 mg/dl) is indicative of:
   A. Traumatic tap
   B. Subarachnoid hemorrhage
   C. Jaundice
   D. Subdural hematoma

5. Penicillin G is the antibiotic of choice for meningitis caused by all of the following organisms *except*:
   A. *Hemophilus influenzae*
   B. *Neisseria meningitis*
   C. *Streptococcus pneumoniae*
   D. *Staphylococcus pyogenes*

6. A 30-year-old male presents with headache and fever. Results of the lumbar puncture suggest meningitis. Which of the following antibiotic choices would be most appropriate?
   A. Ampicillin plus gentamicin
   B. Penicillin G
   C. Ampicillin, gentamicin, plus nafcillin
   D. Chloramphenicol, gentamicin, plus nafcillin

98
Approach to Violence

Select the appropriate letter that correctly answers the question or completes the statement.

1. Patients with which of the following disorders show no propensity toward violence?
   A. Severe depression
   B. Substance abuse
   C. Personality disorders
   D. Paranoia
   E. None of the above

99
Suicide

Select the appropriate letter that correctly answers the question or completes the statement.

1. Correct facts concerning suicide risk include all of the following *except*:
   A. Men have generally higher rates than women.
   B. Whites have generally higher rates than blacks.
   C. Increasing age generally corresponds with increasing risk.
   D. Teenage suicide rates have generally remained unchanged.
   E. While in general suicide rates have remained stable in recent years, unsuccessful attempt rates have increased.

2. For people who repeatedly attempt suicide, which of the following statements is true?
   A. Most people who fail an attempt will actually complete the suicide with the next attempt.
   B. The greatest risk of a repeat suicide attempt is in the first 3 months to a year after the unsuccessful attempt.
   C. Increasing frequency of attempts is not a significant finding.
   D. Increasing lethality in attempts should be ignored in dealing with the suicide patient.
   E. Repeat attempters should receive a cool reception from the emergency department staff in order to decrease the likelihood of positive reinforcement of attention-getting behavior.

3. Which of the persons listed are most likely to successfully attempt suicide?
   A. Obviously psychotic during their attempt
   B. Always depressed when attempting suicide
   C. Only seeking attention from a significant other
   D. May be unusually accident-prone
   E. Don't care if they die

4. Prediction of suicide risk includes all of the following *except*:
   A. The person's psychiatric diagnosis, exclusive of alcoholism or psychosis
   B. The lethality of the chosen method of attempted suicide
   C. Whether the attempter notified another person of his/her attempt
   D. The patient's relative feeling of his/her ability to influence his life
   E. Recent prior attempts

100
Organic Brain Syndromes

Select the appropriate letter that correctly answers the question or completes the statement.

1. A 21-year-old college student taking "speed" for studying is escorted in by his roommates in a very agitated state with visual and auditory hallucinations and complaints of a severe headache. Vitals are blood pressure 140/86, heart rate 110, respirations 26, temperature 102.6°. Suspecting delirium as a presumptive diagnosis, an initial critical action is to:
   A. Obtain prior records for psychiatric history
   B. Contact parents for past drug history
   C. Perform immediate lumbar puncture
   D. Obtain drug screen—urine and serum
   E. Sedate and obtain CT scan of head

2. A 40-year-old male presents with nocturnal wakefulness and being tired all day. This has been present for the past few days. His wife notes that he has become very forgetful lately and has been late to home and work because he cannot remember where he is. The most likely diagnosis is:
   A. Psychotic depression
   B. Dementia
   C. Pseudodementia
   D. Delirium
   E. Ganser's syndrome
3. Of the following, which is most commonly associated with delirium?
   A. Alcohol withdrawal
   B. Seizure disorder
   C. Thyrotoxicosis
   D. Phencyclidine withdrawal
   E. Intracanial infection
4. Neuropathologic changes associated with delirium include all of the following *except*:
   A. Periaqueductal petechiae
   B. Hippocampal neuronal degeneration
   C. Diminished protoplasmic astrocytes
   D. Cerebral edema
   E. Cerebrocortical neuronal degeneration
5. In relation to dementia, all of the following statements are true *except*:
   A. Hallucinations are usually auditory.
   B. Asterixis and myoclonus frequently present.
   C. Vital signs are normal.
   D. Sensorium is usually clear.
   E. Patients present with normal EEG.
6. After establishing a diagnosis of Alzheimer's disease which of the following treatment regimens are of proven benefit?
   A. Acetycholine precursors (lecithin, choline)
   B. Anticholinergic agents
   C. Hydergine
   D. Antidepressants
   E. Physostigmine
7. While evaluating a patient for probable dementia, the single most important area to examine is:
   A. History
   B. Mental status examination
   C. Physical examination
   D. Laboratory and radiologic evaluation
   E. Current medications

101
Thought and Affective Disorders

Select the appropriate letter that correctly answers the question or completes the statement.

1. A 25-year-old female is brought to the emergency department after creating a disturbance at a neighbor's house. On arrival, the patient is shouting and seems paranoid. Which initial response would be most appropriate?
   A. Physically restrain the patient, ideally using 4–5 people
   B. Chemical restraint using injectable haloperidol
   C. Perform history, exam, and laboratory studies to rule out an organic medical disorder
   D. Attempt to establish rapport with the patient by encouraging her to express her feelings
2. Which of the following would be the most appropriate initial treatment during a severe manic episode?
   A. Prompt treatment with high potency antipsychotic agents
   B. Intensive psychotherapy
   C. Lithium, initial doses of 1500–1800 mg per day
   D. Lithium doses of 900–1200 mg per day
3. The psychiatric interview:
   A. Establishes a positive physician-patient relationship
   B. Includes a mental status examination
   C. Aids in establishing a diagnosis
   D. Can be accomplished in a few minutes
   E. All of the above
4. A 56-year-old male is brought to the emergency department by friends for evaluation of recent bizarre behavior. His friends deny any knowledge of past similar behavior and state that the patient has been seeing things. His only significant medical problem is hypertension, for which he is being treated. On arrival the patient appears slightly confused and paranoid. His vital signs are blood pressure 150/90; pulse 104; respiratory rate 16; temperature 99.2°F. Physical examination is normal except that the patient is incontinent of urine. Which of the following statements is most appropriate regarding this patient?
   A. This patient's bizarre behavior, paranoia, and visual hallucinations are probably related to a thought disorder.
   B. This patient should be admitted to rule out a seizure disorder.

C. This patient's behavior is probably related to an organic mental disorder.
D. This patient's behavior is probably related to hypertensive encephalopathy.
E. Immediate psychiatric consultation should be obtained.

5. All the following are true regarding rapid tranquilization *except*:
A. It can be used effectively to control violent behavior in nonpsychotic patients.
B. In the psychotic patient, the main goal in treatment is sedation.
C. An appropriate dose of haloperidol in a 30-year-old psychotic patient is 5–20 mg IM every 30–60 minutes until target symptoms subside or total of 40 mg has been given.
D. The dangers of hypotension and oversedation are minimized with the high-potency antipsychotic agents.
E. Haloperidol, thiothixene, and droperidol have all been successfully used in the United States.

6. A 21-year-old woman is brought to the emergency department by the police after creating a distrubance at a neighbor's house. On arrival the patient is agitated and keeps saying that her body is rotting away. The patient has a poorly kept appearance, seems disorganized, and seems to have auditory hallucinations. She denies suicidal thoughts. After an initial evaluation, you recommend that she be admitted to the psychiatric service but she insists on leaving. All of the following are true *except*:
A. You are liable for assault and battery if you treat a patient against his or her will.
B. You can be sued for negligence if you fail to treat patients who subsequently harm themselves or others.
C. The patient can be admitted to the psychiatric service with careful documentation as to why the patient requires admission.
D. You should initiate involuntary commitment according to prearranged protocols for your hospital.
E. Most states have statutes that provide time-limited involuntary treatment of individuals who need care but are unwilling or unable to accept it.

7. The diagnosis of schizophrenia according to DSM-III is based on research-tested objective criteria that enables the nonpsychiatrist to make the diagnosis with more confidence. Key elements in the diagnosis of schizophrenia include all the following *except*:
A. Continuous signs of illness for a minimum of 6 months.
B. Prior manic or depressive episode
C. Deterioration from prior level of function
D. Absence of organic mental disorder

E. Delusions, auditory hallucinations, and/or loosening of associations

8. A 42-year-old man presents to the emergency department with a complaint of restlessness. The patient describes a feeling of inner tension that is not relieved by activity and is extremely unpleasant. The patient was recently started on thiothixene (Navane) at a dose of 5 mg TID. On examination, the patient is pacing the room but seems oriented with appropriate affect. Which of the following would be most appropriate?
A. Increase Navane dose and obtain prompt psychiatric follow-up
B. Obtain blood and urine for laboratory studies
C. Administer benztropine 1 mg IM
D. Discontinue medication and warn the patient that he may have tardive dyskinesia
E. None of the above

9. The following statements about major depressive episodes are true *except*:
A. Very few patients actually commit suicide.
B. It is related to abnormalities of neurotransmitters and neurogenic receptors.
C. Trazodone (Desyrel) appears safer than standard tricyclics in an overdose.
D. Essential features are the presence of dysphoric mood, making at least four of eight symptoms outlined by DSM-III for 2 weeks or longer.
E. Any medication the patient is taking should be considered as an etiologic agent.

102
Substance Abuse

Select the appropriate letter that correctly answers the question or completes the statement.

1. All of the following are true regarding hydrocarbon vapor abuse *except*:
A. Patients may present with severe muscular weakness resembling Guillain-Barré syndrome.
B. Local neurologic deficits are not associated with hydrocarbon inhalation and their presence should arouse suspicion of another etiology.
C. Inhalation of halogenated hydrocarbons may result in sudden cardiac arrest secondary to cardiac dysrhythmias.
D. Reversible oliguric renal failure has been reported in chronic abusers.

2. Metabolic abnormalities found in chronic toluene abuse include all of the following *except*:
   A. Respiratory alkalosis
   B. Hypokalemia
   C. Hypocalcemia
   D. Hyperchloremia

3. Nitrous oxide inhalation:
   A. May result in sudden cardiac death secondary to direct cardiotoxicity
   B. Causes intense hallucinations that may last for hours following exposure
   C. May result in progressive numbness, paresthesias, and motor weakness resembling multiple sclerosis in chronic abusers
   D. Can cause aplastic anemia with chronic abuse

4. All of the following are true regarding PCP *except*:
   A. Nystagmus, including rotary nystagmus, is a frequent physical finding.
   B. Gastric aspirates may be positive even when PCP has been smoked and in the presence of a negative serum assay.
   C. Stage II intoxication with PCP is usually associated with profound bradycardia and hypotension.
   D. Rhabdomyolysis can occur, leading to myoglobinuria and renal failure.

5. Which of the following would be considered appropriate emergency department treatment for PCP intoxication?
   A. Alkaline diuresis
   B. Thorazine 100–200 mg IM if needed for agitation
   C. Gastric emptying and repeated doses of activated charcoal
   D. Hemodialysis

6. A 27-year-old male homosexual is brought to the emergency department by friends after a syncopal episode following prolonged inhalation of butyl nitrite. He complains of dizziness, headache, and chest pain. He is profoundly cyanotic but only mildly SOB. His vital signs are blood pressure 80/60, heart rate 120, and respiration 26 unlabored. Initial ABGs: pH 7.28, pCO$_2$ 35, pO$_2$ 75. The methemoglobin level is 55%. All of the following would be included in appropriate emergency department management *except*:
   A. High-flow supplemental oxygen
   B. IV RL or NS infusion and Trendelenberg position
   C. Methylene blue 1–2 mg/kg IV bolus
   D. Thiosulfate 1–5 cc/kg IV bolus

7. A 17-year-old white male presents 12 hours following ingestion of an unknown amount of jimsonweed seeds. He is having visual hallucinations, but is only mildly agitated and can be easily controlled with soft restraints. Vital signs are as follows: temperature 101°F, pulse 120, sinus tachycardia, blood pressure 170/100, and respirations 30 unlabored. His skin is dry and flushed, his mouth is dry, and he is complaining of difficulty voiding. Which of the following would be considered appropriate emergency department treatment for this patient?
   A. Ipecac or gastric lavage followed by charcoal
   B. Physostigmine 1–2 mg slow IVP over 2 minutes
   C. Valium prn for agitation
   D. Thorazine prn for psychosis
   E. *A & C*
   F. *B & D*
   G. All of the above

8. All of the following are true regarding LSD *except*:
   A. Accidental overdose with LSD is sometimes fatal secondary to cardiotoxicity.
   B. LSD is often surreptitiously substituted for other street drugs and is sold as cocaine, amphetamine, or mescaline.
   C. Massive overdose can lead to tachycardia, hypertension, hyperthermia, coma, and coagulopathies.
   D. Flashback occurs in approximately 50% of users.

9. A 29-year-old known drug abuser presents to the emergency department in a highly agitated state and rapidly has a generalized seizure followed by coma with dilated pupils, sinus tachycardia, heart rate 140 with multiple PVCs, blood pressure 80, and respirations 40, gasping and irregular. Rectal temperature is noted to be 108°F. Patient is flushed and diaphoretic. There are rales at both bases and bowel sounds are hyperactive. All of the following may be appropriate treatment in this case *except*:
   A. Bolus D50W IV
   B. Naloxone 2 mg IVP
   C. Physostigmine I mg IVP and titrate to effect
   D. Sodium bicarbonate

10. Following aggressive airway management on the patient in question 9, other measures that may be warranted include all of the following *except*:
    A. Iced gastric lavage
    B. Abdominal radiographs
    C. Saline diuresis
    D. Repeated oral doses of activated charcoal following gastric lavage

103
Sexual Assault

Select the appropriate letter that correctly answers the question or completes the statement.

1. True statements concerning sperm examination in a sexual assault victim include all of the following *except*:
   A. Ultraviolet light can help locate semen staining.

B. Supravital dye can help identify sperm in a blood contaminated specimen.
C. Sperm remain motile in the cervix and vagina for 6 to 12 hours.
D. Ejaculation is not necessary to be able to find sperm in the vaginal vault.
E. All of the above.

2. Which statement concerning the legal aspects of sexual assault cases is true?
A. Of those formally accused of rape 25% are convicted.
B. The examiner should elicit a thorough history from both the victim and suspect.
C. The weakest link in a rape case medically is usually the chain of evidence.
D. A woman who is seen after a sexual assault must consent to a legal as well as a medical examination.
E. Any evidence gathered during an evaluation of a sexual assault victim must be turned over to the police.

3. When used as a "morning after pill" for rape victims, diethylstilbestrol has been associated with which of the following effects on the fetus if carried to term?
A. Vaginal cancer
B. Duplication of renal collecting system
C. Arteriovenous malformation of the cerebellum
D. Early macular degeneration
E. Patent ductus arteriosus

4. The tolulene blue dye test can be used:
A. To identify small vaginal lacerations from traumatic intercourse
B. To determine the presence of ejaculate in the vaginal vault
C. Locate semen stains on the body
D. Determine the time of the most recent sexual activity
E. None of the above

5. The primary evidentiary points to be considered in the physical examination of a sexual assault victim include all of the following *except*:
A. Capability of the patient to give consent
B. Use of force
C. Occurrence of vulvar penetration
D. Presence of physical evidence from the rapist or the rape site
E. All of the above

104
Adult Abuse

Select the appropriate letter that correctly answers the question or completes the statement.

1. Approximately what percentage of adult homicides are committed by relatives?
A. 10%   C. 50%
B. 25%   D. 75%

2. Which of the following are true regarding intrafamilial homicides?
A. Men are more likely to be killed by other family members than women.
B. Women are more likely to be killed by other family members than men.
C. Estimates of the number of familial homicides are probably overestimated.
D. There are less than 500 documented murdered wives and girlfriends annually in the United States.

3. Which of the following characterizes the abused female spouse?
A. Typically middle-aged and married for a number of years
B. Financially independent but with very few friends
C. Maintains traditional views of her role in marriage but has consistently poor self-esteem
D. Usually welcomes intervention by friends or medical personnel

4. Older boys that witness domestic violence become particularly prone to which of the following behaviors?
A. Aggressive antisocial behavior
B. Tendency to become withdrawn and anxious
C. Become violent towards their parents
D. Display no adverse reaction

5. According to the cyclic theory of wife abuse, at which phase is the wife unlikely to be responsive to medical or social intervention?
A. Tension-building phase
B. The acute battering phase
C. The gratification phase
D. The learned helplessness phase

6. At what point in the cycle of wife abuse is crisis intervention the most effective?
A. Just as an episode of abuse is beginning
B. Immediately after abuse
C. One to two weeks after the episode of abuse
D. Only when the patient is severely injured and in need of hospitalization

7. An 89-year-old senile white male presents to the emergency department dehydrated and confused after being confined to a single bedroom for 60 days with only occasional food and water. This type of geriatric abuse is an example of:
A. Physical abuse
B. Emotional abuse
C. Active neglect
D. Passive neglect

8. Which of the following is true regarding abuse of the elderly?
   A. Elderly victims are more commonly male than female
   B. Typically the abused patient lives alone
   C. Neglect rather than abuse is a more common problem with the most impaired elderly
   D. Victims are more common in the upper income levels

105
Acid-Base Homeostasis

Select the appropriate letter that correctly answers the question or completes the statement.

1. A 24-year-old patient in respiratory distress presents himself to the emergency department with the following ABGs: pH 7.26, P_{CO_2} 65, P_{O_2} 65, HCO_3, 26. Which of the following statements with regard to the acid-base status are incorrect?
   A. There are virtually no extracellular buffering processes to compensate for his acidosis.
   B. Cardiac output and blood pressure are likely to be severely compromised.
   C. His respiratory disorder has not been chronic in nature.
   D. Administration of oxygen can be given with little concern for inducing CO_2 narcosis.

2. The following acid-base disturbance is most consistent with which of the following diagnoses? pH 7.49, P_{CO_2} 47, P_{O_2} 80, HCO_3, 35.
   A. Respiratory alkalosis
   B. Uncompensated metabolic alkalosis
   C. Chronic respiratory acidosis with renal compensation
   D. Metabolic alkaosis with respiratory compensation

3. Causes of metabolic alkalosis include all of the following except:
   A. Addison's disease
   B. Postchronic hypercapnea
   C. Diuretics
   D. Vomiting
   E. Massive blood transfusions

4. Complications associated with the use of HCO3 in severe metabolic acidosis include all of the following except:
   A. Hypernatremia
   B. Paradoxical CSF alkalosis
   C. Decreased oxygen unloading at the tissue level
   D. Induction of dysrhythmias
   E. Hypokalemia

5. Which of the following is the most important intracellular blood buffer?
   A. Transferrin
   B. Albumin
   C. Hemoglobin
   D. Mucopolysaccharides

6. A 27-year-old diabetic male comes to the emergency department and is found to have a pH of 7.2 and a potassium of 4.0. If you correct the pH, what is his actual serum potassium?
   A. 2.0   C. 4.0
   B. 2.4   D. 5.6

106
Fluid and Electrolyte Balance

Select the appropriate letter that correctly answers the question or completes the statement.

1. Infusion of a hypertonic saline solution will cause which of the following fluid shifts?
   A. ECF contraction and ICF contraction
   B. ECF contraction and ICF expansion
   C. ECF expansion and ICF expansion
   D. ECF expansion and ICF contraction

2. Which of the following is primarily an intracellular ion?
   A. Na+   D. Ca++
   B. CI-   E. HCO_3
   C. K+

3. Which of the following is the normal range for the serum osmolality in mOsm/L?
   A. 250–280   C. 300–310
   B. 285–295   D. 320–330

4. Which of the following substances do not cause significant fluid shifts because of their ability to rapidly equilibrate across cell membranes?
   A. Alcohol   C. Mannitol
   B. Sodium   D. Glucose

5. Which of the following is not a cause of increased insensible fluid losses?
   A. Hyperventilation
   B. Exercise
   C. Hypermetabolic states
   D. Low humidity
   E. Assisted ventilation

6. All of the following changes would increase secretion of ADH *except*:
   A. Decreased plasma osmolality
   B. Hypotension
   C. Stress
   D. Trauma

7. Which of the following is the most likely cause of hyponatremia in the face of urine osmolality greater than 100 mOsm/L (nondilute)?
   A. SIADH
   B. Hyperaldosteronism
   C. Diabetes insipidus
   D. Psychogenic polydipsia

8. Which of the following is the most likely cause of hyponatremia in the face of a urine osmolality less than 100 mOsm/L (dilute)?
   A. SIADH
   B. Hyperaldosteronism
   C. Diabetes insipidus
   D. Psychogenic polydipsia

9. Which of the following is the most common cause of SIADH in which the excess ADH is from an endogenous (posterior pituitary) source?
   A. Pulmonary disease
   B. Postsurgery
   C. Endocrinopathies
   D. Central nervous system disease

10. All of the following statements regarding SIADH are true *except*:
    A. Neoplasms are the most common cause of ectopic ADH production.
    B. Most prominent clinical manifestations are cardiovascular.
    C. Patients are especially apt to have seizures if the Na+ rapidly falls below 120 mEq/L.
    D. The clinical picture is identical to that of water intoxication.

11. A 66-year-old man comes to the emergency department with a 6-month history of crescendo headaches and now notes right-sided weakness. CT scan shows a brain tumor with surrounding edema and mild midline shift. He is fully alert without further complaint, and his vital signs are stable. His serum Na+ is 126 and his urine osmolality is 110. Which of the following would be the most appropriate initial therapy for his hyponatremia?
    A. IV of D$_5$W 100 ml/hour
    B. IV of normal saline 100 ml/hour
    C. IV of hypertonic saline until the Na+ is above 135
    D. IV of D$_5$ normal saline 20 ml/hour

12. All of the following statements regarding diabetes insipidus are true *except*:
    A. Patients usually have any one of a number of neurologic complaints.
    B. It is characterized by decreased ADH production.

C. The etiology is most often idiopathic.
   D. Hypernatremia is the most frequently encountered electrolyte abnormality.

13. Which of the following is the most appropriate treatment for diabetes insipidus?
    A. None
    B. IV normal saline at 100 ml/hour
    C. IV D$_5$W 100 ml/hour
    D. ADH replacement
    E. Fluid restriction

14. Which of the following drugs has *not* been shown to cause nephrogenic diabetes insipidus?
    A. Acetazolamide   C. Amphotericin B
    B. Demeclocyline   D. Lithium

15. All of the following statements regarding aldosterone are true *except*:
    A. It causes Na+ excretion.
    B. It causes K+ excretion.
    C. Levels are increased by angiotensin II.
    D. ECF contraction leads to aldosterone secretion.
    E. Synthesis is decreased by heparin.

16. Which of the following signifies the greatest degree of dehydration?
    A. Decreased sweat production and thirst
    B. Decreased skin turgor and thirst
    C. Decreased skin turgor and dry mucous membranes
    D. Decreased sweat production and decreased urine output

17. Orthostatic hypotensive changes secondary to dehydration usually indicate which of the following total body water deficits?
    A. 10%   C. 30%
    B. 20%   D. 40%

18. Which of the following types of dehydration is most likely in a patient suffering a significant burn injury?
    A. Hypernatremia
    B. Eunatremia
    C. Hyponatremia
    D. None of the above

19. Which of the following is *not* a cause of hypernatremia?
    A. Ingestion of seawater
    B. Diuretic use
    C. Diabetes insipidus
    D. Hypoaldosteronism

20. All of the following are true *except*:
    A. All gastrointestinal fluids have Na+ concentrations lower than that of plasma.
    B. The Na+ concentration of sweat can exceed that of plasma.
    C. Urine formed under the influence of diuretics is hyponatremic relative to plasma.
    D. Diuresis from mannitol and glucose creates a urine hyponatremia relative to plasma.

109

21. All of the following are complications of rapid onset hypernatremia *except*:
    A. Subarachnoid hemmorrhage
    B. Venous sinus thrombosis
    C. Subdural hematoma
    D. Cerebral edema
22. Which of the following is *not* a complication of too rapid water replacement for hypernatremia?
    A. Subdural or subarachnoid hemorrhage
    B. Cerebral edema
    C. CHF
    D. Seizures
23. All of the following are causes of a reduced Na+ concentration relative to plasma water *except*:
    A. Hyperlipemia
    B. SIADH
    C. CHF
    D. Chronic renal failure
    E. Hyperglycemia
24. Which of the following is true regarding hyponatremia?
    A. Drugs are not known to cause hyponatremia.
    B. Na+ concentration below 120 mEq/L is usually associated with severe symptoms.
    C. It decreases aldosterone secretion.
    D. It can cause focal neurologic deficits.
    E. It decreased CSF pressure.
25. An 82-year-old man comes to the emergency department confused, with a blood pressure of 105/78, pulse of 92, and respirations of 18. He is not orthostatic and his mucous membranes are somewhat dry. His Na+ is 112 mEq/L; CBC, K+, Mg, CA, and renal function are normal. Which of the following is the most appropriate treatment of his hyponatremia?
    A. Rehydrate with oral fluids
    B. Hypertonic saline infusion and a central line
    C. Normal saline infusion
    D. Half-normal saline infusion
26. Which of the following will increase K+ excretion?
    A. Increased fluid delivery to the distal renal tubule
    B. Decreased Na+ delivery to the distal tubule
    C. Discontinuing diuretic therapy
    D. Acidosis
27. All of the following statements regarding K+ homeostasis are true *except*:
    A. Paradoxical aciduria results when the kidneys seek to protect the body against hyperkalemia.
    B. K+ and H+ secretion are competitive.
    C. Hormonal regulation of K+ is effected by aldosterone.
    D. Up to a point, the kidneys will preserve K+ homeostasis at the expense of pH homeostasis.
28. Which of the following is a cause of hyperkalemia that leads to a total body deficit of K+?
    A. Diabetes

B. Spironolactone
C. Rhabdomyolysis
D. Hyperaldosteronism

29. Which of the following does *not* contribute to hypokalemia in DKA?
    A. Bicarbonate therapy
    B. Insulin therapy
    C. Renal K+ excretion
    D. Hyperglycemia
30. Why does renal failure contribute to hyperkalemia?
    A. Less K+ is available to the distal nephron for secretion.
    B. Less Na+ is available to the distal nephron to drive K+ excretion.
    C. It increases aldosterone secretion.
    D. The juxtaglomerular apparatus stimulates the renin angiotensin system.
31. A 20-year-old man with non-Hodgkin's lymphoma is seen in the emergency department complaining of a headache and muscle cramps. He is on Tylenol 3 for pain relief but no other medications. He has recently completed first round of chemotherapy without complication. Of the following, which is the most likely cause of his symptoms?
    A. Meningeal carcinomatosis
    B. Hypokalemia
    C. Hyperkalemia
    D. Hypocalcemia
    E. Hypercalcemia
32. The emergency department use of which of the following drugs can result in transient but sometimes significant elevation of the K+ level?
    A. Aminophylline   D. Demerol
    B. Valium   E. Succinylcholine
    C. Lidocaine
33. Which of the following EKG changes are found in hyperkalemia?
    A. Peaked T waves
    B. PR prolongation
    C. QT shortening
    D. All of the above
34. Which of the following EKG patterns can develop in hyperkalemia?
    A. Infarct patterns
    B. Pericarditis
    C. Second degree heart flow
    D. All of the above
35. A 77-year-old man comes to the emergency department feeling weak and short of breath without chest pain. He is on K+ supplementation and is not sure of the dosage. EKG reveals an injury pattern and peaked T waves. Serum K+ is 8.2. Which of the following is the best initial treatment of this patient?
    A. 10 units regular insulin and 250 ml D_{10} KWIV
    B. 20 ml 10% Ca gluconate IV

110

C. 1 amp bicarbonate in 1 l normal saline infusion

D. 10 units regular insulin and 2 amps bicarbonate in one 1 D 10$_{Wnormal\ saline}$ infusion at 250 ml/hour or until symptoms resolve

36. The same patient in question 35 returns to the emergency department the evening of his discharge from the hospital complaining of shortness of breath and swelling in his ankles. His EKG is normal. Which of the following is the most likely etiology for his condition?

A. Na+ overload secondary to Kayexalate
B. Rebound hyperkalemia
C. Hypokalemia
D. Na+ overload secondary to excessive bicarbonate therapy during his hospital stay

37. A 53-year-old patient suffering from Addison's disease comes in with a K+ of 6.6 and complains of weakness. His EKG is normal. Which of the following is the treatment of choice?

A. Normal saline infusion
B. Aldosterone 10 ug IV
C. 9 alpha-fluorohydrocortisone (Florinef) 0.1 mg IV
D. Hydrocortisone 100 mg IV
E. Hydrocortisone 100 mg IM

38. All of the following statements are true regarding gastrointestinal fluid losses *except*:

A. K+ concentration is at least twice plasma for all GI fluids.
B. It leads to secondary hyperaldosteronism.
C. Repeated emesis can lead to hyperkalemia.
D. K+ loss from villous adenomas is small.

39. A 64-year-old man comes to the emergency department with chest pain, and you incidently find his K+ to be 1.8. He is on no medications and has been healthy lately without GI symptoms. Which of the following would *not* be in your differential diagnosis for his hypokalemia?

A. Primary hyperaldosteronism (Conn's syndrome)
B. Lab error
C. Cushing's syndrome
D. Addison's disease
E. Licorice ingestion

40. Which of the following diuretics is *least* likely to cause excessive K+ losses?

A. Aldactone
B. Aldactazide
C. Acetazolamide
D. Furosemide
E. Ethacrynic acid

41. Which of the following primary acid-base disturbances would you most suspect in a patient who is hypokalemic?

A. Metabolic acidosis
B. Metabolic alkalosis

C. Respiratory acidosis
D. Respiratory alkalosis

42. In a patient with hypokalemia, which of the following medications would most concern you?

A. Lasix
B. Verapamil
C. Aldomet
D. Aldactone
E. Lanoxin

43. Which of the following acid-base disturbances can lead to symptoms of hypocalcemia?

A. Metabolic acidosis
B. Metabolic alkalosis
C. Respiratory acidosis
D. Respiratory alkalosis
E. B and D

44. A cachectic 59-year-old man suffering from pain secondary to metastatic carcinoma comes to the emergency department. His albumin is 2.0 from malnutrition. Which of the following choices accurately represents his total ionized Ca++, respectively, in light of his albumin level?

A. Decreased, normal
B. Decreased, decreased
C. Increased, normal
D. Normal, decreased
E. Normal, increased

45. Which of the following carcinomas is the *least* likely to cause hypercalcemia?

A. Colonic
B. Renal
C. Breast
D. Lung

46. Which of the following electrolyte abnormalities potentiates the toxic cardiac effects of digitalis?

A. Hypokalemia
B. Hypocalcemia
C. Hyperkalemia
D. Hypercalcemia
E. A and D

47. A 57-year-old man with multiple myeloma presents with protracted anorexia, nausea, and vomiting. His Ca++ is found to be 15.1. Which of the following modes of therapy is the most appropriate?

A. Lasix 40 mg PO
B. Lasix 40 mg IV
C. 10 units regular insulin IV and a D$_5$ normal saline IV at 250 ml/hour
D. Lasix 50 to 100 mg IV and a normal saline IV at 250 ml/hour after a 500 ml bolus
E. Lasix 40 mg IV and a normal saline IV at 150 ml/hour

48. All of the following are causes of hypocalcemia *except*:

A. Pancreatitis
B. Anticonvulsant therapy
C. Blood transfusions
D. Parathyroid adenoma

49. All of the following statements regarding hypocalcemia are true *except*:
    A. It causes hypoexcitability of neurons.
    B. Few EKG changes are noted.
    C. Clinical manifestations are predominantly neurologic.
    D. Chvostek's sign is positive and demonstrated by ipsilateral facial twitching with percussion of the facial nerve anterior to the ear.

50. A 27-year-old woman is seen 4 days after thyroidectomy with perioral and distal extremity paresthesias, carpopedal spasm, and laryngeal stridor. Which of the following responses would be most appropriate?
    A. Obtain a stat Ca++, Mg++, and electrolytes
    B. Place an IV $D_{5W\ KVO}$ while obtaining the stat labs listed in choice A
    C. 10 ml 10% calcium gluconate IV as soon as you draw her blood
    D. As in C, but wait until you have confirmed your clinical suspicion of a low Ca++ value from the lab

51. All of the following statements regarding magnesium homeostasis are true *except*:
    A. Hypomagnesemia, like hypokalemia and hypercalcemia, predisposes to digitalis toxicity.
    B. Hypermagnesemia leads to hypertension via increased vascular tone.
    C. Hypomagnesemia is common among alcholics.
    D. Diarrhea from any cause can lead to hypomagnesemia.

52. In diabetic ketoacidosis, which of the following electrolytes besides K+ can initially be elevated and then fall precipitously with treatment of this condition?
    A. Mg++   D. Na+
    B. Ca++   E. Fe++
    C. Phosphate

53. Which of the following modes of therapy is indicated for a patient who is hypomagnesemic and having serious cardiac toxicity?
    A. 2 ml 10% magnesium sulfate IV
    B. 10 ml 10T magnesium sulfate IV
    C. 1 amp bicarbonate IV
    D. 10 ml 10% magnesium citrate IV

54. What should be done to prevent hypophosphatemia while treating diabetic ketoacidosis?
    A. Use one-half the usual bicarbonate dose
    B. Use one-half the usual insulin dose
    C. Add potassium phosphate to the IV
    D. Add calcium phosphate to the IV

55. An 80-year-old man arrives from a nursing home with no history other than increasing listlessness. He is afebrile and has trace pedal edema. His Na+ is 118, urine specific gravity is 1.008, urine osmolality is 75, and urine sodium 20. The most probable diagnosis is:
    A. Psychogenic polydipsia
    B. SIADH (neoplasm, drugs, etc.)
    C. Occult or early CHF
    D. Occult liver failure
    E. Renal failure

56. In differentiating causes of hyponatremia, the primary clinical determination should be:
    A. Chief complaint
    B. Current medications
    C. Medical history
    D. State of hydration

57. A 9-month-old female is seen who has apneic spells that the mother relates are brief but worrisome. Further questioning reveals occasional vomiting and slight abdominal distention, which the mother calls new onset of "milk allergy," as well as increasing irritability and infrequent extremity spasms. During a blood pressure check the infant demonstrates carpopedal spasm. Among the tests you astutely order a $Ca+^2$, which is 6. An IV cannot be established. While searching for the underlying cause, your initial treatment is:
    A. PO calcium gluconate
    B. PO calcium lactate
    C. IM calcium chloride
    D. IM calcium gluconate
    E. IM calcium gluceptate

107
Endocrine Disorders

Select the appropriate letter that correctly answers the question or completes the statement.

1. Of the following therapeutic interventions for a patient in thyroid storm, which has the most impact on decreasing morbidity and mortality?
    A. Inhibit thyroid hormone synthesis
    B. Inhibit thyroid hormone release
    C. Prevent peripheral conversion of T_4 to T_3
    D. Inhibit the peripheral effects of thyroid hormone
    E. General supportive measures

2. What would be the therapeutic agent of choice for question 1?

    _____ *B Inderol*

3. With regard to the relationship between uncomplicated hyperthyroidism and thyroid storm, which of the following is true?
    A. Thyroid storm will develop in 6–10% of those with initially uncomplicated hyperthyroidism.
    B. Many of the signs and symptoms of the transition from uncomplicated hyperthyroidism to thyroid

112

storm are due to elevated thyroid hormone and serum catecholamine levels.

C. In opposition to uncomplicated hyperthyroidism, the diagnosis of thyroid storm is based strictly on clinical criteria and its treatment should not await lab confirmation.

D. Differentiation between the two can usually be made on the basis of TFTs.

4. Which of the following is the most common precipitating factor in the development of myxedema coma?

A. Hypoxia
B. Exposure to cold
C. Trauma
D. Congestive heart failure
E. Hypoglycemia

5. Which of the following patterns of TFT (thyroid function test) abnormalities would be most consistent with the clinical diagnosis of myxedema coma? (TT_4 = total T_4, TBG = thyroid-binding globulin, FTI = free thyroid index, TSH = thyroid-stimulating hormone)

A. TT_4 decreased, TBG elevated, FTI decreased, THS elevated
B. TT_4 decreased, TBG decreased, FTI decreased, THS elevated
C. TT_4 decreased, TBG decreased, FTI elevated, TSH elevated
D. TT_4 decreased, TBG elevated, FTI decreased, TSH elevated
E. TT_4 elevated, TBG decreased, FTI elevated, TSH elevated

6. Which of the following statements concerning the treatment of hypothryoidism and its complications is false?

A. The vast majority of cases of hypothyroidism require thyroid hormone replacement—the route and dose administered are determined by the magnitude of the disease.
B. Levothyroxine (T_4) is the replacement hormone of choice in uncomplicated hypothyroidism, whereas triiodothyronine (T_3) is preferred in life-threatening myxedema coma.
C. The single most important therapeutic intervention in the treatment of myxedema coma is the IV administration of thyroid hormone.
D. In a patient with hypothyroidism and hypothermia, active rewarming is usually not indicated.

7. The clinical features and laboratory abnormalities of adrenocortical insufficiency vary according to the location and duration of the lesion producing the disease. Which of the following sequence of laboratory abnormalities is most consistent with chronic primary adrenocortical insufficiency?

A. Decreased glucose, decreased Na+, elevated K+,

elevated ACTH
B. Decreased glucose, decreased Na+, decreased K+, decreased ACTH
C. Decreased glucose, elevated Na+, decreased K+, decreased ACTH
D. Elevated glucose, decreased Na+, decreased K+, elevated ACTH
E. Elevated glucose, elevated Na+, elevated K+, elevated ACTH

8. Primary adrenocortical insufficiency is characterized by all of the following *except*:

A. Inability of the adrenal gland to produce cortisol, aldosterone, or both in spite of an adequate hormonal stimulus
B. Usually becomes manifest when 50% or more of the adrenal mass becomes nonfunctional
C. Elevated ACTH and elevated MSH
D. In the majority of cases is caused by autoimmune or idiopathic processes
E. Is rarely produced by acute adrenal hemorrhage or infarction

9. Concerning the term *functional adrenal insufficiency*, which of the following statements is incorect?

A. It is the most common cause of chronic adrenal insufficiency.
B. It is caused by exogenously administered glucocorticoids that lead to depression of ACTH secretion.
C. It produces a clinical picture consistent with secondary adrenal failure.
D. The degree of adrenal suppression and the expected course of recovery can, in most cases, be predicted on the basis of an accurate and complete patient history.

10. In a patient in whom the diagnosis of acute adrenocortical insufficiency is entertained, which of the following statements does *not* apply?

A. Therapy should be instituted on the basis of clinical impression and before laboratory confirmation is available.
B. Therapeutic and diagnostic interventions should proceed concomitantly.
C. Optimal correction of hypotension will require both glucocorticoid and volume replacement.
D. If the diagnosis of acute adrenocortical insufficiency is unconfirmed, intravenous dexamethasone phosphate should be used for glucocorticoid replacement.
E. Treatment of hypoglycemia should await documented failure of expected glucocorticoid-induced hyperglycemia.

11. Which of the following tests would be most appropriate in attempting to diagnose between primary and secondary adrenocortical insufficiency?
    A. 8-hour ACTH stimulation test
    B. 24-hour urine for 17-hydroxysteroid determination
    C. 48-hour ACTH stimulation test
    D. Dexamethasone suppression test
12. Which of the following therapeutic interventions should be used without delay in a patient with undiagnosed but suspected severe adrenocortical insufficiency?
    A. Intravenous dexamethasone phosphate
    B. Intravenous hydrocortisone hemisuccinate
    C. Intravenous Florinef
    D. Intramuscular cortisone acetate
    E. Subcutaneous glucagon

108
Diabetes

Select the appropriate letter that correctly answers the question or completes the statement.

1. Diabetes:
    A. Is a disorder of glucose metabolism
    B. Has varying degrees of pancreatic beta cell dysfunction
    C. Causes disturbed peripheral tissue glucose uptake and utilization
    D. All of the above
2. All are true of diabetes mellitus *except*:
    A. Approximately 10 million Americans have the diagnosis.
    B. The prevalence has increased 50% in the last 10 years.
    C. One-half of all children with diabetes will die of cardiac disease 25 years after their diagnosis.
    D. One out of every 600 school children have diabetes.
3. All are true about insulin *except*:
    A. High insulin levels are required for the transport of glucose across the cell membrane in muscle.
    B. Insulin promotes passage of certain amino acids across the cell wall.
    C. High levels of insulin are required to inhibit intracellular lipolysis.
    D. The release of insulin is triggered by elevated blood glucose sensed by the beta cells of the pancreas.
4. All of the following statements are true of glucagon *except*:
    A. Glucagon is released by pancreatic alpha cells and its effect is mediated through increasing the activity of adenylcyclase in the liver.
    B. Glycogen breakdown and increasing hepatic gluconeogenesis are two main functions of glucagon.
    C. Glucagon is released in response to hypoglycemia, stress, trauma, infection, exercise, and starvation.
    D. Insulin and glucagon are synergistic in their physiologic effects.
5. Which of the following statements is true?
    A. Type I diabetics are classically elderly, obese, and have poor peripheral sensitivity to insulin.
    B. Type II diabetics have a significant insulin deficiency caused by pancreatic dysfunction.
    C. Type 1 diabetics are more prone to DKA, whereas Type II diabetics are more prone to hyperglycemic hyperosmolar nonketotic coma (HHNC).
    D. Both Type 1 and Type II diabetics usually respond well to oral hypoglycemic agents alone.
6. All of the following statements regarding laboratory values with diabetic patients are true *except*:
    A. False negatives can occur with urine ketone dipstick when ketosis is primarily due to β-hydroxybutyrate.
    B. Anion gap calculations may compensate for falsely low levels of ketosis merely by measuring serum acetone.
    C. The true value of sodium during hyperglycemia may be approximated by adding 1.6 mEq/L to the reported sodium value for every 100 mg/dl glucose above normal.
    D. Acidosis has no effect on calculating serum potassium levels during DKA.
7. All are true of diabetic ketoacidosis *except*:
    A. It most classically occurs in Type II diabetics following the stress of infection or following inadequate insulin administration.
    B. Ketoacidosis is caused by breakdown and release of fatty acids, which are converted to B-hydroxybutyrate and acetoacetate.
    C. Abdominal pain may be present in up to one-half of patients presenting with DKA mimicking an acute abdomen.
    D. Common preceding complaints include malaise, nausea, polydipsia, polyuria, and polyphagia.
8. Physical exam of a patient with DKA commonly reveals:
    A. Depressed sensorium and Kussmaul-Kien respirations
    B. Fruity odor on breath
    C. Clinical dehydration
    D. All of the above
9. A number of other entities may appear similar to DKA and include all of the following *except*:

A. Alcoholic ketoacidosis
B. Intoxication with salicylates, methanol, chloral hydrate, paraldehyde, and cyanide
C. Hyperosmolar coma
D. Narcotic overdose

10. Treatment of patients in DKA includes:
A. Aggressive fluid resuscitation with 0.9% saline
B. Ensuring airway, breathing, and circulation
C. Electrolyte and insulin therapy
D. All of the above

11. All are true statements regarding treatment of DKA *except*:
A. Treatment should be cautious and delayed until laboratory confirmation during pregnancy with DKA.
B. Recent mortality figures have dropped from 40% to under 10% with proper diagnosis and treatment.
C. The most important initial treatment is fluid administration.
D. 0.9% saline may be the fluid of choice for resuscitation, avoiding the possible cerebral edema caused by 0.45% normal saline infusion.

12. A 70-year-old male presents to the emergency department with history of diabetes in DKA. He is awake and alert with blood pressure 90/60 and heart rate 130. Initial treatment would include:
A. 1 liter of 0.9% normal saline in the first half hour followed by fluid administration adjusted according to cardiac status and degree of dehydration
B. 500 cc of 0.9% normal saline over the first hour then 0.9% normal saline at 250 cc/hour
C. 1 liter D5W over the first hour followed by 250 cc/hour of D5W
D. 1 liter of 0.45% normal saline in first half hour followed by 500 cc/hour of D5.45% normal saline

13. The resuscitation of children in DKA, with respect to initial fluid management, should be:
A. 5 ml/kg of 0.9% normal saline over the first hour
B. 10 ml/kg of 0.9% normal saline over the first hour
C. 20 ml/kg of 0.9% normal saline over the first hour
D. 50 ml/kg of 0.9% normal saline over the first hour

14. The following statements are true regarding bicarbonate therapy and DKA, *except*:
A. Acidosis may actually enhance red cell oxygen release, counteracting the 2,3 DPG deficiency in DKA and suggesting caution during $NaHCO_3$ administration.
B. Overly rapid correction of acidosis may cause a paradoxical cerebrospinal fluid acidosis.
C. Because of the severe nature of DKA, and pH below 7.35 should be aggressively corrected.
D. Administration of bicarbonate is suggested below a pH of 7.1 or a serum bicarbonate below 7 mEq/L.

15. The most important *initial* resuscitative therapy is:
A. Insulin   C. IV fluids
B. Glucose and K+   D. HCO_3

16. All of the following are true during resuscitation of patients in DKA *except*:
A. Aggressive volume replacement early in therapy
B. Close electrolyte monitoring including frequent glucose
C. Rapid correction of hyperglycemia with high-dose insulin
D. Close monitoring, including correction of significant acidosis with HCO_3, when needed.

17. The rationale behind slowly dropping the glucose levels in patients with DKA during resuscitation is:
A. Rapid glucose drop can precipitate cerebral edema secondary to rapid changes in serum osmolarity
B. It allows time to do further diagnostic studies
C. To avoid rebound metabolic alkalosis
D. To eliminate the chance of insulin resistance and rebound hyperglycemia

18. Frequent precipitating causes of DKA include:
A. Infection
B. Noncompliance
C. Myocardial infarction
D. All of the above

19. Typical initial values for a patient in HHNC would include:
A. Glucose 300 mg/dl, pH 7.10, osmolarity 290 mOsm/L
B. Glucose 800 mg/dl, pH 7.38, osmolarity 360 mOsm/L
C. Glucose 600 mg/dl, pH 7.0, osmolarity 300 mOsm/L
D. Glucose 175 mg/dl, pH 7.60, osmolarity 365 mOsm/L

20. Hypoglycemia is most commonly caused by which of the following in diabetic patients?
A. Infection
B. Dietary indiscretion
C. Excess insulin administration
D. Dehydration

21. Hypoglycemia can be precipitated in diabetic patients by which of the following?
A. Oral hypoglycemic agents
B. ETOH, salicylates
C. Alteration in insulin dosage
D. All of the above

22. Classically, hypoglycemia presents as:
A. Rapid heart rate, cold clammy skin, anxiety, or sleepiness
B. Hyperthermia
C. Asymptomatic—laboratory diagnosis only
D. Coma

23. Hypoglycemia caused by oral hypoglycemia agents:
    A. Can be prolonged in duration
    B. Should mandate admission and observation
    C. Is particularly common and troublesome with chlorpropamide
    D. All of the above
24. Complications of diabetes include:
    A. Ophthalmologic and neurologic manifestations
    B. Dermatologic and renal manifestations
    C. Cardiovascular complications
    D. All of the above
25. New modalities of therapy for diabetes mellitus include:
    A. New types of insulin and oral hypoglycemic agents
    B. Insulin pumps and pancreatic beta cell transplant
    C. New dietary and exercise recommendations
    D. All of the above

109
Alcohol-Related Disease

Select the appropriate letter that correctly answers the question or completes the statement.

1. Approximately how many alcoholics are there in this country?
    A. 3,000,000
    B. 8,000,000
    C. 12,000,000
    D. 20,000,000
2. A 45-year-old white male presents to the emergency department with a long history of alcoholism and has a history as well of numerous withdrawals on attempting to quit drinking. He demonstrates nearly constant desire for alcohol use and has a long history of failures at detoxification. This patient demonstrates:
    A. Psychologic dependence
    B. Physical dependence
    C. Addiction
    D. Poor coping mechanisms
3. The primary enzyme that breaks down alcohol is:
    A. Alcohol dehydrognase
    B. Aldehyde
    C. Citric acid cycle
    D. Microsomal ethanol oxidizing system
4. Diminished fine motor control in the nonalcoholic is exhibited at what blood alcohol concentration?
    A. 10–20 mg/dl
    B. 20–50 mg/dl
    C. 50–100 mg/dl
    D. 100–150 mg/dl
5. Why is fructose *not* useful in the management of acute alcohol intoxication?

A. It has never been proven conclusively to show an acceleration in decrease in blood ethanol levels.
B. It has severe potential side effects.
C. It may be additive to alcohol in causing severe hypoglycemia.
D. It may precipitate alcohol withdrawal.

6. An alcoholic of 10 years duration presents in the emergency department approximately 24 hours after attempting to quit drinking alcohol. He is complaining of anxiety, inability to sleep at night, and has a gross tremor exhibited. At this time he is suffering from:
    A. Withdrawal seizures
    B. Minor withdrawal
    C. Major withdrawal
    D. Delirium tremens
7. A 45-year-old alcoholic with a long history of alcoholism presents to the emergency department requesting detoxification. He has a history of major withdrawal in the past with seizures. Adequate therapy to prevent seizures in this patient would include:
    A. Benzodiazepine therapy alone
    B. Oral phenytoin for 1 week
    C. Oral benzodiazepine and phenytoin for 5 days
    D. Chronic phenytoin maintenance and benzodiazepine for 5 days
8. In patients with preexisting cardiac disease, what are the cardiac effects of alcohol intoxication?
    A. Increased cardiac output and increased dysrhythmias
    B. Decreased cardiac output and decreased dysrhythmias
    C. Decreased cardiac output and increased dysrhythmias
    D. Increased cardiac output and decreased dysrhythmias
9. In alcoholic hepatitis what is the laboratory test that most closely follows liver function?
    A. Serum glutamic-oxaloacetic transaminase (SGOT)
    B. Prothrombin time
    C. Blood urea nitrogen (BUN)
    D. Glucose
10. Wernicke's encephalopathy is characterized by:
    A. Nystagmus, confusion, and ataxia
    B. Severe amnesia, apathy, and confabulation
    C. Dysconjugate gaze and coma
    D. Rapid response of the mental changes after thiamine
11. Treatment for acute alcoholic rhabdomyolysis is characterized by:
    A. Early physical therapy to prevent contracture
    B. Establishing an acid diuresis to prevent acute renal failure

C. Establishing an alkaline diuresis to prevent acute renal failure

D. Broad-spectrum antibiotics to prevent superinfection

12. The most common bacterial cause of pneumonia in alcoholics is:

A. *Streptococcus pneumoniae*

B. *Klebsiella pneumoniae*

C. Mixed flora

D. Gram-negative rods

13. Typical electrolyte abnormalities in the chronic alcoholic include:

A. Hypokalemia, hypophosphatemia, and hypocalcemia

B. Hyperkalemia, hypophosphatemia, and hypercalcemia

C. Hypermagnesia, hypophosphatemia, and hypocalcemia

D. Hyperphosphatemia, hypercalcemia, and hypermagnesia

14. Alcoholic ketosis is characterized by:

A. Usual occurrence in diabetic alcoholics

B. Usual occurrence in nonalcoholic binge drinking

C. Associated with severe hyperglycemia

D. Usually exhibited by tachypnea, dehydration, ketonuria, and little to no glucose urea

15. Iron deficiency anemia in alcoholics is usually secondary to:

A. Chronic malnutrition

B. Ethanal binding of iron in the diet

C. Small bowel malabsorption

D. Blood loss from the gastrointestinal tract

110
Tricyclic Antidepressants

Select the appropriate letter that correctly answers the question or completes the statement.

1. All of the following EKG abnormalities may be seen with tricyclic antidepressant overdose, *except*:

A. Shortened PR interval

B. Right bundle branch block

C. QT prolongation

D. QRS interval greater than .10 seconds

2. A 23-year-old female is brought to the emergency department by friends 2 hours after ingesting several amitryptyline tablets. She is somewhat sedate but otherwise displays no anticholinergic effects. She says she took a total of twenty 25-mg tablets. Given the history she provides, what would be the best management approach?

A. Refer her directly for psychiatric evaluation since the ingested amount is subtoxic

B. Administer ipecac, activated charcoal and cathartic and await serum amitryptyline and nortryptiline levels to determine further therapy

C. Administer ipecac, activated charcoal, and cathartic but discharge after psychiatric evaluation since the absence of anticholinergic signs precludes a significant ingestion

D. Consider the patient's history and absence of anticholinergic signs unreliable and proceed with definitive treatment and monitoring for at least 6 hours

E. Obtain blood for STAT toxicologic analysis, monitor EKG, and provide definitive management only if plasma tricyclic antidepressant levels exceed 1000 mg/ml

3. Definitive treatment for acute tricyclic antidepressant overdose includes which of the following?

A. Emesis or gastric lavage up to 24 hours after the alleged time of ingestion

B. Physostigmine 2 mg IV push for any patient displaying coma, disorientation, or hallucinations

C. Sodium bicarbonate to control seizures and other CNS manifestations

D. Propranolol as a first-line agent in controlling hemodymanically significant supraventricular tachycardias

E. Lidocaine as a first-line agent in management of ventricular tachycardias

4. A 35-year-old male is being evaluated following an alleged ingestion of 1.25 g of imipramine. ECG monitor shows a QRS interval of 0.12 seconds, and he has frequent PVCs and short runs of ventricular tachycardia. Initial management of his cardiac disturbance should include which of the following?

A. Lidocaine 1 mg/kg bolus then infusion 2–4 mg/min

B. Phenytoin 500–1000 mg IV at a rate not to exceed 50 mg/min

C. Sodium bicarbonate 0.5–3.0 mEq/kg to maintain pH of 7.45

D. Physostigmine 1–3 mg slow IV push

E. Propranolol 1 mg bolus every 5 minutes to a maximum of 5 mg

5. Which of the following is the drug of choice for tricyclic antidepressant-induced seizures?

A. Phenytoin

B. Valium

C. Phenobarbital

D. Physostigmine

E. Sodium bicarbonate

6. Each of the following statements concerning tricyclic antidepressant overdose is true *except*:
   A. Major pharmacologic activities include sedation, anticholinergic activity, and amelioration of depression.
   B. Excretion of tricyclic antidepressants in gastric and bile secretions through enterohepatic circulation make repeated doses of activated charcoal important in treatment of tricyclic antidepressant overdoses.
   C. Structurally, they resemble the phenothiazines.
   D. Physostigmine is the specific antidote in tricyclic antidepressant poisoning and is used to control both cardiac and CNS toxic manifestations.

111
Tranquilizer Overdose

Select the appropriate letter that correctly answers the question or completes the statement.

1. Which of the following statements regarding tranquilizer overdose is correct?
   A. Benzodiazepines, as a group, account for the most deaths attributed to tranquilizer overdoses.
   B. Phenothiazines have a low therapeutic index, accounting for frequent deaths in adult overdose.
   C. Most lithium overdoses result from routine therapy due to its narrow margin of safety.
   D. Most tranquilizer overdoses occur in well-educated men in the middle to upper socioeconomic class.
   E. Most tranquilizer overdoses occur in women in the middle to upper socioeconomic class.

2. A 32-year-old female presents to the emergency department comatose with miotic pupils, depressed deep tendon reflexes, and rectal temperature of 32°C. A few drops of ferric chloride are added to a urine sample and a reddish brown color develops. The patient most likely has ingested which of the following?
   A. Benzodiazepine
   B. Meprobamate
   C. Lithium
   D. Phenothiazine
   E. Haloperidol

3. A 28-year-old male, recently started on Haldol, presents with acute onset of dysphagia. Which therapeutic trial should be performed?
   A. Physostigmine 1–4 mg slow IV push
   B. Physostigmine 0.5 mg slow IV push
   C. Benztropine 20 mg IV over 2 minutes
   D. Diphenhydramine 1–5 mg/kg IV up to a maximum of 50 mg over 2 minutes
   E. None of the above; obtain a psychiatric consultation

4. A 20-year-old female has been given appropriate treatment and 6 hours of observation in the emergency department following an overdose of tranquilizers. Psychiatric consultation is complete. The patient is alert and shows no signs of systemic toxicity. She can now be discharged unless the agent was which of the following:
   A. Benzodiazepine
   B. Thioridazine
   C. Chlorpromazine
   D. Haloperidol
   E. Thiothixene

5. The following are true concerning acute dystonic reactions *except*:
   A. Symptoms range from mild dysphagia to bizarre posturing.
   B. They can be a frequent event in young people experimenting with drugs.
   C. Treatment should be continued on an oral regimen for at least 24 hours.
   D. Dystonia is a dose-related event with phenothiazines or butyrophenones.
   E. Treatment is usually with benztropine or diphenhydramine IV or IM.

6. All the following would be indicated following phenothiazine overdose *except*:
   A. Abdominal x-ray
   B. Gastric lavage
   C. ECG
   D. Hemodialysis
   E. Acidifying the urine

7. All of the following characterize benzodiazepine overdose *except*:
   A. In a 3-month period, 1 in 10 Americans takes diazepam for tension or anxiety.
   B. Benzodiazepine prescriptions should be limited to an amount that would not be lethal if taken at one time.
   C. Mixed ingestions with benzodiazepines are common.
   D. Deaths from benzodiazepine overdoses are relatively common because they are involved in more overdoses than any other class of drug.
   E. If significant symptoms appear in patients with apparent benzodiazepine ingestion, additional agents should be sought.

8. Phenothiazines are characterized by all of the following *except*:
   A. Phenothiazines decreases the seizure threshold.
   B. Phenothiazines produce a quinidine-like effect on the heart.
   C. Seizures secondary to phenothiazines are usually treated with diazepam and short-acting barbiturates.
   D. Phenothiazines like lithium have a very narrow margin of safety.

E. Phenothiazines can cause prolongation of the PR and QT intervals.

9. All the following characterize lithium overdose *except*:
A. There is very narrow margin of safety.
B. Patients must be admitted to the hospital to be observed for symptom progression.
C. Hemodialysis is not beneficial.
D. There is usually a good correlation between serum lithium levels and symptoms.
E. Osmotic and saline diuresis increase renal lithium clearance.

10. In managing hypotension resulting from phenothiazine overdose, each of the following treatment modalities may be appropriate *except*:
A. Trendelenburg positioning
B. Isotonic fluids
C. Methoxamine 10–20 mg IV
D. Epinephrine 0.5–1.0 mg of 1:10000 solution IV
E. Dopamine 15–30 µg/kg/min

11. For which agent might hemodialysis be useful in the event of massive overdose?
A. Benzodiazepine
B. Thioridazine
C. Chlorpromazine
D. Hydroxyzine
E. Meprobamate

112
Sedative-Hypnotics

Select the appropriate letter that correctly answers the question or completes the statement.

1. Overdose with which of the following sedatives responds well to forced diuresis with saline and furosemide?
A. Ethchlorvinyl
B. Meprobamate
C. Glutethimide
D. Methaqualone

2. All of the following are true regarding severe intoxication with chloral hydrate *except*:
A. It may produce a variety of skin manifestations including purpura, bullae, and erythema multiforme.
B. It may cause primary supraventricular tachycardia or ventricular dysrhythmias.
C. It may cause a paradoxical CNS excitation with agitation and psychosis prior to coma.
D. It responds well to aqueous hemodialysis or charcoal hemoperfusion.
E. It may cause severe gastritis with hematemesis and gastric necrosis.

3. A 2-year-old child has ingested an entire bottle, approximately 25 tablets, of Sominex, an over-the-counter sleep aid. You could expect to find all of the following clinical manifestations *except*:

A. Agitation and hallucinations
B. Flushed dry skin and dry mouth
C. Seizures
D. Bradycardia and hypotension

4. Which subclass of sedative hypnotic agents is responsible for the majority of drug-related deaths in this category?
A. Meprobamate (carbamates)
B. Barbiturates
C. Benzodiazepines
D. Chloral hydrate (chloral derivatives)
E. Methaqualone

5. All of the following are potential physiologic effects of barbiturate toxicity *except*:
A. Hyperthermia   *Hypo*
B. Respiratory depression
C. Noncardiac pulmonary edema
D. Venodilitation with hypotension
E. Negative inotropic effect on myocardium

6. Skin findings in the comatose patient suggestive of barbiturate overdose and present in up to 50% of patients dying of barbiturate overdose include:
A. Petechiae
B. Diffuse macullar rash affecting palms and soles
C. Intense erythema of the trunk and extremities
D. Clear vessicles and bullae at skin pressure sites
E. Eczematoid reaction involving the face, chest, and abdomen

7. The initial treatment of cardiovascular collapse associated with barbiturate overdose consists primarily of:
A. Volume expansion with monitoring of central venous pressures or pulmonary capillary wedge pressures
B. MAST trousers
C. Dopamine infusion
D. Rapid infusion of 1000 cc of isotonic fluid containing 2 mEq/kg sodium bicarbonate
E. Norepinephrine infusion

8. Forced alkaline diuresis for enhancing barbiturate excretion in the overdosed patients is most likely to be effective for:
A. Thiopental
B. Amobarbital
C. Phenobarbital
D. Pentobarbital
E. Secobarbital

9. Which of the following is characteristic feature of methaqualone overdose generally not associated with other sedative-hypnotic agents?
A. Profound cardiovascular depression
B. Symmetric pyramidal tract signs such as hypertonicity and hyperreflexia
C. Coma
D. Noncardiac pulmonary edema
E. Cerebellar signs such as nystagmus and ataxia

10. A 28-year-old female presents to the emergency department 1 hour after ingesting approximately 6 g of methaqualone. She is comatose, has shallow respirations, and displays hyperreflexia and intermittent seizures. Blood pressure is 70/40. Appropriate management measures might include all *except*:
    A. Forced diruesis to enhance renal excretion
    B. Volume expansion and pressors if necessary
    C. Endotracheal intubation and ventilatory support
    D. Gastric lavage and activated charcoal
    E. Hemodialysis or charcoal hemoperfusion

113
Narcotics

Select the appropriate letter that correctly answers the question or completes the statement.

1. Which of the following narcotics may be associated with a more prolonged duration of clinical intoxication in the overdose patient due to its slow metabolism?
    A. Codeine
    B. Propoxyphene
    C. Morphine
    D. Meperidine
    E. Methadone

2. All of the following statements regarding clinical manifestations in narcotic overdose are true *except*:
    A. Respiratory depression is nearly always the cause of death.
    B. Noncardiogenic pulmonary edema is common and universally present in fatal cases.
    C. Narcotics cause vasodilatation with resultant relative hypovolemia and orthostatic hypotension.
    D. Narcotics depress myocardial contractility and the resultant cardiovascular collapse causes profound hypotension.
    E. Miosis is typical; however, meperidine may dilate the pupils.

3. Which statement regarding noncardiogenic pulmonary edema in narcotic overdose is true?
    A. Pulmonary edema is thought to be the result of a hypersensitivity reaction.
    B. It is probably the result of hypoxia with resultant pulmonary vascular constriction and capillary damage.
    C. While usually seen in overdoses, pulmonary edema is also associated with an idiosyncratic reaction to therapeutic doses.
    D. It develops as a direct result of myocardial depression and elevates pulmonary capillary wedge pressures.
    E. It is generally not seen in heroin overdoses.

4. A 28-year-old known narcotic abuser presents with clinical manifestations of narcotic overdose. In the emergency department he sustains a grand mal seizure. The narcotic *most likely* implicated is:
    A. Heroin
    B. Morphine
    C. Meperidine
    D. Codeine
    E. Hydrocodone

5. The most common dermatologic manifestations of narcotic overdose is (are):
    A. Flushed skin, pruritis, and urticaria
    B. Multiple vesicles and bullae over pressure points
    C. Multiple bruises and petechiae
    D. An intensely pruritic eczematous reaction
    E. Erythema multiforme

6. Naloxone differs from previously synthesized narcotic antagonists in that:
    A. Naloxone has only weak agonist activity at opioid receptors in the brain.
    B. Naloxone may produce analgesia, respiratory depression, and miosis.
    C. Naloxone is a weak competitive antagonist at opioid receptors in the brain.
    D. Naloxone is less potent, therefore antagonistic activity dominates at opioid receptors in the brain.
    E. Naloxone is devoid of any agonist activity at opioid receptors in the brain.

7. All of the following are characteristic clinical manifestations in narcotic overdose *except*:
    A. Stupor and coma
    B. Respiratory depression
    C. Pink frothy sputum
    D. Dilated pupils
    E. Needle tracks

8. You are managing a suspected narcotic overdose and large doses (total 15 mg) of naloxone have been required to achieve a clinical response. The agent involved is most likely among which of the following?
    A. Pentazocine, propoxyphene, codeine
    B. Pentazocine, propoxyphene, morphine
    C. Heroin, morphine, codeine
    D. Hydrocodone, pentazocine, propoxyphene
    E. Opium power, morphine, meperidine

9. The appropriate pediatric dose of naloxone is which of the following?
    A. 0.1 mg/kg to a total dose of 0.5 mg/kg
    B. 0.01 mg/kg to a total dose of 0.20 mg/kg
    C. 0.001 mg/kg to a total dose of 0.4 mg
    D. 0.001 mg/kg to a total dose of 0.005 mg/kg
    E. 0.01 mg/kg to a total dose of 0.4 mg

10. A 34-year-old narcotic addict has been stabilized after presenting with a methadone overdose. Narcotic reversal has been achieved with an initial dose of 0.8 mg naloxone IV. To prevent redevelopment of narcotic overdose symptoms, the most reasonable approach would be to do which of the following?

A. Give 2 mg naloxone IM for prolonged effect
B. Repeat small IV doses of naloxone as needed when symptoms develop
C. Support ventilation but give no more naloxone since repeated administration will precipitate withdrawal
D. Begin a continuous infusion of naloxone IV at 0.4–0.8 mg/hour
E. Begin a continous infusion of naloxone IV at 4.0–8.0 mg/hour

11. Which of the following narcotics does not cross the blood-brain barrier and the placenta equally?
A. Meperidine
B. Methadone
C. Codeine
D. Heroin
E. Morphine

12. Which of the following narcotics is fat-soluble and is therefore stored in body tissues?
A. Propoxyphene
B. Morphine
C. Heroin
D. Oxycodone

13. In terms of cardiovascular effects, which of the following narcotics is the safest?
A. Propoxyphene
B. Meperidine
C. Morphine
D. Codeine

14. In symptomatic propoxyphene overdose, what is the minimum observation time?
A. 6 hours
B. 12 hours
C. 24 hours
D. 36 hours

15. Which of the following narcotics is contraindicated in infants?
A. Codeine
B. Diphenoxylate
C. Meperidine
D. Morphine

16. Which narcotic drug overdose has *not* been reported to produce pulmonary edema?
A. Pentazocine
B. Propoxyphene
C. Heroin
D. Methadone

17. All of the following statements about propoxyphene overdose are true *except*:
A. Convulsions occur commonly.
B. Pulmonary edema is common in severe cases.
C. Psychotic reactions lasting 3 to 4 days can occur.
D. Death is uncommon unless doses greater than 120 mg/kg are ingested.   35 mg/kg

18. The appropriate initial dosage of naloxone in a child weighing 13 kg who is suspected to be symptomatic from a narcotic ingestion is:
A. 0.01 mg
B. 0.13 mg
C. 8.0 mg
D. 13.0 mg

19. All of the following statements are true about the abstinence syndrome *except*:
A. The abstinence syndrome has a typical course and evolves over a period of hours and days rather than minutes.

B. Naloxone administered to a narcotics addict causes an intense withdrawal syndrome that begins within 5 minutes.
C. Symptoms include lacrimation, rhinorrhea, insomnia, vomiting, diarrhea, and gooseflesh.
D. Treatment consists of administering narcotics to correct and reverse the syndrome.

114
Salicylates and Acetaminophen

Select the appropriate letter that correctly answers the question or completes the statement.

1. All of the following statements regarding absorption of salicylates in overdose are true *except*:
A. Peak serum levels of most salicylate products occur within 2–4 hours.
B. Two-thirds of an ingested dose is absorbed in 1 hour.
C. Peak levels tend to occur sooner in ingestion of enteric-coated tablets.
D. Large doses of orally administered salicylates may result in delayed gastric emptying due to pylorospasm and concentrations in the stomach.
E. Although the low pH in the stomach favors gastric absorption, most salicylate is absorbed in the small intestine.

2. All of the following are typical metabolic consequences of salicylate intoxication *except*:
A. Hyperglycemia and glucosuria
B. Ketonemia and ketonuria
C. Hypothermia
D. Hyperventilation and respiratory alkalosis
E. "Anion-gap" metabolic acidosis

3. The most common acid base disturbance seen in older children and adults with salicylate toxicity is:
A. Pure metabolic acidosis
B. Respiratory alkalosis with metabolic acidosis
C. Respiratory alkalosis with metabolic alkalosis
D. Pure respiratory alkalosis
E. None of the above

4. Which of the following electrolyte disturbances is most commonly seen in salicylate toxicity:
A. Hyperkalemia
B. Hypokalemia
C. Hypernatremia
D. Hyponatremia
E. Hyperchloremia

5. A 7-year-old female diabetic, who has been despondent recently regarding her diabetes and the conflict it creates between her and her parents, presents after she admitted taking a bottle of aspirin. She is fully alert but is complaining of tinnitus and nausea. She has been taking her insulin lately, is on no other medications, and has no other medical problems. Her vital signs are blood pressure 118/70, pulse 102, respirations 26. Which of the following glucose values are most likely in this patient on admission?

   A. 66   C. 220
   B. 105   D. 520

6. Which of the following blood gas panels is most likely in the patient in question 5?

	pH	pO$_2$	pCO$_2$	HCO$_3$
A.	7.30	97	35	low
B.	7.51	102	22	nl.
C.	7.40	95	39	nl.
D.	7.49	86	40	up

7. You wish to quickly confirm the history of a salicylate ingestion in the patient in question 5. Which of the following tests is of help?

   A. Magnesium oxide test
   B. Aluminum hydroxide test
   C. Ferric chloride test
   D. Iron oxide test

8. Which of the following treatment plans is most appropriate for the patient in question 5?

   A. Ipecac, charcoal, cathartic, IV of D5 LR with 40 mEq/L KCl to maintain good urine output
   B. Gastric lavage, charcoal, cathartic, IV of D5 LR to maintain good urine output
   C. Ipecac, charcoal, cathartic, IV LR with 40 mEq/L KCl to maintain good urine output
   D. As in C above but maintain IV at TKO

9. Your initial salicylate level was drawn 2 hours after ingestion and found to be 50 mg/dl. What would you conclude?

   A. It indicates a severe ingestion.
   B. It indicates an insignificant ingestion.
   C. As in A, a protocol for dialysis should begin.
   D. It indicates a moderate ingestion.
   E. It is too early to make a conclusion.

10. Which of the following is the greatest obstacle in our ability to alkalinize the urine in significant salicylate ingestions?

    A. Respiratory alkalosis
    B. Renal failure
    C. Renal tubular acidosis
    D. K+ depletion
    E. Ongoing depletion of bicarbonate

11. Which of the following statements regarding chronic salicylate ingestion is true?

    A. The most common problems result from gastric intolerance including erosive gastritis and GI blood loss.
    B. Presenting symptoms of chronic salicylism may mimic myocardial infarction, DKA, encephalitis, or alcoholic ketoacidosis.
    C. Physiologic changes in the elderly that decrease salcylate metabolism and excretion can result in salicylate toxicity.
    D. In chronic salicylate ingestions, the salicylate level does not correlate with ABG assessment or with the patient's level of consciousness.
    E. All of the above are true.

12. The potentially toxic dose and potentially lethal dose of salicylate is:

    A. 200 mg/kg and 500 mg/kg, respectively
    B. 100 mg/kg and 200 mg/kg, respectively
    C. 500 mg/kg and 1000 mg/kg, respectively
    D. 50 mg/kg and 200 mg/kg, respectively
    E. The severity of toxicity and potential lethalness cannot be estimated by the ingested dose.

13. All of the following therapeutic endeavors in the management of a serum salicylate overdose are correct *except*:

    A. In a comatose or convulsing patient, itubation and gastric lavage are indicated.
    B. Activated charcoal should be administered.
    C. Isotonic saline or RL with 5% dextrose should be given to correct dehydration and then a urine output of 2–3 cc/hour should be maintained.
    D. 40 mg of potassium should be given with the initial infusion and then supplemented based on laboratory values. This should be followed by urine alkalinization.
    E. Forced alkaline diuresis should be instituted to enhance salicylate excretion.

14. Which of the following drugs when taken is in combination with or prior to a toxic ingestion of acetaminophen is particularly hazardous?

    A. Barbiturates   D. Alcohol
    B. Narcotics   E. *A* and *D*
    C. Benzodiazepines

15. Which of the following acetaminophen levels in µg/ml are consistently associated with hepatic damage?

    A. Greater than 300 at 4 hours and 45 at 15 hours
    B. Greater than 120 at 4 hours and 50 at 12 hours
    C. Greater than 50 at 4 hours and 120 at 12 hours
    D. Greater than 300 at 4 hours and 120 at 12 hours

16. A 30-year-old male presents following the ingestion of Tylenol 8 hours previously. What would you expect his initial complaints to be if it was not a mixed ingestion?

    A. CNS depression
    B. Hyperreactive and agitated
    C. Abdominal pain, mainly right upper quadrant

D. Anorexia, nausea, vomiting
E. Diaphoresis, tremors, confusion

17. Which of the following treatment modalities is not effective acetaminophen overdose?
A. Charcoal
B. Forced diuresis
C. Cathartics
D. Hemodialysis

18. Which of the following is the correct initial dose of Mucomyst (N-acetylcysteine) for acetaminophen overdose?
A. 140 mg/kg
B. 140 mg/kg diluted 1:3 in a soft drink
C. 70 mg/kg diluted 1:3 in a soft drink
D. 140 mg/kg twice q 1 hour

19. A patient arrives at the emergency department 2 hours following the ingestion of an unknown amount of acetaminophen. An acetaminophen level drawn immediately after arrival indicates a serum level of 60 mg/ml. Which of the following statements best describes the significance of the acetaminophen level?
A. This is a toxic level and N-acetylcysteine therapy should be instituted without delay
B. This level is non-toxic but should be reported at 4 hours to determine if the level has risen into a toxic range.
C. Since acetaminophen is rapidly absorbed, the 2-hour level is adequate estimate of the potential for hepatic toxicity.
D. Serum levels are not reliable indicators of the potential toxicity of acetaminophen ingestion; plasma half-life will need to be calculated.
E. This ingestion might not be toxic in an adult but would likely result in hepatotoxicity in a young child.

20. A patient has ingested 25 g of acetaminophen and several OTC cold medications 1 hour prior to arrival at the emergency department. He has not vomited and is alert with stable vital signs. APAP levels must be sent out and won't be available until the following day. General management should include:
A. Gastric lavage, activated charcoal followed by cathartic
B. Gastric lavage, activated charcoal, and cathartic but N-acetylcysteine only if APAP levels return in toxic range
C. Gastric lavage, activated charcoal and cathartic, then re-lavage until clear then give N-acetylcysteine
D. Gastric lavage, cathartic, and N-acetylcysteine but withhold charcoal
E. Gastric lavage followed by N-acetylcysteine, then activated charcoal 1 hour later

115
Hallucinations

Select the appropriate letter that correctly answers the question or completes the statement.

1. A 34-year-old male presents with a neighbor who heard him screaming "they're going to get me" and other paranoid-type delusions. There is no history of obvious drug ingestion or empty drug bottles, and the neighbor knows no post medical history. The vital signs are blood pressure 170/100, heart rate 125, respirations 29, and temperature 99°F. The patient is extremely agitated and frightened. Which of the following would *not* be included in your differential?
A. Acute psychotic break
B. Cocaine intoxication
C. LSD
D. Mixed drug intoxication
E. Glutethimide overdose

2. A 5-year-old male is brought to the emergency department by his parents who state he ate some wild mushrooms 2 hours prior to admission and now is "acting strange." The patient complains of abdominal pain. A sample mushroom was brought in with the patient. Poison control identifies the mushroom as *A. muscaria*. With this information you:
A. Give 1 mg atropine IV
B. Intubate and lavage via nasogastric tube
C. Give Valium 5 mg po
D. Observe for 6–12 hours then discharge
E. Admit to pediatric ICU

3. Which is *not* associated with intravenous marijuana use?
A. Severe abdominal pain
B. Death
C. Hypotension
D. Acute renal insufficiency
E. Rhabdomyolysis

4. A 19-year-old male is brought to the emergency department by the police with a history of PCP ingestion. The patient is initially agitated and is restrained by the police officers. After haloperidol 10 mg IM the patient quiets down. Five minutes later the patient becomes stuporous then becomes comatose. You do all of the following *except*:
A. Intubate and place IV D5W TKO
B. Thiamine 100 mg IV, dextrose 50 gm IV, naloxone 2 mg IV
C. Gastric lavage then nasogastric suction
D. Urine acidification to increase renal elimination
E. Watch for hyperthermia, siezures, and bronchospasm

5. The most common serious medical complication of PCP toxicity is:
   A. Bronchospasm
   B. Myoglobinuric renal failure
   C. Grand mal seizures
   D. Acute hypertension (greater than 140/90
   E. Hyperthermia

116
Stimulants

Select the appropriate letter that correctly answers the question or completes the statement.

1. Which of the following therapeutic measures is *not* recommended for treatment of amphetamine or cocaine overdoses?
   A. Phentolamine for hypertensive emergencies
   B. Lidocaine for ventricular dysrhythmias
   C. Ammonium chloride
   D. Phenothiazines for hyperthermia
   E. Mannitol or furosemide

2. Which of the following statements is incorrect regarding cocaine?
   A. Death from cocaine toxicity results from CNS and adrenergic stimulation.
   B. Toxic psychosis is a common presentation and usually involves visual or tactile hallucinations.
   C. Urine drug screen for metabolites are positive for up to 36 hours after use.
   D. Peripheral effects include hypertension, tachycardia, sweating, mydriasis, and cardiac dysrhythmias.
   E. Propranolol, 1 mg IV, is the primary treatment for the cardiac manifestations of cocaine overdose.

3. A 34-year-old white male "yuppie" presents with complaints of weight loss, insomnia, restlessness, and blurred vision. His PMH is negative. Which of the following physical findings are *not* more consistent with stimulant abuse rather than with primary depression?
   A. Chronic fatigue
   B. Perforated nasal septum
   C. Cycloplegia
   D. Tics
   E. Exopthalmos

117
Corrosives

Select the appropriate letter that correctly answers the question or completes the statement.

1. All of the following may be indicated following acute alkali ingestion *except*:
   A. Milk
   B. Steroids
   C. Nasogastric or orogastric aspiration
   D. Careful history on the quantity, concentration, and nature of the agent
   E. Cricothyrotomy or tracheostomy

2. Which of the following is true concerning corrosive ingestion?
   A. Alkalis produce a rapidly penetrating coagulative necrosis.
   B. Acids produce a liquefactive necrosis.
   C. Alkalis are the offending agent about 10 times as often as acids.
   D. Steroids are generally not recommended for alkali ingestion.
   E. Cathartics and absorbants are beneficial in corrosive ingestion.

3. Which of the following would be indicated following acute acid ingestion?
   A. Gastric aspiration
   B. Dilution and neutralization
   C. Syrup of ipecac
   D. Prophylactic antibiotics and steroids
   E. Blind nasotracheal intubation

118
Hydrocarbons

Select the appropriate letter that correctly answers the question or completes the statement.

1. In which of the following hydrocarbon ingestions should the stomach *not* be emptied?
   A. Benzene
   B. More than 1 ml/kg gasoline
   C. Lubricating oil
   D. More than 1 ml/kg lighter fluid
   E. *A* and *C*

2. Which of the following are potential complications of hydrocarbon ingestions to consider in management?
   A. Pulmonary edema
   B. ARDS

C. Metabolic acidosis
D. Neurologic dysfunction
E. All of the above
3. Which of the following is the most likely from acute hydrocarbon toxicity?
A. Ventricular arrhythmias
B. Aspiration pneumonitis
C. Hepatic necrosis
D. Bloody diarrhea
E. Seizures

119

Acute Iron Poisoning

Select the appropriate letter that correctly answers the question or completes the statement.

1. The pharmokinetics of iron:
A. Involves binding to the protein ferritin for transportation to other cells
B. Proceeds via first order kinetics
C. Involves storage as hemosiderin and use in hemoglobin synthesis in the bone marrow
D. Involves transformation of the ferrous to the ferric form in GI mucosal cells
2. The pathophysiology of iron involves:
A. Uncoupling of mitochondrial oxidative phosphorylation
B. A direct toxic effect on GI mucosa
C. Free iron being an intracellular toxin
D. The total free serum iron level exceeding the transferrin binding capacity
E. All of the above
3. Laboratory studies can help elucidate which of the following metabolic abnormalities in iron toxicity?
A. Hyperglycemia and metabolic acidosis
B. Leukopenia
C. Coagulopathy
D. Metabolic acidosis
4. After ingesting toxic doses of iron, patients most frequently present with:
A. Hepatic failure
B. Coma
C. Hepatic necrosis
D. Vomiting
5. The diagnosis of severe iron poisoning:
A. Can be excluded if the serum iron level is less than 300 µg/dl 3–5 hours postingestion
B. Should involve a determination of the amount of elemental iron ingested

C. Can be excluded if the first voided urine is of normal color after a challenge dose of deferoxamine
D. Cannot be aided by abdominal x-rays
6. A 22-year-old male presents to the emergency department in a stuporous state. His friend presents you with a bottle of iron-containing vitamins. Initial treatment includes:
A. Gastric emptying with ipecac to ensure complete removal of aggregated tablets
B. Stomach lavage utilizing hypertonic phosphage solution to create insoluble aggregates in the gut
C. Mixing four amps of 8.4% HCO_3 with 1 l of water for subsequent gastric lavage
D. Surgical consultation for removal of a likely iron bezoar
7. After an argument with her boyfriend, a 16-year-old female took a handful of vitamins containing iron. Her management is predicated on:
A. The presence of radiopaque tablets in the gut on abdominal flat plate
B. A knowledge of the amount of elemental iron ingested
C. The total level of serum iron and the serum iron to IBC ratio
D. Abnormal glucose and leukocyte values
E. All of the above
8. A vitamin containing ferrous sulfate 325 mg was ingested by a 20-kg child. It is determined that 15 tablets are missing from the previously full bottle. Ferrous sulfate 325 mg is 22% elemental iron. Which of the following statements is true?
A. Deferoxamine given orally will bind iron in the gut, preferentially the ferrous form.
B. 10.5 g of deferoxamine would bind all of the elemental iron in the total number of missing tablets.
C. A protective effect is exerted at the cellular level by extracellular iron chelation when deferoxamine is given IV.
D. A and C
E. B and C
9. Ingestion of elemental iron may lead to moderate or serious toxicity in which of the following situations?
A. Ingestion of 17 mg/kg of elemental iron by an 18-month-old child
B. Ingestion of 6 tablets of ferrous sulfate (325 mg each) by a 30-lb toddler
C. Ingestion of 935 mg of elemental iron by a 49-kg male
D. None of the above

120
Fever of Unknown Origin

Select the appropriate letter that correctly answers the question or completes the statement.

1. All the following statements are true *except*:
   A. Febrile infants less than 60 days old have a low incidence of occult bactermia (less than 5%).
   B. Most febrile infants less than 60 days old have no identifiable source of infection.
   C. Patients with temperatures over 41.1°C have a 50% rate of bacteremia.
   D. Bacteremia may occur in infants less than 2 months of age in the absence of fever.

2. Which of the following laboratory results is most indicative of serious bacterial infection?
   A. The presence of band cells
   B. C-reactive protein less than 10 mg/l
   C. Erythrocyte sedimentation rate greater than 25 mm/hour
   D. WBC count greater than 10,000/mm^3

121
Acute Bacterial Meningitis

Select the appropriate letter that correctly answers the question or completes the statement.

1. Organisms commonly seen in meningitis in older infants (2 months to 1 year) include all of the following *except*:
   A. *Hemophilus influenzae* type B
   B. *Escherichia coli*
   C. *Streptococcus pneumoniae*
   D. *Neisseria meningitidis*

2. Family members and intimate contacts of a child with meningococcal disease should receive which of the following medications?
   A. Ampicillin
   B. Rifampin
   C. Chloramphenicol
   D. None of the above

3. It would generally be agreed that a lumbar puncture is mandatory in which of the following instances?
   A. A 3-year-old who is febrile had a brief generalized seizure, but now appears well and who has an otitis media
   B. A 2-year-old with mumps parotitis who has mild

nuchal rigidity, but who otherwise appears well and has no alteration of his sensorium
   C. A 6-year-old who is febrile, has mild nuchal rigidity, otitis media, and presently appears ill
   D. All of the above

4. Appropriate antibiotic therapy for meningitis in a newborn is:
   A. Nafcillin and chloramphenicol
   B. Ampicillin and chloramphenicol
   C. Nafcillin and gentamicin
   D. Ampicillin and gentamicin

5. Appropriate antibiotic therapy for meningitis in a child over 2 months of age is:
   A. Nafcillin and chloramphenicol
   B. Ampicillin and chloramphenicol
   C. Nafcillin and gentamicin
   D. Ampicillin and gentamicin

6. Following a diagnosis of meningitis, a patient who is in impending shock with new onset seizure activity should receive what anticonvulsant regimen?
   A. No anticonvulsant
   B. IM diazepam 0.2 mg/kg
   C. IV diazepam 0.1 mg/kg
   D. IV phenobarbital 50 mg/kg
   E. IV diazepam 0.2 mg/kg followed by diphenylhydantoin

7. Further definitive resuscitation in a patient with meningitis and shock who is unresponsive to initial rehydration attempts should include:
   A. Whole blood infusion type-specific
   B. IV vasopressor agents
   C. Plasmanate volume expander
   D. Apply MAST trousers
   E. Lumbar puncture to therapeutically reduce increased intracranial pressure causing the shock-like state

122
Ear Infections

Select the appropriate letter that correctly answers the question or completes the statement.

1. Which is the most common pathogen resulting in otitis media in all pediatric age groups?
   A. *Staphylococcus aureus*
   B. Group A beta hemolytic *Streptococcus*
   C. *Streptococcus pneumoniae*
   D. *Hemophilus influenzae*

2. Gram-negative enteric pathogens may cause otitis media in which age group?
   A. Newborn   C. 6-month-old
   B. 2-month-old   D. 1-year-old

3. The most reliable criterion for acute suppurative otitis media is:
   A. Bulging tympanic membranes
   B. Hyperemic tympanic membranes
   C. Exquisite tenderness to otoscopic examination
   D. Fluid from the external auditory canal
   E. History of chronic suppurative otitis media
4. All of the following are indications for tympanocentesis *except*:
   A. Otitis media in the ill newborn
   B. Recurrent otitis within 2 weeks
   C. Chronic treatment failure of 20 days antibiotics
   D. Otitis in a child with leukemia
   E. Pyrexia and otalgia persisting despite 2 days treatment with antipyretic and antibiotic
5. All the following are common causes of acute suppurative otitis media *except*:
   A. *Streptococcus pyogenes*
   B. *Streptococcus pneumoniae*
   C. *Hemophilus influenzae*
   D. *Pseudomonas aeruginosa*
   E. *Neisseria catarrhalis*

123
Croup and Epiglottis

Select the appropriate letter that correctly answers the question or completes the statement.
1. Fever may be seen with all of the following *except*:
   A. Croup
   B. Botulism
   C. Epiglottitis
   D. Ludwig's angina
2. Home management of croup is advocated with the use of:
   A. Oral ampicillin
   B. Rectal chloralhydrate
   C. Humidified air
   D. Oral steroids
   E. Epinephrine inhaler (Primatene)
3. In which age group does epiglottitis typically occur?
   A. 3 to 7 months   D. 1 to 2 months
   B. 3 to 7 years   E. Birth to 1 year
   C. 1 to 2 years
4. Croup is characterized by:
   A. Barky cough
   B. Prostration, toxic appearance
   C. *Hemophilus influenzae* type B
   D. All of the above
   E. *A* and *B*
5. When endotracheal intubation is not readily available, acceptable initial therapy for suspected worsening of epiglottitis in an infant includes:
   A. Cricothyroidotomy
   B. Immediate IV establishment
   C. Bag-mask ventilation
   D. Stat cross table soft tissue x-ray
   E. Blind endotracheal intubation
6. Which radiologic feature is characteristic of laryngotracheobronchitis (croup) on an AP soft tissue radiograph of the neck?
   A. Aryepiglottic edema
   B. "Steeple" or "pencil" sign
   C. Distended hypopharyngeal airspace
   D. Obliteration of laryngeal ventricles
   E. Tonsillar hypertrophy

124
Asthma and Bronchiolitis

Select the appropriate letter that correctly answers the question or completes the statement.
1. Which one of the following statements is true regarding asthma?
   A. Isoetharine is a long-acting bronchodilator relative to metaproterenol.
   B. Older children with a peak expiration flow rate (PEFR) of greater than 65% of the predicted value may be discharged even if still wheezing.
   C. Isoetharine should be administered prior to discharge.
   D. The pCO_2 is often normal during acute asthma attacks.
2. Which one of the following complications might be anticipated in an asthmatic who is experiencing his or her first attack?
   A. Tension pneumothorax
   B. Pneumomediastinum
   C. Ventilatary failure
   D. Adrenal suppression
3. Which one of the following statements is incorrect regarding asthma?
   A. Patients with $PaCO_2$ over 40 or PaO_2 under 70 with oxygen are candidates for Intensive Care Unit admission.
   B. The diagnosis of bronchiolitis is generally reserved for patients less than 1 year of age.
   C. Bronchiolitis rarely responds to epinephrine.
   D. Pneumomediastinum may occur in 5% of asthmatics.

125
Pneumonia

Select the appropriate letter that correctly answers the question or completes the statement.

1. A mother brings her 2 1/2-year-old daughter to the emergency room with a cold. She states this is the fifth cold in the last year or so and that the child had pneumonia last year. You should advise:
   A. That is normal for a child less than 5 years old.
   B. Her daughter needs a work-up for cystic fibrosis.
   C. The history suggests a primary immune deficiency that needs further evaluation.
   D. This is too many colds for a child this age, but only close observation and no work-up are required.
2. The following are all likely symptoms of pneumonia in a neonate *except*:
   A. Decreased muscle tone
   B. Productive cough
   C. Anorexia
   D. Tachypnea
3. All health care workers involved in the initial assessment of the child with pneumonia should rapidly identify:
   A. Patient wit underlying debilitating illness
   B. Patient with compromised host defenses
   C. Patient with respiratory distress and/or impending respiratory failure
   D. All of the above
4. After evaluating a 3-year-old you feel he has an uncomplicated viral pneumonia. You should:
   A. Admit child for observation
   B. Prescribe PO penicillin to prevent superinfection with pneumococcus
   C. Instruct parents on supportive measures they can take at home, then discharge patient
   D. Give one shot of a long-acting penicillin and discharge
5. A 6-week-old infant with protracted pneumonia and staccato cough has symptoms characteristic of which etiologic agent?
   A. *Chlamydia trachomatis*
   B. *Herpesvirus hominus*
   C. *Bordetella pertussis*
   D. *Mycoplasma pneumoniae*
   E. *Streptococcus pneumoniae*
6. All of the following maneuvers are indicated to facilitate pulmonary clearing in a seriously ill child with pneumonia *except*:
   A. Segmental postural drainage
   B. Mechanical ventilation
   C. Bronchodilator therapy
   D. Nonnarcotic antitussive (i.e., dextromethorphan)
   E. Needle aspiration of empyema
7. An uncomplicated bacterial pneumonia in a 5-year-old is *best* treated initially as an outpatient with:
   A. Procaine penicillin 25,000 U/kg IM
   B. Tetracycline 50 mg/kg PO
   C. Erythromycin 40 mg/kg PO
   D. Ampicillin 40 mg/kg PO
   E. Amoxicillin 20 mg/kg PO

126
Diarrheal Disease

Select the appropriate letter that correctly answers the question or completes the statement.

1. A distinguishing characteristic of *Yersinia enteritis* from the other types of bacterial gastroenteritis is:
   A. The abrupt onset of diarrhea
   B. More common in the winter months
   C. Usually greenish colored stools
   D. Self-limited
   E. Associated with crampy abdominal pain
2. Which of the following is *not* characteristic of *Shigella* enteritis?
   A. Abrupt onset of diarrhea
   B. Vomiting
   C. Soaring fever
   D. Crampy abdominal pain
3. After taking an appropriate history including diet, recent travel, and drug exposure, you decide that a patient most likely has *Salmonella* enteritis. Which of the following is consistent with this?
   A. Abrupt onset of diarrhea, high fever, paucity of vomiting
   B. Sporadic epidemics in early infancy, high volume of watery fecal-smelling stool
   C. Transient fever, protracted vomiting, loose stools with mucus
   D. Self-limited disease lasting 3 days, abrupt onset, slimy green malodorous stool with blood, no fever
4. Which pathogen would a child with diarrhea most likely have in the winter months?
   A. Rotovirus
   B. *Yersinia*
   C. *Shigella* and *Salmonella*
   D. *E. coli*
5. All of the following are true of *Shigella* enteritis *except*:
   A. Antibiotics can decrease the amount of diarrhea in enteritis but do not alter the duration of infectivity.

B. Appropriate antibiotics for treatment of extraintestinal disease associated with enteritis may be life-saving.

C. A definitive diagnosis can be made by isolation of the organism from stool or blood.

D. It is appropriate to try to isolate a specific pathogen in enteritis.

Match the items on the right with their associated items on the left.

  _C_   6. *Campylobacter*
  _B_   7. *Shigella*
  _A_   8. Enteropatho-
            genic *E. coli*

A. Bismuth sub-salicylate
B. Trimethoprim plus sulfame-thoxazole
C. Erythromycin

127

Cardiac Disease in Children

Select the appropriate letter that correctly answers the question or completes the statement.

1. Midface hypoplasia, short palpebral fissure, and ventricular septal defect are all components of which clinical syndrome?
   A. Fetal hydantoin syndrome
   B. Down's syndrome (trisomy 21)
   C. Fetal alcohol syndrome
   D. Congenital rubella

2. Cyanosis is a component of all but one of the following congenital cardiac anomalies. Which one?
   A. Coarctation of the aorta
   B. Tetralogy of Fallot
   C. Transposition of the great vessels
   D. Ebstein's anomaly

3. Which of the following findings is most indicative of significant cardiac disease?
   A. Central cyanosis
   B. Congestive heart failure
   C. Associated dysmorphic features
   D. Failure to thrive

4. Which one of the following congenital cardiac diseases are characterized by obstruction of right ventricular outflow tract, dextroposition of the aorta, right ventricular hypertrophy, and ventricular septal defect?
   A. Tetralogy of Fallat
   B. Ebstein's anomaly
   C. Truncus arteriosus
   D. Eisenmenger's syndrome

128

Child Abuse

Select the appropriate letter that correctly answers the question or completes the statement.

1. Which one of the following statements regarding child abuse is *not* true?
   A. 50% of fractures in children under 1 year of age are due to child abuse.
   B. Subdural hematomas in infants under 15 months of age may be due to shaken baby syndrome.
   C. Homicide accounts for less than 1 in 100 deaths in children younger than 18 years of age.
   D. Polle's syndrome is characterized by parental inducement of the child's illness or parental fabrication (Munchausen's syndrome by proxy).

2. Which of the following statements is true?
   A. 1–2% of all childhood injuries seen in the emergency department are due to child abuse.
   B. 25% of women and 10% of men have been victimized by childhood sexual abuse.
   C. Exsanguination is the most common cause of death from child abuse.
   D. Childhood sexual abuse victims rarely require prophylactic antibiotics.

Comprehensive Review

Select the appropriate letter that correctly answers the question or completes the statement.

1. A 35-year-old trauma patient presents with tachycardia, normal blood pressure, a narrowed pulse pressure, and cool moist skin. Which of the following is the most accurate conclusion?
   A. He has lost 25% of his blood volume.
   B. He has lost greater than 25% of his blood volume.
   C. He has lost 15% of his blood volume.
   D. He has lost up to 25% of his blood volume.
   E. He has lost up to 40% of his blood volume.

2. All of the following could be attempted in an 8-kg infant in which peripheral IV access has been unsuccessful *except*:
   A. Intraosseous line
   B. Subclavian line
   C. Venous cutdown
   D. External jugular line

3. A patient's response to acute blood loss includes a neuroendocrine reflex mediated by baroreceptors in the heart and great vessels. Which of the following best characterizes this process?
   A. A drop in the mean blood pressure stimulates the parasympathetic pathways.
   B. Epinephrine is released from nerve endings in the heart and great vessels.
   C. Norepinephrine and epinephrine are both released from nerve endings in the heart and great vessels.
   D. Epinephrine is secreted from the adrenal medulla.

4. Which of the following leaves its stinger at the site of injury?
   A. Honey bee   C. Wasp
   B. Fire out   D. Hornet

5. Posterior epistaxis is uncommon in the pediatric population. When encountered it is easily treated and once stopped requires no further investigation. True or False? Provide explanation to substantiate.
   A. True
   B. False

6. A 24-year-old male presents to the emergency department with history of stab wound to the left neck. EMT's state initial vitals are stable although he is oozing blood even with direct pressure. In the department he suddenly develops tachypnea, tachycardia, and hypotension with equal breath sounds bilaterally. You should:
   A. Perform needle thoracentesis on the left since he is exhibiting a tension pneumothorax
   B. Consult a surgeon since he is more than likely exsanguinating
   C. Place him in the left lateral decubitus position and Trendelenburg

D. Start two more large-bore IV's (total of 4), making sure he has venous access contralateral to the injury

7. In a victim of high speed trauma whose chest x-ray is suggestive of widened superior mediastinum, which is the most reliable indication for aortography?
   A. Fractured first or second rib
   B. Pneumomediastinum
   C. Obscure aortic knob
   D. Left hemothorax

8. A 22-year-old 37-week pregnant female falls off a first story balcony sustaining a right femur and right pelvis fracture. The fetus remained stable and was delivered by normal vaginal delivery. At the time of delivery, what is the most commonly noted injury sustained by the fetus from the accident?
   A. Mental retardation
   B. Kidney damage
   C. Pelvis fractures
   D. Skull fractures
   E. Fetal death

9. Which of the following factors is most contributory to bladder injury in blunt trauma?
   A. Carcinoma of the bladder
   B. Full bladder
   C. Pregnancy
   D. Pelvic fracture

Match the items on the left with the appropriate items on the right.
   _____10. Hydrogen Sulfide   A. Bitter almonds
   _____11. Nitrogen Oxide   B. Rotten eggs
   _____12. Hydrogen cyanide   C. Red-brown gas

Select the appropriate letter that correctly answers the question or completes the statement.

13. A 37-year-old male presents 12 hours after he woke up to find his hands swollen, red, and covered with huge blisters but he is able to move the fingers. Apparently he was drunk and was crawling on his hands looking for his car keys which he dropped (it was 10°F outside.) Which of the following best classifies the severity of the cold injury?
   A. 1st degree
   B. 2nd degree
   C. 3rd degree
   D. 4th degree
   E. You cannot tell for sure

14. A 5-day-old black male is brought to the emergency department by his mother on a warm summer day because of a cough and "not feeling well." He is listless and his rectal temperature is 34.1°C. The disease process that should be ruled out first in this setting is:
   A. Hypopituitarism
   B. Septicemia

C. Intracranial hemorrhage

D. Hypothyroidism

E. Hypoadrenalism

15. Which of the following drugs has been found useful in reversing neurotransmitter blockage in treating delirium?

A. Physostigmine
D. Scopalamine

B. Tripelenamine
E. Amantadine

C. Homatropine

16. A 37-year-old male presents to the emergency department drowsy and somnolent brought in by a concerned friend. There was an empty pill bottle beside the couch where he was sleeping. He has been seeing a psychiatrist but the friend does not know whether he was on any medication. The patient is not cooperative and it is questionable whether his information would be reliable. Vitals are stable but he continues to doze off and does not have gag reflex. Which of the following approaches would be most reasonable?

A. Ipecac emesis, 50–100 g charcoal, and a cathartic

B. Ipecac emesis and a cathartic

C. Gastric lavage, 50–100 g charcoal, and a cathartic

D. Nasotracheal intubation then as in C above

17. Which of the following is generally *not* associated with the clinical presentation of glutethimede overdose?

A. Potential for development of cerebral edema and increased intracranial pressure

B. Anticholinergic symptoms

C. Prolonged and cyclic coma

D. Flaccid muscle tone and hyporeflexia

E. Pinpoint, unreactive pupils

18. A 30-year-old male drug addict with multiple needle tracks is brought to the emergency department comatose, with shallow respirations, miosis, and pink frothy sputum. Initial management should be performed in which of the following sequences?

A. Naloxone 0.4 mg, intubate and ventilate, administer 25 g glucose IV

B. Intubate and ventilate, administer 25 g glucose IV, naloxone 0.4 mg IV

C. Intubate and ventilate, naloxone 0.4 mg IV, Lasix 20 mg IV

D. Naloxone 0.4 mg IV, intubate and ventilate, Lasix 20 mg IV

E. Intubate and ventilate, administer 25 g glucose IV, naloxone 4 mg IV

19. What is the toxic ingredient in oil of wintergreen?

A. Naphthol

B. Methyl salicylate

C. Methyl alcohol

D. Codeine

20. A 14-year-old male presents with a 4 cm contaminated laceration of his hand. You are concerned because he has dirty soil within the wound. On questioning his immune status you find he has received only two previous tetanus immunizations. He should receive the following from you:

A. 0.5 ml dT only

B. 0.5 ml dT plus 250 units of Hyper-Tet

C. 250 units of Hyper-Tet only

D. 0.5 ml dT plus prophylactic antibiotics to cover clostridia

21. Cribriform plate fracture can be manifested clinically as:

A. CSF rhinorrhea
C. Septal hematoma

B. Enophthalmos
D. Malocclusion

22. Which of the following medications can be used to treat SIADH?

A. Acetazolamide
C. Tetracycline

B. Lasix
D. Demeclocycline

23. A 71-year-old man comes to the emergency department feeling "run down" but without chest pain or shortness of breath. His blood pressure is 146/97, pulse is 59, and respirations are 15. EKG shows first degree heart block, flattened T waves, and slight QT prolongation. He cannot remember what medications he is on. Which of the following electrolyte abnormalities are most likely in this patient?

A. Hypokalemia
C. Hyponatremia

B. Hyperkalemia
D. Hypercalcemia

24. A patient has muscle cramps, irritability, and positive Chvostek's and Trousseau's signs. You are highly suspicious of hypocalcemia, but what other deficiency can clinically mimic hypocalcemia?

A. K+
D. Mg++

B. HCO_3
E. Fe++

C. Phosphate

25. A 12-month-old male has had a lower fever, mild diarrhea, and fussiness for 5 days. Up to now, the mother had thought these were a result of the unusually hot summer. The infant appears lethargic and dehydrated. Temperature is 100.5°F rectally with a Na+ 160. IV fluids are initially given quickly as a fever work-up is in progress. This work-up (minus a lumbar puncture) is fruitless. After a 5-hour delay the patient is finally admitted but suffers a brief seizure while leaving the department. Your main concern is:

A. Immediate lumbar puncture

B. Cerebral edema

C. Febrile seizure

D. Occult head trauma from child abuse

26. A 75-year-old lady presents with a 1-day history of crampy abdominal pain associated with nausea and some diarrhea. She has a history of congestive heart failure that is treated with Digitalis and Lasix. She has no other medical problems. She is in mild distress with a temperature of 100.5°F, pulse of 112, blood pressure of 110/60. The abdomen shows diffuse tenderness without guarding or rebound. Stool is 3+ hemotest postive. The bowel sounds are slightly decreased. The most likely radiographic finding would be:
    A. Free air beneath the diaphragm
    B. Distention of the small bowel with multiple air fluid levels
    C. Calcification in the epigastric area
    D. Gas in the bowel wall
    E. Blurring of the psoas shadows bilaterally

27. Currant jelly stools due to mucosal hemorrhage and increased mucous production is typical of which entity?
    A. Regional enteritis
    B. Intussusception
    C. Sigmoid volvulus
    D. Salmonellosis
    E. Large bowel obstruction

28. The radiographic finding of gas in the bowel wall would be highly suggestive of:
    A. Ulcerative colitis
    B. Regional enteritis
    C. Amebic abscess
    D. Mesenteric vascular occlusion
    E. Intussusception

29. A previously healthy 8-month-old presents with a sudden onset of abdominal pain associated with one episode of vomiting. The parents relate that the child seemed okay for 15 minutes then had another attack of pain. He had a normal physical exam. The most likely diagnosis is:
    A. Intussusception
    B. Pyloric stenosis
    C. Sigmoid volvulus
    D. Incarcerated hernia
    E. Hirschsprung's disease

30. All of the following are true of an amebic abscess of the liver *except*:
    A. Increased incidence in the homosexual population
    B. History of diarrhea
    C. Trophzoites found in the stool
    D. X-ray and laboratory results are similar to a pyrogenic abscess
    E. Amebic hepatitis may precede abscess formation

31. A 32-year-old woman presents with a sudden onset of abdominal pain with nausea and vomiting. She had a similar episode 3 months ago and was told that her amylase was high. There is no history of alcohol use or any other medications. Physical examination shows temperature 100°F, pulse 110, and blood pressure 110/75. She has diffuse tenderness over the abdomen with decreased bowel sounds. Amylase is now 1,200. WBC count is 11,500. Management of this patient should include IV fluids, nasogastric suction, and analgesics along with:
    A. Early endoscopy
    B. Antibiotics IV
    C. Exploratory laparotomy
    D. IV cimetidine
    E. Ultrasound of the abdomen

32. The amylase:creatinine clearance ratio is elevated greater than 5 in all of the following *except*:
    A. Burns
    B. Diabetic ketoacidosis
    C. Acute pancreatitis
    D. Chronic pancreatitis
    E. Macroamylasemia

33. Alpha-fetoprotein would be expected to be elevated in:
    A. Hepatoma
    B. Inflammatory bowel disease
    C. Pancreatic carcinoma
    D. Peptic ulcer disease
    E. Hepatitis B

34. All of the following are causes of hyperacute T waves on the electrocardiogram that can mimic acute myocardial ischemia *except*:
    A. Idiopathic hypertrophic subaortic stenosis
    B. Hyperkalemia
    C. Subarachnoid hemorrhage
    D. Left bundle branch block
    E. All of the above

35. A 35-year-old male comes to the emergency department complaining of a several day history of increasing nausea without abdominal pain. He has recently been diagnosed as having a peptic ulcer by an upper GI series and started on cimetadine with initial improvement clinically. He persists in drinking one six-pack of beer per day as well as smoking two packs of cigarettes per day. He is a well-controlled asthmatic on long-term theophylline. The best diagnostic test now would be:
    A. Stool for occult blood
    B. Gastric endoscopy
    C. Theophylline level
    D. Serum amylase
    E. Ultrasound of gallbladder

36. Kerley B lines seen on a chest X-ray are indicative of:
    A. Pulmonary embolus
    B. Aspiration
    C. Pulmonary contusion
    D. Congenital heart disease
    E. Congestive heart failure

37. A 18-year-old male is brought to the emergency department after an accidental overdose of heroin. He is comatose with pinpoint pupils and a respiratory rate of 5. Which are the most likely blood gases on this patient while breathing room air?
   A. Po_2 85, $PcoO_2$ 35, pH 7.32
   B. Po_2 70, Pco_2 58, pH 7.28
   C. Po_2 40, Pco_2 40, pH 7.4
   D. Po_2 50, Pco_2 55, pH 7.37
   E. Po_2 55, Pco_2 52, pH 7.41

38. A 40-year-old female is brought to the emergency department with a complaint of syncope and left-sided chest pain. On physical examination, a low-pitched, rasping, diamond-shaped systolic murmur is heard at the second right intercostal space. 12 lead EKG reveals no acute changes. What is your initial impression?
   1. Rule out acute myocardial infarction
   2. Could represent mitral valve prolapse
   3. Aortic stenosis
   4. Mitral stenosis
   A. 1, 2, and 3
   B. 1 and 4
   C. 1 only
   D. 3 only
   E. 2, 3, and 4

39. Electrical alternans with 1 to 1 total atrial/ventricular complexes is pathognomonic of which condition?
   A. Pulmonary emboli
   B. Atrial septal defect
   C. Cardiac tamponade
   D. Sick sinus syndrome
   E. Hyperkalemia

40. A previously healthy 25-year-old black female presents with a several day history of generalized malaise, fever, and headache. Her family says she "hasn't been acting right." As you enter the room to see the patient, she has a generalized grand mal seizure followed by a postictal period. Her vital signs are temperature 102.4°F, pulse 115, and blood pressure 140/108. Heent: Pupils are equal and reactive, fundi, and benign. Neck: supple; chest: clear to auscultation and percussion; cardia: regular rhythm without murmurs; abdomen: decreased bowel sounds without tenderness or masses; and extremities: a diffuse petechial rash greatest over the forearms. Laboratory data are as follows: WBC count: 15,800; H/H: 10/22; platelets: 40,000; sodium: 135; potassium: 4.4; chloride: 102; HCO_3: 10; BUN: 55; and creatinine: 3.5. Review of the smear shows multiple fragments. This disease process is most likely to be:
   A. Thrombotic thrombocytopenia purpura
   B. Diffuse intravascular coagulation
   C. Idiopathic thrombocytopenia purpura
   D. Massive overdose of heroin

   E. None of the above

41. A 26-year-old white female collapses in a supermarket. She has previously been in good health. Vital signs are pulse 130, blood pressure 60/0, respirations 24. The most likely cause of this patient's condition is:
   A. Bleeding peptic ulcer
   B. Ruptured ectopic pregnancy
   C. Rupture of congenital aneurysm
   D. Massive pulmonary emboli
   E. Mitral valve prolapse with rupture of mitral valve leaflets

42. A 54-year-old woman complains of abdominal pain nausea, and vomiting without diarrhea. She has a history of frequent urinary tract infections as well as increased blood pressure. She had a total abdominal hysterectomy 10 years ago. Her x-ray film is shown in Figure 1. The most likely diagnosis at this point would be:
   A. Perforated ulcer
   B. Pancreatitis
   C. Small bowel obstruction
   D. Nephrolithiasis
   E. Regional enteritis

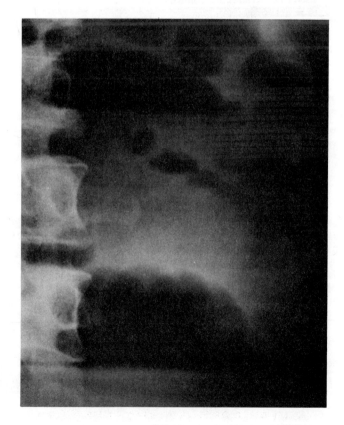

Fig. 1.

Match the blood gas measurements on the right with their associated items on the left.

_____43. A previously heal-
thy 50-year-old
who sustains a pul-
monary embolism
after routine
surgery

	pH	P_{CO_2}	P_{O_2}
A.	7.47	32	78
B.	7.38	44	60
C.	7.39	60	55
D.	7.45	26	50
E.	7.30	55	55

_____44. A 26-year-old
with a severe
asthma attack
lasting 24 hours
who is diaphor-
etic and using
accessory muscles
of respiration

_____45. A patient with
severe chronic
bronchitis who is
currently at his
baseline level
of function

_____46. A patient with
chronic bronchitis
who is in acute
decompensation
from an upper
respiratory tract
infection

_____47. A previously
healthy young
patient with
marked respiratory
distress after
severe gastric
aspiration

Select the appropriate letter that correctly answers the question or completes the statement.

48. A 65-year-old man is transported to the ED after complaining of a headache followed by a seizure. He has a history of hypertension and adult onset diabetes mellitus, as well as a smoking history of 1 pack per day. His medications include Aldomet, hydrochlorothiazide, and chloropropamide. Vital signs are blood pressure 300/170, pulse 130, and temperature 100°F. He is postictal, beginning to arouse. Pupils are equal, and fundi are not seen well. The neck is supple, and he moves the left side more than the right. The breath sounds are equal with clear lung fields. The best initial step in managing this patient would be:
   A. CT scan
   B. Lumbar puncture
   C. Nitroprusside
   D. $D_{50}W$

E. Intubation

49. A 50-year-old chronic alcoholic with a sudden onset of chest and abdominal pain after vomiting blood-tinged material is seen in the ED. He is in moderate distress, clammy, with a blood pressure of 90/60, and a pulse of 125. He is diaphoretic with some left upper quadrant tenderness but no guarding or rebound. Chest x-ray film shows a small left pleural effusion. The most likely diagnosis is:
   A. Boerhaave's syndrome
   B. Mallory-Weiss tear
   C. Aspiration of vomitus
   D. Hemorrhagic gastritis with perforation
   E. Acute pancreatitis

50. A 2-month-old boy with projectile vomiting of 2 days duration is seen in the ED. He is afebrile and does not appear dehydrated. The parents are unsure about his last stool. Physical examination reveals a small, nontender mass palpable in the epigastrium. The most likely diagnosis is:
   A. Intussusception
   B. Pyloric stenosis
   C. Gastric volvulus
   D. Congenital biliary atresia
   E. Gastric bezoar

51. What is the most common cause of the abnormality shown in the x-ray film in Figure 2?
   A. Peptic ulcer disease
   B. Abdominal ulcer disease
   C. Cholecystitis
   D. Inflammatory bowel disease
   E. Mesenteric vascular occlusion

52. A 30-year-old woman comes to the ED complaining of a sudden onset of epigastric and right upper quadrant abdominal pain. She has some nausea but no vomiting or diarrhea. She is taking a "fluid pill" for blood pressure and uses aspirin 2 to 3 times a week for headaches. She has been taking oral contraceptives for 8 years. Her pulse is 120 and blood pressure is 80/60. There is tenderness over the epigastrium and right upper quadrant without guarding or rebound, and the bowel sounds are diminished. Pelvic examiniation reveals no abnormalities. Stool hemotest is negative, hemoglobin is 9, WBC is 12,400, and amylase is normal. The most likely diagnosis is:
   A. Erosive gastritis
   B. Acute pancreatitis
   C. Ruptured ectopic pregnancy
   D. Acute appendicitis
   E. Ruptured liver cell adenoma

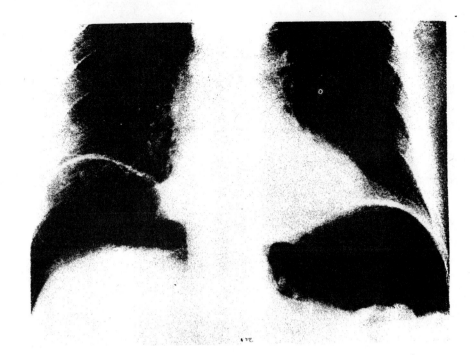

Fig. 2.

53. A patient is admitted to the cardiac care unit after a myocardial infarction. A Swan-Ganz catheter is inserted, and initally the wedge pressure is 12 with a pulmonary artery diastolic pressure of 12 also. The nurse calls you to see the patient because his pulmonary artery diastolic pressure is now 20, while his wedge pressure remains at 12. The most likely reason for this acute elevation of pulmonary artery diastolic pressure is:

A. Equipment malfunction
B. Papillary muscle rupture
C. Decreased ventricular compliance
D. Pulmonary emboli
E. Development of ventricular aneurysm

Match the items on the right with their associated items on the left. Each answer may be used once, more than once, or not at all.

____ 54. Hyperthyroidism
____ 55. Constrictive pericarditis
____ 56. Wolff-Parkinson-White syndrome
____ 57. Idiopathic hypertrophic subaortic stenosis
____ 58. Prolapsing mitral valve

A. Atrial fibrillation unresponsive to usual medication
B. Congestive heart failure with a small heart on x-ray film
C. A young woman with atypical chest pain and palpitations
D. The most common cause of sudden death in young athletes
E. Wide QRS on sinus rhythm with a narrow QRS while in supraventricular tachycardia

ANSWERS

1

Introduction

No questions.

2

Life and Death

No questions.

3

Approach to Patient in Emergency

No questions.

Because Chapters 1, 2, and 3 are of a general nature, no questions were prepared for this material. To assist your review and make it easier to obtain additional information on any topic, the chapter numbers of this book correspond to the chapter numbers in *Emergency Medicine: Concepts and Clinical Practice*, edited by Rosen, Baker, Braen, Dailey, and Levy. Also, the correct answer and rationale for each question includes the page number from the 2-volume text for further consulation.

4
Airway Management

1. **C**, Page 43.
   All of the drugs except sodium bicarbonate may be given through the endotracheal tube, in addition to steroids, naloxone, and isoetharine (Bronkosol). Sodium bicarbonate, levarterenol, and calcium preparations are contraindicated because of the large volume required and theoretical possibility of surfactant inactivation, atelectasis, or tissue necrosis occurring.
2. **A**, Page 46.
   The cricoid cartilage ring is the narrowest segment of the infant airway (the glottic aperture is the narrowest in the adult), increasing the risks of obstruction from subglottic stenosis, scarring, granuloma formation, and ulceration. Cuffed tubes should not be used in children under 12 years old.
3. **B**, Pages 60–61.
   The use of the EOA places stress on the cervical spine. At present there is no evidence that the device is safe in the setting of potential or confirmed cervical spine trauma, especially if these patients are not in full respiratory arrest. Consequently, the EOA should not at present be considered an adequate airway device for the trauma patient.
4. **A**, Pages 63–64.
   Tracheostomy is a relatively difficult procedure even under ideal conditions and should not be used in the setting of emergency airway intervention. Exceptions to this rule are the infant who cannot be intubated (when cricothrotomy is not recommended because of the small cricothyroid space and narrowest luminal diameter being at the level of the pediatric cricoid), severe laryngotracheal trauma with loss of landmarks, or tracheal transection in which the distal trachea retracts into the mediastinum. Cricothyrotomy would be the emergency procedure of choice in the other patients.

5
Intubation and Muscle Relaxation

1. **D**, Page 73.
   Blind nasotracheal intubation is indicated when direct laryngoscopy is difficult or impossible, cervical spine integrity is in question, or possible long-term ventilation is anticipated. The procedure is contraindicated if there is a coagulopathy or anticoagulation, basilar skull fracture involving the cribiform plate, nasal obstruction, upper airway obstruction or friable tumor, acute epiglottitis, or upper airway foreign body. Advantages over orotracheal intubation include reduced cervical spine manipulation, better toleration by an awake patient, less depression of swallowing mechanism, better tube fixation; fewer oropharyngeal secretions, and less kinking. The main disadvantage is its failure rate, which ranges from 5–20%.
2. **D**, Pages 69–73.
   Endotracheal intubation is indicated to protect the airway from obstruction or aspiration, or to treat respiratory failure and hypoventilation. A curved laryngoscope blade (MacIntosh) is inserted into the voleculla while a straight blade (Magill) is inserted under the epiglottis. Bacteremia occurs transiently in 16% of patients intubated nasotracheally. High residual volume endotracheal tube cuffs (low-pressure) are actually more preferable than high-pressure, low residual volume cuffs because of less tracheal ischemia and reduced aspiration with low-pressure cuffs.
3. **C**, Page 74.
   A term newborn requires a 3.5-mm internal diameter tube. A premature infant requires a 2.5-mm tube. Required tube size may be estimated by the following formula:

$$\frac{\text{age in years} + 16}{4} = \frac{\text{tube size}}{\text{internal diameter}}$$

or

$$\frac{\text{age in years} + 4}{4} = \frac{\text{tube size}}{\text{internal diameter}}$$

4. **A**, Pages 74–77.
   The three parameters listed in A indicate that extubation should be successful. The patient should be awake and free of sedation when extubated. While Sellick's maneuver has been used to prevent aspiration, it is contraindicated if the patient is actively vomiting because of the risk of esophageal rupture. Premedication with lidocaine is often used but has not been shown to blunt the cardiovascular response to endotracheal intubation.
5. **E**, Pages 77–81.
   Succinylcholine is a depolarizing neuromuscular blocking agent that may cause hyperkalemia transiently, but especially in patients with severe burns, massive trauma, sepsis, head injury, or motor neurologic deficit. Vercuronium bromide, atracurium besylate, pancuronium bromide, and d-tubocurare are all nondepolarizing agents and have a reduced effect on serum potassium.

6
Cardiac Arrest

1. **B**, Page 86.
   Usually only 4 to 10 minutes elapse between cardiac arrest and brain death. With CPR this time constraint may be extended to 12 to 16 minutes. The other statements are correct.
2. **C**, Page 91.
   The jaw thrust requires the least amount of cervical hyperextension and is the safest maneuver in a patient with suspected neck injury.
3. **D**, Pages 102–104.
   The initial treatment of monitored ventricular fibrillation is defibrillation with 200 W-sec. If unsuccessful, a repeat defibrillation at 200 W-sec should be performed.
4. **A**, Pages 104–106.
   Epinephrine, oxygen, and bicarbonate should be given for persistent ventricular fibrillation. Lidocaine is given as indicated. Atropine is not indicated.
5. **B**, Page 109.
   Excess sodium bicarbonate causes CSF acidosis, increased hemoglobin binding of oxygen, hypokalemia, and hyperosmolality.
6. **C**, Pages 84–85.
   Calcium chloride is the drug of choice. Calcium gluconate requires metabolism to ionic form. Glucose and insulin work more slowly and epinephrine and bicarbonate are used for cardiac arrest alone.
7. **C**, Page 115.
   Isoproterenol is a weak vasoconstrictor. The three other statements are true.
8. **A**, Pages 115–116.
   Dopamine causes renal, mesenteric, coronary, and cerebral vasodilation at doses of 1 to 10 µg/kg/min. At 10 to 20 µg/kg/min it exerts both alpha and beta effects, whereas at doses over 20 µg/kg/min its effects are predominantly alpha. Norepinephrine increases both preload and afterload, thereby increasing myocardial oxygen demand. Methoxamine is almost exclusively an alpha agonist.
9. **C**, Pages 116–118.
   All but procainamide, which has unpredictable effects, are indicated in digitalis toxicity. Bretylium is generally contraindicated in digitalis toxic arrythmias, but it has been used successfully after other agents have failed. Dilantin is considered the drug of choice for digitalis toxicity.
10. **D**, Page 119.
    Electromechanical dissociation is not an indication for pacing. The other arrhythmias may not be amenable to pacing.
11. **B**, Pages 120–121.
    A patient who is pulseless after penetrating trauma should undergo immediate thoracotomy for hemostasis as well as open chest massage. Intubation should be carried out first.
12. **A**, Page 124.
    Appropriate size ET tube for a 4-year-old is 5.0 to 5.5. A formula for ascertaining tube size requirement is: (age + 16)/4 = tube size (in mm).

7
Brain Resuscitation

1. **C**, Pages 147–148.
   The cerebral blood flow obtained when CPR is initiated is inversely proportional to preceding arrest time. Fifty percent of normal cerebral blood flow can be obtained when CPR is initiated within 2 minutes of ventricular fibrillation. If CPR is not initiated until 5 minutes, only 28% of cerebral blood flow can be achieved. This is one reason widespread lay training in basic CPR is so important.
2. **B**, Page 149.
   Hyperventilation is very important in the management of increased intracranial pressure as after a head injury. Postischemic encephalopathy is not associated with increased intracranial pressure and hyperventilation is of no proven value. All the other listed answers are important to maintain an optimal environment for maximal neurologic recovery.
3. **C**, Page 145.
   Global brain ischemia produces regionally scattered focal ischemic changes, not the diffuse homogeneous damage that might be expected. While it was first thought that after 4–6 minutes of anoxia, irreversible brain damage occurs, now neurons have been proven viable after 60 minutes of complete anoxia. Immediately after resumption of flow following cardiac arrest, CNS blood flow is increased for 15–30 minutes, then it decreases markedly. The etiology of the decrease in CNS blood flow is debated, but it is not due to increased intracranial pressure.
4. **A**, Page 144.
   Neurologic function will be progressively diminished as cerebral blood flow decreases with the higher functions (memory, coordination) waning first. As the cerebral blood flow decreases below 35% of normal, all functions cease and a flat EEG ensues. However, cellular viability is maintained as long as the cerebral blood flow is 20% of normal. It is unclear how much cerebral blood flow even the best cardiopulmonary resuscitation can maintain.

5. **E**, Pages 151–153.

Succinylcholine is an important adjunct to control patient irritability and facilitate intubation but is not postulated to have any direct effect on neuronal recovery. All of the other answers are being studied as potential therapies for postischemic encephalopathy.

6. **E**, Page 152.

Most studies have demonstrated beneficial effects of the calcium channel blockers in postischemic encephalopathy. All of the answers are postulated as beneficial effects with these agents. Clinical trials currently are underway using calcium blockers in cardiac arrest survivors.

8
Multiple Trauma

1. **C**, Page 168.

Hypotension in the context of trauma must be aggressively treated with lactated Ringer infusion through 2 large bore catheters wide open. If no response is detected, O negative blood should be given followed by type specific or typed and cross-matched blood when available and simultaneously the trauma surgeon should be contacted and the operating room prepared.

2. **B**, Page 168.

This lack of response indicates the need for immediate blood transfusion and additional IV lines for continued lactated Ringer's infusion while the arrangements mentioned above are being made. In this situation, waiting for fully typed blood is not recommended.

3. **E**, Page 165.

As noted above, further diagnostic tests are contraindicated when a patient is in shock and needs an operation. It is the emergency physician's responsibility to effectively communicate to the surgeon just how urgent the situation is.

4. **C**, Page 170.

Peritoneal lavage is contraindicated in an unstable hypotensive patient. A portable chest x-ray should be taken while the initial phase of resuscitation is under way and can provide valuable information. It is preferable to have the nasogastric tube inserted prior to chest x-ray because nasogastric deviation is a sign of possible aortic pathology.

5. **A**, Page 167.

A respiratory rate of 10 with apnea following trauma is an indication for intubation, providing there is no immediately resolvable situation such as upper airway obstruction due to dentures, tongue, or other object.

6. **C**, Page 167.

Once breathing has ceased, nasotracheal intubation should not be attempted because the epiglottis will not open adequately. If there is a possibility of cervical spine injury, orotracheal intubation should not be performed due to manipulation required during the procedure.

7. **A**, Page 167.

Cricothyrotomy is much preferred over tracheostomy due to its increased morbidity and technical difficulty.

8. **C**, Page 171.

It is the transferring physician who must be sure the patient is adequately prepared for transfer and the correct arrangements have been made for their safe arrival to the receiving institution. The consultant at the receiving hospital has the responsibility of scrutinizing the care given and insisting that the patient be stabilized prior to transfer.

9. **D**, Page 172.

This child displays no sign of injury or instability. Vital signs are normal for his age. Thus, observation and a complete examination are indicated.

10. **C**, Page 168.

Clotting problems in trauma patients are often overlooked. They are a result of the washout phenomenon or DIC. Either way, fresh frozen plasma is the treatment of choice due to its effectiveness and availability. Some authorities recommend fresh frozen plasma after each 5 units of transfused blood.

11. **B**, Page 165.

The pneumonic ABC for airway, breathing, and circulation is the correct order of priorities and must always be adhered to. Obviously, these interventions can be made simultaneously if the trauma team is well-prepared and coordinated.

12. **A**, Page 160.

The blood pressure can remain normal despite up to 25% blood loss. One should treat the patient, not the lavage results. If the patient is hypotensive, aggressive fluid therapy is required. There is no blood pressure cut off for venous cutdowns but should be reserved for those not responding to initial fluid therapy.

13. **E**, Page 170.

Priapism is sustained penile erection and loss of rectal tone may be the only sign of a spinal cord injury. Diaphragmatic breathing indicates thoracic spine injury as intercostal muscles are supplied by the thoracic cord.

14. **B**, Page 175.

Besides the pelvis, a chest x-ray and cervical spine film should be done in this context. This should not slow the patient's resuscitation or his or her transit to the operating room if proper planning is done.

15. **E**, Page 168.

Banked blood is low in Factors V, VIII, and platelets. Infusion of crystalloid along with banked blood that is stored at 4°C can cause a significant hypothermia.

16. **C**, Page 170.

Cardiac tamponade requires need for pericardiocentesis and possible thoracotomy depending on the condition of the patient.

17. **B**, Page 172.

Patients with penetrating trauma who arrest en route to the hospital or in the emergency department have the best prognosis and are most like to benefit from emergency thoracotomy. All of the others have very poor prognosis and thoracotomy is not recommended.

18. **B**, Page 173.

0.5–1.0 ml/kg/hour is the minimum urine output and can be used as a guide for resuscitation.

9

Hemorrhagic Shock

1. **B**, Pages 179–180.

Shock is not an all-or-none phenomenon, but rather a continuum in which not all cells are affected to the same degree. The hydraulic model is a useful analogy for conceptualizing the shock state.

2. **C**, Page 181.

According to the Frank-Starling relationship, an increase in end diastolic volume is associated with an increase in cardiac output. However, peripheral vascular resistance is increased at the expense of cardiac output since cardiac output is proportional to the arterial blood pressure divided by total peripheral vascular resistance. Mild blood losses can be countered by the above processes without affecting the physiologic condition of the patient.

3. **C**, Page 181.

In the kidney, salt and fluid retention is stimulated, while urinary output any GFR is decreased. Arteriolar constriction like shock itself is a heterogenous process in which the blood flow to the brain and heart occurs at the expense of blood flow to essential organs.

4. **C**, Page 182.

Despite successful resuscitation, capillary leaks may continue for 36–48 hours. Injured mitochondria cannot utilize increasing amounts of oxygen that might be available. A change to anaerobic metabolism results in lesser amounts of ATP, thus causing failure in the ATP sodium-potassium pump and leakage of sodium into the cell and potassium into the interstitium.

5. **A**, Page 183.

Metabolic acidosis has a beneficial effect via shifting the oxyhemoglobic dissociation curve to the right, thus displacing oxygen more readily from the blood to the tissues. Detrimental effects include an increased sensitivity to catecholamines and a reduced cardiac output.

6. **C**, Page 183.

Stroke volume, contractility, and myocardial oxygen interaction are decreased. Hemorrhagic necrosis of the heart occurs.

7. **A**, Page 184.

Gastrointestinal motility is decreased rather than augmented during shock. Other complications are as shown.

8. **D**, Page 185.

It is uncommon for placenta previa to present with hypovolemic shock with the first episode of bleeding. Hypovolemic shock may present as syncope or cardiac arrest with rhythms other than ventricular fibrillation or asystole.

9. **D**, Page 185.

Systolic blood pressure may decrease; however, diastolic blood pressure may increase or stay the same. The other answers are characteristics of compensated shock.

10. **B**, Page 186.

In some patients peripheral arterial constriction can maintain the mean blood pressure at the expense of a markedly decreased cardiac output.

11. **A**, Page 187.

In the well-conditioned athlete the normal resting pulse may be bradycardic; however, an appropriate rise in heart rate occurs in response to shock. Bradycardia is also seen as a preterminal event in head injury, and when using beta blockers. Vagal stimulation due to anxiety, pain, or stress may also occur.

12. **A**, Page 190.

In whole blood clotting factors, leukocytes and platelets are found in reduced amounts. Potassium levels are increased, and albumin and serum proteins are found in an isotonic medium.

13. **C**, Pages 190–191.

Full cross-matching typically takes 45 minutes. Stored blood does contain 2,3 DPG, a substance that augments the delivery of oxygen to peripheral tissues. It is uncommon for a major reaction to occur to type-specific blood. Autotransfusion, while compatible, has increased coagulopathy.

14. **C**, Pages 192–194.

The liver readily converts lactate to bicarbonate even in hypotensive states. Dextrose is not needed in shock where glucose levels are already elevated due to circulating catecholamines. Lactated Ringer's is useful in acidosis and has not been proven to be detrimental in ARDS.

15. **B**, Pages 188–191.

Lactated Ringer's is the initial fluid of choice. O-negative blood typically is immediately available for profound shock. Type-specific is usually available within 20 minutes. Fresh-frozen plasma is usually required after significant transfusion to correct clotting abnormalities. Inotropic agents such as dopamine are required only after hypovolemia has been corrected.

16. **A**, Pages 195, 196.

During cardiac tamponade, a low CVP measurement may occur in the setting of hypovolemia. Serial CVP measurements are a good way to monitor fluid replacement, and in the absence of cardiac or pulmonary disease, they correlate well with left ventricular pressure and diastolic pressure. Actual pressure measurements tend to normalize prior to correction of the volume deficit.

17. **D**, Page 197, 198.

While mannitol and steroids may be helpful in preventing acute tubular necrosis, they should be given only after correction of a volume deficit.

10
Anaphylaxis

1. **D**, Page 203.

Anaphylactoid reactions are clinically similar to anaphylaxis; however, they do not require prior exposure or sensitization such as that seen with radiopaque contrast media or medications such as aspirin or nonsteroidal antiinflammatory drugs.

2. **C**, Page 206.

Atropine is an anticholinergic agent that works by decreasing cAMP levels. Theophylline increases cAMP levels by preventing the breakdown of cAMP through inhibition of phosphodiesterase.

3. **B**, Page 206.

Histamine receptor stimulation causes contraction of intestinal smooth muscle.

4. **C**, Page 203, 210.

The fatality rate of penicillin is about 500 deaths per year and parenteral administration results in most of these. Bee stings are second with 100 deaths per year. Radiopaque contrast media is an anaphylactoid reaction.

5. **A**, Page 215.

The extremity should be placed in the dependent position to reduce venous and lymphatic drainage.

6. **C**, Pages 214, 215.

The patient with vasovagal syncope usually has bradycardia as opposed to tachycardia with anaphylaxis.

7. **D**, Page 215.

In a mild reaction, subcutaneous administration is the route of choice. The correct dose is 0.01 cc/kg of the 1:1,000 solution. The 1:10,000 solution is used for intravenous administration.

8. **C**, Page 218.

Epinephrine increases myocardial oxygen consumption and should be used with caution in elderly patients and in those with known coronary artery disease.

9. **C**, Page 222.

A rise in IgC antibody levels, also called "blocking" antibodies, results in protection against anaphylaxis. This is the mechanism that results with hyposensitization immunotherapy.

10. **B**, Page 223.

Garments that fit close to the body should be worn to prevent the insect from becoming trapped and stinging defensively.

11. **D**, Page 224.

Risk factors for an anaphylactoid reaction include increased age, a prior severe reaction, a history of atopy or asthma, dehydration, renal or hepatic dysfunction, and cardiac disease.

12. **C**, Page 225.

Pretreatment with prednisone and Benadryl significantly reduces the frequency and severity of radiopaque contrast media reactions. Nonionic radiopaque media has a much less disruptive effect on endothelium and reduces the severity of the reaction. Epinephrine would be used if a reaction developed.

11
Blood and Blood Component Therapy

1. **B**, Page 234.
   Patients A and C should receive a fluid challenge of 2 liters of crystalloid prior to contemplating a blood transfusion. If clinical condition and/or vital signs deteriorate during crystalloid therapy, then blood should be given at once. Patient B requires aggressive resuscitation, including STAT transfusion of 2 units of O-negative blood. Only in the most serious, immediately life-threatening situations should a patient be given O-negative blood before crystalloid/colloid or type-specific blood. Properly cross-matched blood is always the best choice for blood replacement, when possible.

2. **D**, Page 236.
   It was found that some O blood had significant titers of A and B antibodies. As a result blood is now tested and categorized as "low titer" if antibody titer is *less* than 1:200 in normal saline.

3. **C**, Page 236.
   Blood loss up to 1,000 cc may cause mild tachycardia but is in general compensated for by vasoconstriction. Losses over 1,000 cc result in orthostatic hypotension. Losses of 1,5000–2,000 cc cause decreased cardiac output, end organ dysfunction, and diminished arterial pressure.

4. **B**, Page 238.
   Platelets at 24 hours retain only 50% functional capacity and at 72 hours have no normal function. Whole blood is stored at 4°C, allowing RBCs to retain metabolic activity for about 100 days. Aranulocytes, however, lose their functional activity within 24 hours. Factor V activity falls to 50% within 3 to 5 days, while Factor VIII activity falls to 50% within a week. Plasma potassium and hydrogen levels rise, causing hyperkolemia and acidosis. There is no appreciable change in albumin, gamma globulin, or other coagulation factors.

5. **B**, Page 239.
   aPTT is a good measure of Factor VIII therapy and activity in the acute care setting.

6. **D**, Page 239.
   Fresh-frozen plasma (2 to 3 ml/kg) is indicated in cases of active bleeding associated with vitamin K dependent factor deficiency. Vitamin K alone corrects too slowly and whole blood is not indicated here. Protamine sulfate is a heparin antagonist.

7. **D**, Page 240.
   Salt-poor is confusing terminology in that these solutions contain 100 to 160 mEq/L of sodium.

8. **A**, Page 240.
   Because fever is also a sign of intravascular transfusion reaction, one cannot assume this patient is having an uncomplicated febrile reaction. Transfusion must be stopped immediately and work-up initiated.

9. **C**, Page 241.
   Rapid infusion of whole blood may precipitate citrate toxicity—especially in a patient with liver failure. Muscle tremors and prolonged QT segment require immediate treatment with 1 to 10 g of a 10% solution of calcium chloride. High citrate levels cause cardiac arrest if untreated.

10. **B**, Page 244.
    Cryoprecipitate is rich in fibrinogen and Factor VIII.

11. **C**, Page 245.
    Spontaneous bleeding does not usually occur until level drops below 20,000/mm³. Between 40,000 and 100,000/mm³ platelets may predispose to bleeding with injury and surgery.

12. **C**, Page 245.
    One unit will raise the platelet count by about 5,000/mm³. As a general rule, 1 unit of platelets given per each 7 kg of body weight raises the platelet count by 50,000.

13. **A**, Pages 240–243.
    Complications of transfusions include hypocalcemia, hemolysis, fever, allergic reactions, hyperkalemia or hypokalemia, citrate toxicity, hypothermia coagulopathies, and altered hemoglobin function.

14. **B**, Page 239.
    Administration of PRBCs reduces citrate load and minimal serum is contained in PRBC. Prophylaxis with calcium chloride may cause hypercalcemia and is not indicated. Bicarbonate is likewise not indicated.

12
Coma

1. **B**, Pages 251–254.
   ICP of 0 to 15 is normal. The Cushing reflex includes increased systolic blood pressure, bradycardia, and bradypnea and is more pronounced in children. Normal CPP is greater than 50.

2. **C**, Page 256.
   The initial step is hyperventilation. A PaCO₂ of less than 20 will produce anaerobic metabolism and is deleterious. A PaCO₂ of 25 to 28 is ideal. All other measures are secondary in reducing ICP.

3. **B**, Pages 256–257.
   Choices *A, C,* and *D* should be given to all patients

in coma. Dexamethasone has no place in initial management of coma but is used to treat cerebral edema.

4. **D**, Page 263.

Conjugate eye movement is opposite the direction of head rotation (oculocephalic reflex). With deepening coma the oculovestibular reflex persists while the oculocephalic reflex may be blunted. The corneal reflex involves the fifth and seventh cranial nerves.

5. **C**, Pages 262–263.

The patient's head should be elevated 30°. Water must be at least 7°F lower than body temperature. The oculovestibular response persists for 2 to 3 minutes hence one should wait at least 5 minutes before testing the opposite ear. After irrigation, the fast component of nystagmus is away from the irrigated ear in the awake patient.

6. **B**, Page 382.

Components of the Glasgow Coma Scale include all of the choices except pupillary response.

7. **C**, Page 252.

Uncal herniation produces ipsilateral pupillary dilatation and either ipsilateral *or* contralateral hemiparesis. Loss of the corneal reflex precedes apnea, which is a preterminal event. Ocular reflexes may persist despite ipsilateral 3rd nerve palsy and hemiparesis.

8. **D**, Pages 262–263.

Nystagmus in response to caloric testing implies an intact cortex. Active resistance to eye opening and closing is highly suggestive of a conversion reaction.

13

Chest Pain

1. **C**, Pages 271–273.
2. **B**, Pages 271–273.
3. **D**, Pages 271–273.
4. **C**, Pages 271–273.
5. **A**, Pages 271–273.

Proximal dissection of the aorta can cause a new murmur of aortic insufficiency, involve the coronary arteries and produce acute ischemia, even an infarction, and cause life-threatening cardiac tamponade. Neither of these would present with a low hematocrit even if there is leaking of an aneurysm, which is rare; there would not be enough time for the acute blood loss to be reflected in the hematocrit, which takes 8 to 12 hours. Hypertension is a major risk factor for each, more so for aortic dissection. Even when an acute infarction is the initial manifestation of coronary artery disease, most people will admit to symptoms before the acute event. A dissection comes on suddenly with

maximal pain at the onset without prior warning. *Most* dissections are misdiagnosed as ischemic heart disease on their initial presentation. To help make the correct diagnosis, a careful physical examination with particular attention to differences in the pulses or a diastolic murmur and chest x-ray looking for a widened mediastinum are helpful.

6. **D**, Page 272.

While variant angina and esophageal spasm are often readily relieved with nitroglycerin, at times the neural compression syndrome may be relieved, although the cause is unknown. Mitral valve prolapse is seldom relieved by nitroglycerin and may be worsened if the vasodilatation causes less ventricular filling and more strain on the papillary muscles.

7. **C**, Page 273.

Diagnoses based on the effects of a therapeutic challenge are unreliable, because of both a placebo effect and the possibility of coincidental pain relief as from simultaneously administered oxygen, relief of anxiety, etc. Cardiac enzymes, although helpful in CCU, are seldom useful in the emergency department largely because of a 12-hour time lag. The electrocardiogram is a valuable tool to determine coronary artery disease, but many other conditions, even esophageal disease, may cause an abnormal EKG. A completely normal EKG, especially if obtained during an episode of pain, is very unusual with significant coronary artery disease.

8. **C**, Page 272.

Typically, visceral pain is vague, diffuse, poorly localized, of at least 2–3 minutes in duration. Sharp or stabbing pain, well localized, lasting less than 30 seconds, is seen very infrequently. All of the other listed conditions are associated with myocardial ischemia fairly often.

9. **B**, Page 272.

Pericarditis is often pleuritic in nature, aggravated by coughing, swallowing, and changes in position. It can mimic pleurisy exactly but is much more likely to be relieved by sitting up and leaning forward. The diagnosis is confirmed by an EKG with diffuse S-T segment elevation with an upward concavity and/or a pericardial rub.

10. **A**, Page 272.

Classically, princemetal's variant angina occurs at rest and is associated with transient S-T segment elevation rather than depression typical of classic angina pectoris. It is believed to be due to spasm of the coronary arteries and can lead to an infarction. Nitrates and calcium channel blockers are effective treatments, but beta blockers may theoretically worsen the syndrome by allowing unopposed alpha stimulation of the coronary arteries if there is a compensatory increase in circulating adrenergic levels.

14
Headache

1. **D**, Pages 279–280.
   In addition to the structure in choices A, B, and C, the dural base of the skull and the dural arteries are also sensitive. The cranium, brain parenchyma, most of the dura, arachnoid, and the pia mater do not have sensation to pain.

2. **D**, Pages 280, 281, 284.
   Acute onset suggests a vascular headache. The headache caused by tumor usually has gradual onset with a recent change in frequency or duration noted by the patient.

3. **D**, Pages 280–282.
   In addition to those listed, headaches associated with glaucoma and hypoxia secondary to COPD tend to awaken people.

4. **D**, Pages 282–283.
   Localized tenderness of scalp and neck do not necessarily mean the patient has a muscle contraction headache. Such tenderness may represent a reaction to pain. This finding is therefore nonspecific.

5. **A**, Pages 282–285.
   Oculomotor and abducent nerves are most commonly affected by increased intracranial pressure or inflammation.

6. **C**, Page 287.
   Studies have shown that 130 mm Hg diastolic is the level at which patients become symptomatic.

7. **C**, Pages 284, 289.
   At the time of acute exacerbation the headache is very severe and "boring." Before this stage the patient may have intermittent mild headaches.

8. **B**, Pages 284, 289.
   Although a low grade anemia and leukocytosis may be present, these are not as characteristic as the substantially elevated sedimentation rate in the patient with temporal arteritis.

9. **B**, Pages 284–285.
   Initially migraines are classically unilateral.

10. **C**, Page 285.
    Generally less intense than the classic migraine, ophthalmoplegic migraines may last 3 to 5 days. Palsies of the muscles served by the III, IV, and VI cranial nerves may occur which explains the finding of pupillary dilatation (mydriasis), diplopia, and external strabismus.

11. **C**, Pages 285–287.
    In itself diabetes mellitus is not a contraindication. However, the resulting peripheral vascular disease may contraindicate the use of these drugs.

12. **D**, Page 285.

Cluster headaches are more common in males, they are chronic, awaken people after 2 to 3 hours of sleep, last 30 to 90 minutes, lack any prodrome, and are typically unilateral.

13. **B**, Page 285.
    The patient described may have atlantoaxial subluxation. If this is missed, quadriplegia could result. Rheumatoid arthritis and ankylosing spondylitis patients are at risk for this problem. X-ray films of the cervical spine would show a gap of 3 mm or more between the posterior part of the atlas and the anterior border of the odontoid process.

14. **C**, Page 285.
    While a thrombotic CVA may cause hemiplegia, retinal hemorrhage is usually not seen. A subdural hematoma causes hemiplegia only as a preterminal event. The retinal hemorrhages exclude a diagnosis of hemiplegic migraine. Subarachnoid hemorrhage is the most common cause of CVAs in the 20- to 40-year-old age group.

15. **C**, Pages 284, 289.
    Temporal arteritis is acute in onset with a history of acute exacerbations and remissions. Therapy must be begun immediately if biopsy is not readily available. Intraocular pressure measurement is required to rule out glaucoma. Untreated cases of temporal arteritis often involve the contralateral eye within 6 weeks of initial presentation.

16. **B**, Page 285.
    Ophthalmoplegic or hemiplegic migraines are rarely components of classic migraines. Subarachnoid hemorrhage may mimic these symptoms, especially if recovery is incomplete. Only 10% of all migraines are classic and ergot alkaloids often are successful in their treatment.

15
Pain Control: Anesthesia and Analgesia

1. **A**, Pages 296–297.
   Nitrous oxide provides effective pain relief during myocardial infarction. Because it may increase intracranial pressure, it is contraindicated in patients with head injury. It diffuses readily into closed spaces and is thus contraindicated in patients with bowel obstruction or pneumothorax.

2. **D**, Pages 300–302.
   Epinephrine is contraindicated in tissues supplied by end arteries such as fingers, toes, penis, and skin flaps. It maybe used on mucous membranes to slow bleeding, although absorption of the anesthetic is unaltered.

3. **C**, Pages 303–305.
   Propoxyphene has only agonist opiate activity. The others have mixed activity.
4. **B**, Page 300.
   Lidocaine is an amide and procaine is an ester. There is no cross-reactivity. Allergic reactions to local anesthetics are rare, but when they do occur they are in response to esters. Chlorprocaine is an ester as is Novocaine (procaine). Cocaine is inappropriate for local infiltration.

16
Fever

1. **C**, Pages 310–311.
   Achlorhydria is often present in patients with high fevers; gastric acid secretion is resumed when the fever resolves. Leukocytes demonstrate maximum phagocytic activity between 38°C and 40°C. Fever does seem to directly inhibit certain viruses such as coxsackie and polio. During fever there are decreased levels of circulating iron, which is thought to be beneficial because many microbes need iron for growth and reproduction.
2. **B**, Pages 302, 316–317.
   Fever in the first 8 weeks of life is always cause for alarm. In one study 15% of infants with a rectal temperature over 38°C were found to be bacteremic, most with group B streptococcus. These bacteremic infants could not be distinguished from their nonbacteremic peers by the degree of fever, WBC counts, or the presence or absence of a localized source of infection. Any child with a fever in the first 8 weeks of life should be hospitalized and have a complete septic work up.
3. **C**, Page 310.
4. **D**, Page 310.
5. **E**, Page 310.
6. **A**, Page 310.
7. **B**, Page 310.
8. **A**, Page 309.
   At rest, 60% of body heat is eliminated by radiation, and convection accounts for 12–15% of total heat loss. In a warm environment, radiation and convection become more important. Vaporization is most effective in a dry, cool environment.
9. **C**, Page 313.
   Crushing's syndrome causes a leukocytosis with a left shift. All of the other situations cause a leukocytosis with *no* left shift.

17
Poisoning

1. **B**, Page 330.
   Nasotracheal rather than orotracheal intubation is the treatment of choice for a comatose patient with absent gag reflex. Oxygen, glucose, and Narcan are always indicated. A fluid bolus rather than pressor agents is the first step in the treatment of a hypotensive poisoned patient since the hypotension is much more likely to be secondary to loss of vascular resistance rather than myocardial depression.
2. **A**, Page 332.
   Bradycardia may result from muscarinic agents (pilocarpine and Amanita mushrooms), cholinesterase inhibitors (organophosphates), beta blockers, and cardiac glycosides. Tachycardia is characteristically produced by sympathomimetics (amphetamines, cocaine) and anticholinergics (atropine, tricyclic antidepressants).
3. **B**, Page 332.
   Benzodiazepines, narcotics, and barbiturates may cause respiratory depression. Hydrocarbons and caustics may cause hypoxia and thus tachypnea. Strychnine can cause a global hyperexcitability, while salicylism is known for initial respiratory alkalosis and secondary metabolic acidosis both producing tachypnea.
4. **B**, Page 333.
   Phencyclidine (PCP) is the only drug known to cause both vertical and horizontal nystagmus.
5. **A**, Page 333.
   Barbiturate burns are vesiculobullous lesions that occur with intravenous abuse of the drug. Organophosphates cause hyperactive gastrointestinal motility and hyperhidrosis. Urinary retention is characteristic of atropinism.
6. **D**, Page 336.
   Drug screens typically take several hours to complete and are not capable of detecting many substances. They are frequently reported long after therapy has been initiated but can be occasionally helpful—when the toxic substance has not been identified from historical sources or initial laboratory studies.
7. **A**, Page 337.
   Urinary retention is seen in anticholinergic poisoning. The other answers typify cholinergic poisoning (SLUDE), with parasympathetic overdrive.

8. **B**, Page 338.

This once widely held view has been challenged by recent studies.

9. **C**, Pages 340–341.

There is no absolute contraindication to charcoal; however, its lack of efficacy in treatment of alkali, mineral acids, and ferrous sulfate has established. There have been reports of mechanical complications with charcoal if aspirated. Its usefulness in enterogastric and enterohepatic recirculation has been shown.

10. **D**, Page 343.

The elimination of acetaminophen is not enhanced by forced diuresis.

11. **D**, Page 345.

The antidote to anticholinergics is physostigmine. Bicarbonate may also be helpful. Pralidoxime (PAM) is useful in organophosphate toxicity.

12. **B**, Pages 345–348.

Nitroprusside may cause methemoglobinemia treated with 1% methylene blue solution. Heavy metals, not lithium, are treated with the chelating agent EDTA. Extrapyramidal reactions are treated with Benadryl.

18
Treatment of Wounds

1. **B**, Pages 363–365

A, *C*, and *D* are all known risk factors for increased chance of infection. Also devitalized tissue, foreign bodies, subcutaneous sutures, and high-velocity missile injuries are known risk factors. Although time since injury is always an important factor and differs in regards to risk of infection with various body areas, it has been shown that wounds have increased risk of infection if older than 4–8 hours. Therefore, a wound only 2–3 hours old can usually be safely repaired with primary closure.

2. **D**, Page 364.

Although healing occurs fairly rapidly in regard to epithelization and collagen synthesis, you must consider ultimate strength and integrity. Collagen synthesis peaks at about day 7 with greatest healing mass occurring around 3 weeks. However, ultimate strength of the wound is only 15–20% of end result at 3 weeks and only 60% at 4 months. A halfback frequently encounters direct force to his arms of sufficient magnitude to disrupt his healing wound; therefore, he has a high likelihood of recurring injury if returning to full contact within 4 to 6 months.

3. **C**, Pages 364, 365.

Allergies to local anesthetics are rare, but this history must be taken. The esters include procaine (Novocaine), tetracaine, and benzocaine. The amides used are lidocaine and bupivacaine (Marcaine). As well, multidose vials of the amides contain methylparaben, an ester, as a preservative. Cardiac lidocaine contains no methyparaben. Cross-reactivity does not exist between the amides and esters. Thus, in this case an amide like cardiac lidocaine would be the safest alternative. If a question still exists, a test dose of 0.1 ml should be given with observation for reaction over 30 minutes. Also, aqueous diphenhydramine (Benadryl) provides effective local anesthesia.

4. **A**, Pages 366, 368.

B, *C*, and *D* are all effective means to cleanse wounds. Betadine scrub solutions are toxic to tissues and therefore are not used. Simply soaking the wound is ineffective since a scrub with a small-pore sponge or high-pressure irrigation must be used. Also, the importance of debridement of devitalized tissue cannot be overemphasized. Hydrogen peroxide or alcohols should not be used and providone-iodine solutions of greater than 5% are also toxic to tissues and defense mechanisms.

5. **B**, Page 368.

The location of the wound, time since injury, amount of devitalized tissue, mechanism of injury, and whether or not contamination is present are all factors entering a decision on type of closure. Wounds in close proximity to bursae as well as blunt-force mechanism to the feet have a high propensity toward infection; therefore, delayed primary closure should be considered. Clean facial wounds can usually be safely primary closed up to 12 to 18 hours out. Wounds on areas of the body without exceptional blood supply should best be closed with delayed primary closure if older than 4 to 8 hours. If doubt exists, delayed primary closure in 3 to 4 days should be used since risk of infection is decreased and total healing time is unaffected.

6. **D**, Pages 368, 369.

PDS is an excellent monofilament absorbable suture. Also Dexon and Vicryl are absorbable. Cutting needles are used for skin closure, whereas noncutting are used for organ repair or subcutaneous suturing. *C* is a correct statement. *D* seems to be correct, but it must be remembered that subcutaneous sutures increase risk of infection; therefore, they should not be used on hands or feet. When used in other areas they should be kept to a minimum.

7. **A**, Page 370.

B, *C*, and *D* are situations in which one could not be faulted for using prophylactic antibiotics. Although *A* seems correct and much controversy now exists in this area, there seems to be no rationale for antibiotics since the initial bacteremia would have already occurred by the time the patient presents for treatment. Irrigating antibiotic solutions do decrease infection and topical antibiotics have a beneficial effect on wound healing; therefore, they should be used. Also, delayed primary closure should be considered in *B*, *C*, and *D*.

8. **C**, Pages 370–371.

Keeping tissue moist and preventing scab formation speed overall healing process. Therefore, topical antibiotics and transparent semiocclusive dressings should be used initially. If scab formation occurs, the scab should be swabbed with dilute hydrogen peroxide daily until the scab separates. Facial sutures should be removed in 3 to 5 days and replaced with steri-strips. Suture removal on scalp at 7 to 10 days, trunk at 7 to 10 days, extremities 10 to 14 days, and joints at 14 days. Also, the patient should return in 48 hours for recheck of high risk wounds. If redness, increased pain, swelling, fever, or red streaking occurs, the patient should return for rechecks.

19

Head Trauma

1. **E**, Page 377.

Narcotic overdose and hypoglycemia are particularly important because they are easily treated and potentially fatal. It is important to keep these in mind, especially in cases where there are no witnesses available. D50 and Narcan should be given when there is doubt as to the exact cause of the comatose state.

2. **E**, Page 378.

Classically, as the uncus herniates it compresses the ipsilateral 3rd cranial nerve, causing ipsilateral pupil dilatation and contralateral weakness because the pyramidal tract decussates below this level. However, occasionally the shift will be great enough to cause compression on both sides leading to any combination of the above findings.

3. **D**, Page 380.

This reflex may be a clue to increased intracranial pressure; however, it is often a late finding.

4. **E**, Page 380.

Cushing's reflex refers to the rise in blood pressure and fall in pulse as a response to increased intracranial pressure. It is a late finding and an unreli-

able aid in the diagnosis of a rising intracranial pressure.

5. **B**, Page 382 (Table 19–1).

One point is given for the minimal response in each of the three categories making 3 the minimum score. The maximum score is 16.

6. **B**, Page 381.

All of the choices are important, but history of a deterioration in the level of consciousness is particularly alarming and mandates swift evaluation and interpretation.

7. **D**, Page 382 (Table 19–1).

Speech = *3*, eye opening = *3*, motor = *5* = 11.

8. **B**, Pages 381–382.

The Glasgow Coma Scale presupposes head injury alone, but the required responses can be affected by other injuries or conditions, e.g., hypotension, alcohol intoxication, spinal cord damage, etc. Thus, the score may be inappropriately low.

9. **E**, Page 381.

Patients with facial injuries who are awake with no cervical trauma can be transported sitting. However, this patient may not be capable of reporting cervical pain. After cervical immobilization, he should be transported prone, or on his side—not supine. Intubation or cricothyroidotomy is not indicated.

10. **C**, Page 382.

Orotracheal intubation with inline traction is preferred. Nasotracheal intubation requires a breathing patient. Cricothyroidotomy should be reserved for patients in whom intubation is impossible. EOA may be useful, but is not preferred.

11. **D**, Page 382.

First priority in this patient is to put a cervical collar on him. Anyone who needs a cervical spine series needs cervical collar.

12. **B**, Page 383.

Trauma patients with an immobilized C-spine are at great risk for aspiration and immediate steps must be taken in the event of vomiting. Turning of the head or removal of the collar is contraindicated for obvious reasons. Intubation may be necessary but never prior to adequate suctioning and evacuation of the emesis. Log-rolling to the left with full stabilization of the entire spine is the method of choice while suctioning.

13. **A**, Page 383.

Prevertebral soft tissue swelling is often overlooked but is a valuable clue to cervical spine injury. It is caused by hematoma and swelling of the soft tissues overlying the damaged bone.

14. **A**, Pages 383, 384.

The patient should be intubated and hyperventilated to protect the airway and lower intracranial pressure. Because of apparent hypovolemia, the patient should be vigorously fluid-resuscitated, and diuretic therapy is not appropriate until this is accomplished. A CT, rather than skull x-ray, is indicated.

15. **D**, Page 384.

Maintaining mild hypocapnia is effective in decreasing the intracranial pressure through a vasoconstrictive effect on the cerebrovascular bed.

16. **E**, Pages 392, 393.

Patients with structured brain damage are more likely to have posttraumatic seizures, especially penetrating trauma and depressed skull fractures.

17. **A**, Page 385.

For status epilepticus, Dilantin is second line treatment behind Valium, not phenobarbital, which can alter the mental status and is therefore less desirable in this setting.

18. **B**, Page 389.

Commonly, the only radiographic sign of a basilar skull fracture may be a blood/air interface in the sphenoid sinus.

19. **E**, Page 389.

The major risk is infection, not the leak itself. Antibiotics that cross the blood brain barrier may be beneficial. Lumbar puncture is not indicated unless the patient develops a fever.

20. **E**, Page 390.

The classic description of epidural hemorrhage is that of a short period of unconsciousness, lucid interval, and then deterioration. However, a significant number present in other ways.

21. **B**, Pages 390, 391.

Subdural hemorrhage is six times more common than epidural, and acute subdurals have a mortality of 60–80% compared with 25–50% for epidurals.

22. **D**, Page 380.

Classically, epidurals are caused by laceration of the middle meningeal artery as it courses under the temporal bone, but torn sinuses or communicating veins can also cause life-threatening epidural hematomas.

23. **D**, Page 391.

Generally, as the hematoma ages, it becomes isodense between day 7 and day 21 and then hypodense.

24. **C**, Page 390.

Significant hemorrhage can occur from any scalp laceration. It is important to close the galea in scalp lacerations because if not, the action of the muscles attached to it may open the wound.

25. **B**, Page 389.

Blood-air interface in the sphenoid sinus may be the only sign of basilar skull fracture. Antibiotics may be indicated in patients with CSF leak, but not routinely in basilar skull fractures.

26. **A**, Pages 383, 384.

While the patient probably requires intubation, a lateral film alone does not clear the cervical spine. Therefore, orotracheal intubation should be deferred until AP and odontoid views are obtained.

27. **A**, Page 386.

NMR is excellent for demonstrating posttraumatic intracranial pathology, including subacute subdural hematomas not seen on CT. Second choice would be CT with contrast. The other choices are too invasive or insensitive.

28. **D**, Page 380.

Classically, subdurals are caused by rupture of bridging veins, but they can also be caused by arteriolar bleeding or delayed bleeding from organizing vessels around the clot.

29. **D**, Page 387.

The patient should stay with a responsible adult and be observed for 24 hours. Warning signs and symptoms should be explained to both the patient and observer.

30. **C**, Page 386.

Intoxicated patients with head trauma but without obvious neurologic deficits should have cervical and skull radiographs. An alcohol level should be drawn, which gives a rough indication of how long it will take for the patient to improve, assuming the alteration in mental status is due to only intoxication.

31. **D**, Page 388.

A wide variety of disturbances in neurologic function, e.g., confusion, are sufficient to make this diagnosis. Postconcussion syndromes, e.g., anatomic headache, may occur.

20

Facial Trauma

1. **C**, Page 396.

Direct pressure will usually control bleeding in facial trauma. Blind clamping may result in damage to important nearby structures.

2. **C**, Page 396.

Shock as a result of facial trauma is extremely rare and additional sources should be sought. Hemorrhage can be controlled with direct pressure. Choices A, B, and D can be present secondary to facial trauma and must be considered.

3. **B**, Page 397.

Extraocular muscles are innervated by cranial nerve III, IV, and VI, while the others are seen with the VII or facial nerve.

4. **B**, Page 397.

Diplopia on upward gaze can indicate the presence of an orbital blowout fracture.

5. **C**, Pages 398, 406.

Submental view gives the best view of the zygomatic arch. Mandibular fractures are best seen on panoramic view. The Water's view shows the maxilla, maxillary sinuses, orbital floor, inferior orbital rim, and zygomatic bones.

6. **D**, Page 398.

Following appropriate irrigation and debridement, facial wounds without significant contamination or crush injury may be closed primarily up to 24 hours later.

7. **D**, Page 399.

Epinephrine is used to prolong the anesthesia time and decrease vascular bleeding. However, in areas of the ear or nose it may cause necrosis and should not be used.

8. **B**, Page 400.

After proper anesthesia, the area is scrubbed to remove any embedded material. Foreign debris remaining after wound closure will be incorporated into the dermis, a condition known as traumatic tattooing. Removal of the material at a later date is difficult.

9. **C**, Page 403.

A septal hematoma should be incised to allow drainage. Untreated, it will result in necrosis of the septal cartilage. The others are more likely to be seen with specific facial fractures, such as blowout fracture of the eye.

10. **D**, Page 404.

Excising perpendicular to the skin results in a bald area. Shaving the eyebrow would destroy the landmarks necessary for an accurate closure.

11. **A**, Page 404.

The parotid gland, parotid duct, and facial nerve are important structures between the tragus of the ear and the mid-cheek. Injury in this area should prompt evaluation of these structures.

12. **A**, Page 406.

LeFort II, Le Fort III, and nasoethmoid may result in a cribriform plate fracture with associated dural leak, but a Le Fort I fracture involves only the maxilla at the level of the nasal fossa.

13. **D**, Pages 407–408.

Malor flattening is seen in a zygomatic tripoid fracture as well as B and C. In an isolated orbital floor fracture, though, depression of the malar emimence is not seen.

14. **A**, Page 410.

The reverse is performed when relocating a temporomandibular joint dislocation. Initially, downward pressure is applied to unlock the condyles. Finally, posterior pressure is applied.

15. **C**, Page 410.

An avulsed tooth should be held by the crown. Wiping the tooth clean removes a membrane important in successful reimplantation. A is the best choice, but B and C are also acceptable.

16. **B**, Page 410.

Reimplantation after 2 hours results in only minimal tooth survival.

17. **C**, Pages 411, 412.

C is the most common site of posterior bleeds and supply mainly coming from external carotid system. A is the most common site of anterior bleeds. B is supplied by internal carotid circulation and D is untrue. Also, C is usually on the lateral wall and difficult to identify.

18. **D**, Pages 411–413.

Both A, B, and C must be considered, particularly in the pediatric population. D is a cause of posterior epistaxis and, although uncommon, is usually seen in adults. This can be a cause of massive epistaxis, usually with history of trauma to temporal region or lateral orbit. Also, anticoagulants, hypertension, neoplasm, and coagulopathy must be considered in adults. As well, foreign body should be considered in unilateral epistaxis, especially in children.

19. **B**, Pages 411, 412.

B as well as ethmoid labyrinth and maxillary fractures must be sought after to decrease morbidity and mortality. Clinical exam can usually distinguish these. A and C are unlikely, and D should never be considered.

20. **A**, Pages 414, 415.

Silver nitrate cautery is usually successful in a dry field and holding contact for 20–30 seconds. More than one stick may be necessary, and the chance of B occurring is virtually zero, although increased with electrocautery. No cautery should be attempted in C, rather, reversal of the condition with fresh frozen plasma. D should usually be done after hemostasis is obtained; however, nasal packing is indicated if the source cannot be indicated. Also, Gelfoam or Oxycel may be used to attempt hemostasis.

21. **B**, Page 417.

Although bilateral anteriorly packed nosebleeds are occasionally admitted, this in not a criteria. If admitted, it is usually for sedation and observation. The other three conditions must be admitted for the following reasons. Hypoxemia and CO_2 retention occur with A as well as possible acute airway obstruction. Fresh-frozen plasma must be given to C. D, as well as severe associated hypertension (190/120), those requiring transfusion, and extremely debilitated patients should also be admitted.

21
Neck Injuries

1. **B**, Page 419.
   Answers *A*, *C*, and *D* are fundamental principles of prehospital care. The physician must be aware that rapid transport may indeed be the most important aspect of prehospital care in neck injuries. Answer *B* is controversial since recent data do not support rigid cervical immobilization in penetrating trauma (i.e., gunshot wound without neurologic deficit or stab wound). Prone or sitting positions may be better tolerated in regards to clearing of blood, vomitus, and secretions.

2. **A**, Page 421.
   PTV is an acceptable alternative to other airway management for periods not exceeding 30 minutes; however, it is contraindicated in complete upper airway obstruction since it may cause fatal air embolism. It is preferred with a 12–14-gauge catheter entering the superior aspect of the cricothyroid membrane. Using an interposed Y-connector and oxygen at 15 liters per minute, the 4-connector is occluded for 1 of every 5 seconds to allow exhalation. *B* prevents later increases in morbidity and mortality. *C* is obvious; beware of contained hematomas in region of cricothyroid membrane since these should not receive cricothyrotomy. *D* is correct and is used to avoid straining or gagging, which may cause a hematoma to rupture, if required prehospital nasotracheal intubation may be performed.

3. **C**, Pages 422, 423.
4. **A**, Pages 422, 423.
5. **D**, Pages 422, 423.
6. **B**, Pages 422, 423.
   Most are self-explanatory. Horner's syndrome should be ipsilateral to the lesion. If phrenic nerve injury is present, fluoroscopy should reveal an immobile hemidiaphragm. Accompanying *B* in laryngeal fractures is stridor, dyspnea, dysphonia, pain, and tenderness. The most common thyroid cartilage fracture is vertical anterior from thyroid notch to cricothyroid membrane. Beware that complete avulsion of trachea from larynx may be present. Look for loss of cartilaginous landmarks and flattening of anterior profile of neck with inability to palpate thyroid cartilage.

7. **B**, Page 423.
   With injury distal to the thyroid cartilage and respiratory compromise, disruption of the trachea must be considered. A cricothyrotomy may allow descension of the distal stump into the mediastinum. Subcutaneous air also suggests that saliva has reached the deep tissues; therefore, antibiotics are indicated.

Also, subcutaneous air in children may further compromise the airway. Short-term steroids are recommended for blunt laryngeal trauma without fracture; however, they should also be considered if the patient does not require surgical correction.

8. **A**, Page 424.
   The description of signs and symptoms is classic for esophageal injury. Disruption can be rapidly fatal; therefore, minimum required work-up in the emergency department is esophagoscopy, water soluble esophagogram repeated with barium if negative. Small tears are difficult to identify; therefore, a single test should never be relied on to exclude the diagnosis.

9. **D**, Pages 424, 425.
   Gentle probing may rupture a hematoma or introduce air embolism—lacerations do heal well and puncture wounds should not be sutured; however, *B* is incorrect as the work-up would not be complete. Carotid artery injuries often present delayed neurologic features secondary to thrombotic occlusion around an intimal tear or mural contusion. *D* is a vital part of the exam that is frequently omitted, but if a bruit is missed, morbidity and/or mortality dramatically increases secondary thrombotic and/or embolic episodes. Cerebral angiography should be obtained early.

10. **D**, Pages 425, 426.
    The zones are defined as follows: Zone 1—below sternal notch, Zone II—between sternal notch and angle of the mandible, Zone III—above angle of the mandible. All Zone I injuries should receive preoperative aortography to determine surgical approach. All Zone III injuries should be evaluated with selective carotid angiograms. Zone II injuries can usually be readily explored; however, in select cases angiography may be helpful. A Zone I injury with unresponsive hypotension should be suspected of having massive intrathoracic hemorrhage and may require thoracotomy for proximal vascular control.

11. **B**, Page 426.
    The statement is essentially true except that it is recommended that primary closure occur within 12–18 hours. If beyond this or grossly contaminated, closure should be delayed for 72 hours. Also, do not forget routine tetanus prophylaxis with toxoid and/or tetanus immune globulin (Hyper-Tet).

12. **B**, Page 427.
    Tardieu's spots are petechial hemorrhages arising from increased venous pressure cephalad to the ligature. They are found in skin as well as subconjunctival areas. *C* is a true statement as well as *A*. Immobilization and/or cervical spine films are not required in most cases, the exception being a hanging with significant force from a fall.

13. **D**, Pages 427, 428.

Respiratory complications are the cause of the majority of mortalities. Airway obstruction, bronchopneumonia, aspiration pneumonia, and ARDS must all be observed for and treated aggressively. It is believed that ARDS in this setting is secondary to a centroneurogenic lesion. PEEP, fluid restriction, and components of *B* above are all recommended for cerebral edema and/or ARDS. Dilantin may prevent ischemic damage by preventing seizures and possibly retarding the development of ARDS. Narcan and calcium channel blockers are also being tested in this area. Steroids have no proven benefit in treatment of cerebral edema or centroneurogenic ARDS.

22
Spinal Injury

1. **C**, Pages 432, 433.

Answers *A*, *B*, and *D* are the three common categories of spinal cord injury mechanisms. Spinal artery embolism is rare, although thrombosis may occasionally be seen with lower cervical dislocation and subsequent thrombosis of the anterior spinal artery.

2. **A**, Pages 433, 434.

Maximal neurologic deficit usually appears over a several hour course primarily due to changes as described in *B*. Answers *C* and *D* are considered cornerstones of therapy and should always be kept in mind to yield maximal prognosis.

3. **C**, Pages 438, 439.

The anterior column is supported by anterior and posterior longitudinal ligaments. The posterior column is supported by nuchal ligament complex, capsular ligaments, and ligamenta flava. Mechanically stable injuries should lead one to suspect neurologic instability especially if a component of *C* is present. You must prove that the injury is not a neurologically unstable one; incidence in *D* is quoted at 14%.

4. **B**, Pages 438, 439 (Table 22–1).

In a study of 384 cases, various percentages with neurologic deficit are quoted in Table 22–1 as 27%, 56%, 11%, and 19%, *A* through *D*, respectively. It is important to note association of two of the following three: fracture, dislocation, and evidence of ligamentous disruption, an association that may be very subtle.

5. **C**, Page 439.

The correct sequence one would take to obtain adequate radiographs would be *C, A, D, B*. Oblique views can also lend usefulness in this situation. Of course, time restraints must be taken into account and

if a question arises in a head-injured patient undergoing CT examination of head, C-spine cuts could also be obtained. Also, it must be emphasized that inadequate visualization of C_6–T_1 results in increased morbidity and more successful litigation.

6. **B**, Page 445.

In assessing possible high cervical injury in a child, the posterior cervical line attaching base of spinous processes C_1 to C_3 should be used; if base of C_2 spinous process lies greater than 2 mm behind posterior cervical line, Hangman's fracture should be suspected. Normal predental space in a child is less than 5 mm (3 mm in an adult). Normal distance in *C* is less than 7 mm in adult or child. Normal distance in *D* is 14 mm in children younger than 15 years of age and less than 22 mm in adults. Be aware that in children less than 2 years of age expiratory films can give false retropharyngeal widening.

7. **D**, Page 445.

This injury is unstable and must be dealt with immediately by a neurosurgeon. The patient must remain immobilized and further studies will not aid unless other injury is suspected. Be aware that shadow lines, nonfusion in children, and congenital anomalies all may mimic fracture of the odontoid.

8. **C**, Pages 445, 452.

Although unlikely with this history and exam, unilateral facet dislocation must be considered. Oblique films help to differentiate this from torticollis, a purely muscular disorder. Simultaneous flexion and rotation cause contralateral facet dislocation with the superior facet riding forward over the tip of the inferior facet. Mechanical stability is the rule but obliques are necessary to evaluate the intervertbral foramen.

9. **B**, Page 447.

B occurs usually after a direct blow to the spinous process from a club, karate chop, etc. It is considered stable and not associated with any neurologic impairment. The other statements are all true. In unilateral facet dislocation, a rotational injury, the displacement of superior vertebral body is less than 50% of the AP diameter of the inferior involved vertebral body.

10. **D**, Page 457.

The fracture described is a Hangman's fracture, which occurs usually as a result of deceleration and severe hyperextension although unstable. Cord damage is usually minimal as AP diameter of neural canal is greatest at this level. Also, bilateral pedicle fractures allow decompression. Prevertebral swelling may lead to respiratory obstruction, which is your next concern. The lesion in *C* is stable in flexion and unstable in extension; it may also be associated with a central cord syndrome.

11. **A**, Page 460.

Cervical and lumbar regions are the most common sites of vertebral compression fracture since these areas straighten at time of impact. *D* and *B* are true and are related; *C* is true and is also termed a blowout fracture of C_1 with resultant fractures of anterior and posterior arches as well as disruption of transverse ligament.

12. **D**, Page 461.

D usually indicates a lower cervical injury since phrenic nerve from C_{3-4} innervates the diaphragm, whereas the intercostal muscles are innervated by thoracic nerves. Spontaneous muscle fasciculations suggest decreased inhibitory impulses from injured spine; therefore, fasciculations occur in muscles innervated by section of cord just above injury. Horner's syndrome (ptosis, miosis, anhydrosis) is secondary to disruption of cervical sympathetic chain, usually C_7-T_2. *C* was described by Maroon in young football players.

13. **B**, Page 462.

B must be frequently assessed because if the cervical region is involved, respiratory failure should be anticipated. *A* describes an upper motor neuron (spinal cord) lesion, whereas *D* describes a lower motor neuron (nerve root or cauda equina) lesion. *C* indicates a 50% chance of functional motor recovery. It is improtant to note that *C* or *D* may be presentation of spinal shock. Also, it should be remembered that light touch is a posterior column function and pain sensation (pinprick) is an anterior spinothalamic tract function.

14. **A**, Page 462.

Perianal region is S_{2-4} sensory dermatome, whereas the lateral foot is S_1 dermatome. Persistent perianal sensation is a sign of sacral sparing and indicates a partial lesion with possible functional recovery. The other three associations are correct.

15. **B**, Pages 462, 465.

B describes outcome results of complete lesions, and occasionally spinal shock mimics a complete lesion. Return of only some function occurs in less than 24 hours. *A* describes a central cord syndrome in which grater than 50% will become ambulatory. *C* describes a Brown-Sequard syndrome (or hemisection) in which prognosis is good and surgery unnecessary. *D* describes an anterior cord syndrome that has preservation of posterior column functions of position, touch, and vibration; surgical intervention should be strongly considered.

16. **D**, Page 468.

In confirmed cases of spinal injury, placement of traction devices is occasionally indicated in the emergency department. Gardner-Wells tongs are the most easily applied because placement is rapid and simple,

and does not require calvarial drilling. Placement should be slightly posterior to bilateral pinnae. *A* is true since the device is monitored by an automatic pressure sensitive pin. Both *B* and *C* are true and self-explanatory.

17. **C**, Pages 469, 470.

Spinal cord injury and subsequent respiratory arrest is an indication for cricothyrotomy in this situation because edema or epidural hematoma spread is more than likely causing phrenic nerve dysfunction. *A* should be performed only in a patient spontaneously breathing, unconscious, or conscious with use of topical anesthesia and by a physician skilled in this maneuver. *B* is performed only if mild-to-moderate respiratory distress is present. *D* should be performed following airway management.

18. **A**, Page 470.

Normal pulse or bradycardia are usually seen secondary to unopposed vagal tone. *B* is present without peripheral signs of vasoconstriction. In elderly or congestive heart failure, dopamine may be substituted for *D*. Also, it should be remembered that nasogastric tubes should be placed in spinal injuries because ileus is common.

19. **B**, Page 470.

Mannitol and other osmotically active agents have not been proven beneficial in treating edema in this injury. *A* is done to prevent stress/gastric ulceration, *C* to limit edema and subsequent neurologic deficit progression, and *D* to prevent bladder overdistension and/or monitoring of urine output. Also, sheepskin should be used early to prevent pressure necrosis in denervated skin.

23
Pulmonary and Chest Wall Injuries

1. **C**, Page 473.

Use of binders, belts, and restrictive dressings should not be used; they promote hypoventilation, subsequent atelectasis, and pneumonia.

2. **C**, Page 478.

Pulmonary contusion is described as lung parenchymal damage with edema and hemorrhage without pulmonary laceration. Most commonly caused by motor vehicle accidents. There is an increased pulmonary membrane permeability.

3. **D**, Page 479.

Pulmonary contusion occurs within minutes, apparent on x-ray, is localized to a lobe or segment, and lasts 48–72 hours. Adult respiratory distress syndrome develops 24–72 hours and tends to be diffuse.

4. **D.**

   Fractures 1–2 ribs can cause serious injury. Fifty percent of cases have avulsion of aorta distal to the subclavian artery. All are seen except *D*.

5. **B**, Pages 476–478.

   Commonly missed injury resulting from blunt trauma is often associated with pulmonary contusions. It alters respiration adversely, with a paradoxical motion of the chest wall. Flail segment paradoxically moves inward on inspiration and outward on expiration. Three or more adjacent ribs are fractured at two points.

6. **A**, Page 479.

   A widening $P(A-A)O_2$ indicates a decreased pulmonary diffusion capacity of the contused lung. No increase occurs before clinical changes occur.

7. **E**, Page 480.

   These injuries are infrequently life-threatening; only 4% are severe lacerations. They are usually associated with hemopneumothorax, multiple fractures, and hemoptysis. These will require thoracotomy.

8. **D**, Page 478.

   Kinetic injury is dissipated into underlying tissue. Patients will have relatively innocuous-appearing nonpenetrating injury. The heart, liver, spleen, and spinal cord have been shown to be vulnerable to injury. All victims must be closely observed.

9. **D**, Page 482.

   Tube thoracostomy has the potential complications of hemothorax, pulmonary edema, bronchopleural fistula, pleural leaks, empyema, subcutaneous emphysema, and ipsilateral pneumothorax.

10. **E**, Pages 478, 479.

   Pulmonary contusion is present in 30–75% of patients with blunt chest trauma, usually automobile accidents. It is also caused by shock waves of an explosion in air or water and by high velocity missiles.

24
Vascular and Cardiac Injuries

1. **C**, Page 488.

   The most common sign of a myocardial contusion is sinus tachycardia. Chest pain may occur immediately but is usually delayed, occurring from 24 hours to 3 days after initial injury.

2. **E**, Page 488.

   The contused heart at autopsy has a discrete area of hemorrhage often located in the anterior wall of the right ventricle or atria, and is usually subendocardial

in nature but may extend in a pyramidal transmural fashion. A contusion may cause coronary thrombosis, but this usually occurs in the already diseased atheromatous vessel.

3. **A**, Page 494.

   The most common symptom found is retrosternal or interscapular pain present in about 25% of patients with an aortic injury.

4. **A**, Page 494.

   Most tears of the ascending aorta occur within the pericardium leading to the development of a pericardial tamponade, and therefore one sees the physical finding of pericardial tamponade.

5. **D**, Page 494.

   Sympathetic afferent nerve fibers located in the area of the aortic isthmus capable of causing reflex hypertension as a response to a stretching stimulus have been discovered and explain the high incidence of generalized hypertension.

6. **C**, Page 489.

   The most common sign of a myocardial contusion is sinus tachycardia. This sign is present in approximately 70% of patients with documented myocardial contusions.

7. **A**, Page 492.

   The clinical presentation of a patient who has sustained a myocardial rupture is usually that of a cardiac tamponade. Of great assistance in the early identification of these injuries is the monitoring of the central venous pressure in all patients with severe trauma admitted to the emergency department.

25
Acute Pericardial Tamponade

1. **C**, Pages 501, 502.

   As intrapericardial pressure and volume are increased, there is an initial rise in venous pressure while arterial pressure is maintained. This will often be reflected in neck vein distension and elevation of CVP greater than 15-cm H_2O.

2. **D**, Pages 502, 503.

   A and *B* are helpful if present but are uncommon and nonspecific. *C* may be helpful if there is a large enough volume of pericardial fluid involved. However, ultrasound is not usually readily available and is not therapeutic. *A* properly performed pericardiocentesis in a patient who is deteriorating may prove diagnostic and therapeutic.

3. **D**, Pages 503.

   Even in this critical setting, management of the airway is still the first priority.

26
Esophageal and Diaphragmatic Injuries

1. **C**, Pages 508, 509.
2. **A**, Pages 508, 509.
3. **F**, Pages 508, 509.
4. **B**, Pages 508, 509.
5. **E**, Pages 508, 509.
   1. The mid-esophagus is an unusual site for perforation except as a complication of the EOA. 2. Endoscopic perforation tends to occur near the esophageal introitus distally or at the site of preexisting disease, especially caustic burns. 3. In children less than 4 years of age, the cricopharyngeal narrowing is the usual point of foreign body impaction. 4. The esophagus is weakest distally in the left posterior aspect, and this is the common site of emetic and pressure-induced rupture. 5. Both nasotracheal intubation and passage of Ewald tube can result in esophageal perforation at the pyriform sinus.
6. **D**, Pages 508–509.
   While more than 80% of spontaneous esophageal ruptures occur in intoxicated middle-aged males, usually with retching against a closed cricopharyngeal muscle, intoxication also predisposes to esophageal foreign bodies, due to loss of oral tactile sensation. Since spontaneous rupture results in almost instantaneous massive mediastinal contamination, normal vital signs and CXR hours after the event makes foreign body more likely.
7. **D**, Page 511.
   Spontaneous pneumomediastinum is probably due to extreme valsalva maneuvers and is clinically benign. It generally occurs in younger patients and low-grade fever may be present. There are no associated pulmonary infiltrates, pleural effusions, or mediastinal air fluid levels.
8. **B**, Page 507.
   In the absence of esophageal disease, it is very unusual for a foreign body perforation to occur anywhere outside the following three levels: The cricopharyngeal muscle, the left mainstem bronchus, and at the gastroesophageal junction.
9. **C**, Pages 513, 514, 516.
   The chest x-ray can be normal in 20–40% of cases and is often nonspecific, therefore necessitating serial examinations.
10. **B**, Page 514.
    Diaphragmatic injuries can mimic each of the choices listed (especially in the delayed phase) except renal colic.
11. **B**, Pages 512–514.

Both large and small diaphragmatic tears do not heal spontaneously, because of visceral herniation and negative pressure gradient. 85% of patients will progress to the obstructive stage within 3 years. Repair of all diaphragmatic tears should be considered.

12. **D**, Pages 514, 516, 517.
    Diaphragmatic injury may increase the false *negative* rate of peritoneal lavage. Lavage may be falsely negative in isolated diaphragmatic injury and when the injured abdominal structure is herniated through the diaphragm into the chest. The presence of a diaphragmatic tear would preclude a "false" positive lavage.

27
Abdominal Trauma

1. **A**, Page 519.
   Blunt injuries carry a greater mortality because of the increased difficulties of diagnosis and the common association with severe concomitant trauma to multiple intraperitoneal organs and extraabdominal systems.
2. **B**, Page 521.
   Free intraperitoneal air is not an indication for laparotomy in stab wounds to the abdomen because this may be from introduction of air from outside with the penetrating implement. Since a significant number of stab wounds do not reach the peritoneum, local wound exploration is a useful technique prior to peritoneal lavage.
3. **C**, Pages 520–524.
   Stabbing trauma has a lower incidence of intraperitoneal injury, making selective management with serial observation, wound exploration, and peritoneal lavage the main modalities in stable patients. Peritoneal lavage is more accurate and has more stringent criteria for stabbing trauma. The mortality of gunshot trauma is higher than stabbing trauma.
4. **C**, Page 526.
   In the Davis et al. series, the physical findings most associated with internal injury are abdominal tenderness and guarding in 75% of patients. Peritoneal signs of rebound tenderness and rigidity occur in 28% of patients. Pain and blood on rectal examination is uncommon.
5. **B**, Page 519 (Table 27–1).
   Because it is the largest and heaviest solid organ in the abdomen and because of its fixation, the liver is the most commonly injured organ in penetrating

trauma. This occurs with a 37% incidence, followed by small bowel (26%), stomach (19%), colon (16.5%), and spleen (7%).

6. **D**, Pages 520–521.

   In stabbing trauma, implements in situ are most safely removed in the operating room, except when the implement impedes the emergency department resuscitation.

7. **D**, Pages 523, 524.

   Local exploration of wounds is not indicated in cases of gunshots because of the greater technical difficulty and hazard in visualizing extensive missile tracks and the tendency to underestimate the degree of damage. All the other responses are appropriate managements.

8. **B**, Page 526 (Table 27–4).

   The spleen is the most commonly injured organ with an incidence of 41%. In nearly two-thirds of these cases it is an isolated injury. The next organ injured is the liver at 19%.

9. **D**, Page 527.

   In injuries attributed to shoulder-lap seatbelts, the most common injury is rib fractures, while abdominal injuries have a low incidence. A solitary lap seatbelt results most commonly in abdominal injuries.

10. **C**, Page 529.

    When hypotension accompanies significant blunt trauma and is unexplained, one should assume intraperitoneal hemorrhage until proven otherwise. A head injury alone does not explain shock except in the preterminal stage or with very small infants.

11. **D**, Page 530.

    The amylase serum level is an unreliable test for pancreatic injury because hyperamylasemia can be found in patients who used narcotics, alcohol, and various other drugs. In a study of hyperamylasemia and blunt trauma, the cause was due to pancreas in 8%, other intraabdominal organs in 59%, and no injury was noted in 33%.

12. **B**, Page 531 (Fig. 27–4).

    A rupturing of a hollow retroperitoneal viscus can be detected by a stippling pattern, outlining the duodenum, kidney, or psoas muscle.

13. **C**, Pages 531, 533.

    The ultrasound is of limited value for thoracic lesion since visualization is obscured by the ribs and sternum. Other uses of ultrasound are in diagnosis of abruptio placentae, hemorrhage or enlargement of the pancreas, subcapsular hematomas, and intraperitoneal and retroperitoneal fluid collections.

14. **D**, Page 529.

    Pain referred to the testicles is compatible with a retroperitoneal injury and occurs most commonly with urogenital and duodenal injuries.

15. **C**, Page 537.

    The gravid uterus offers some protection to in-traperitoneal organs, thus the incidence of maternal deaths is extremely low. The rate of fetal mortality is considerable, ranging from 50–75%. Fetal injury is increased proportionately with the duration of pregnancy and uterine size.

16. **C**, Page 537.

    In the third trimester a vena caval compression may occur if the patient lies supine, resulting in a reduced preload and cardiac output. If spinal injuries are not suspected, the patient should be placed laterally or at a slight tilt.

17. **E**, Page 538.

    A maternal hemorrhage may cause a 10–20% reduction in uterine perfusion and may further delay the maternal signs of hypotension. In this instance fetal monitoring may reveal distress and a decrease in fetal heart tones, which may be a sign of imminent maternal shock.

18. **B**, Page 540.

    This is Kehr's sign of splenic rupture. Referred pain to the left shoulder tip occurs with this sign and is increased if the left upper quadrant is palpated after patient is in Trendelenburg position for a few minutes. This increases the pooling of blood next to the left diaphragm, causing phrenic nerve irritation.

19. **B**, Page 522.

    The dome of the diaphragm extends under the ribs and often is involved in penetrating chest trauma. Since this injury is associated with a minimal hemorrhage or free air as in other abdominal organ trauma, the criteria for lower chest wounds is reduced.

28
Genitourinary Trauma

1. **D**, Page 551.

   One report shows 6–68% of all renal injury admission as penetrating with the remaining 92–94% as blunt.

2. **C**, Page 551.

   IVP demonstrates an intact capsule, only intrarenal extravasation of dye, and disruption of pelvicaliceal system. However, it is possible to get extrarenal dye extravasation if there is an associated cortical tear with the caliceal laceration.

3. **D**, Page 552.

   Both may present without hematuria but with signficant morbidity and mortality if not diagnosed. It is due mainly to an abrupt cessation in urine production and flow.

4. **A**, Page 553.

This solution is given rapidly intravenously in the adult. Also, in adults 100 ml of a 60% solution may be used. In children, 2 ml/kg of body weight of 50% Hypaque solution is used.

5. **E**, Page 554.

All of the above represent renal compromise in one form or another, whether it is from decrease in renal blood flow, obstruction secondary to calculi, or intrinsic renal disease, making the kidney more susceptible to injury.

6. **B**, Page 555.

Abdominal pain following trauma and a positive peritoneal lavage do not necessarily require an IVP provided there are no other signs or symptoms referrable to the GU tract.

7. **E**, Page 555.

Unilateral enlargement of a kidney could be secondary to edema, which can also obliterate the psoas shadow. Spine scoliosis, loss of psoas shadow, and displaced bowel are all signs of retroperitoneal hemorrhage or urine extravasation.

8. **A**, Page 556.

Any patient in shock must first be stabilized prior to angiography.

9. **E**, Page 559.

Class I and II lesions can be treated nonsurgically with close observation in the hospital and bedrest. Antibiotics are indicated in Type III lesions, which are being treated nonsurgically.

10. **E**, Page 559.

Deep renal parenchymal and collecting system lacerations (Class III) will require surgery if there is significant hemorrhage, vascular injury, or urinary extravasation. Otherwise, it is up to the surgeon to operate on Class III lesions. Class I and II lesions do not require surgery.

11. **A**, Page 559.

According to some authors, hydronephrosis is more prevalent by far in the general population, and predisposes to traumatic rupture of the ureter or pelvis.

12. **B**, Page 559.

7.5% is a figure from one large study and is low enough that one may not sufficiently be suspicious of renal injuries. The liver is the most likely intrabdominal organ to be injured in penetrating trauma.

13. **C**, Page 561.

Children's kidneys are relatively larger, increasing the risk for injury. Ossification centers in the 10th and 11th ribs do not close until the second decade, thus their rib cage offers less protection.

14. **A**, Page 561.

Since traumatic injuries are rare, significant abdominal trauma must occur. Therefore, since the small intestines are the most mobile organ in the abdomen, with blunt, acceleration, and deceleration injuries, the small intestines and its mesentery are most susceptible to injury.

15. **B**, Page 562.

In almost all cases of blunt trauma, avulsion is at the ureteropelvic junction and 32% of ureteral injuries present without hematuria. These injuries are not associated with any particular clinical picture and cause few symptoms.

16. **C**, Page 562, 563.

Retrograde ureterography has greater concentration of dye because it is not diluted with urine for better delineation of injury. All ureteral injuries should be repaired surgically.

17. **D**, Pages 563, 564.

Intraperitoneal ruptures are life-threatening, requiring surgical repair and suprapubic catheter drainage.

18. **E**, Page 564.

The obturator fat line can be displaced by a pelvic hematoma, and ileus can be due to extravasated urine.

19. **B**, Page 564.

Self-explanatory.

20. **D**, Page 567.

Meatal blood is highly suspicious for urethral injury. Passage of rubber tube should not be attempted if blood is present. Urethrogram is indicated with meatal blood.

21. **B**, Page 567.

Posterior urethral tears demonstrate a complete transection of the urethra at the prostatic apex, and thus the patient is not able to void. The prostate is high-riding and boggy due to hematoma. They are almost always caused by auto or motorcycle accidents and are frequently associated with pelvic fractures.

22. **D**, Page 566.

This injury is caused by straddle-type injuries where the urethra is crushed against the inferior border of the pubic bone. They maintain a good urinary stream. Only rarely will sphincter spasm occur preventing voiding.

23. **E**, Page 567.

Incontinence results from injury to the urogenital diaphragm and bladder neck. Stricture formation depends on extent of injury, presence of infection, and length of time urethral stent left in place. Potency is influenced entirely by degree of damage to vessels and nerves.

24. **A**, Page 569.

Beyond 6 hours local reshaping is the standard therapy.

25. **C**, Page 569.

May be treated surgically, involving hematoma evacuation, suturing of tunica albuginea, and pressure dressing. Also may be treated nonsurgically with bedrest, early ice packs for 2 -48 hours, then heat, a pressure dressing, and sometimes a Foley catheter.

26. **A**, Page 569.

Self-limiting disease most often caused by vigorous intercourse. It presents as a firm, nontender, cordlike structure that will resolve on its own in 4–8 weeks if not further traumatized.

27. **E**, Page 569.

The fibrotic area of the carpora cavernosum urethra causes decreased penile distensibility with subsequent painful curved erections.

28. **B**, Page 570.

80% of testicular dislocations are found in the abdominal wall. Careful examination of the scrotum is important in trauma victims since the scrotum may not appear empty due to hematoma.

29. **B**, Page 570.

In pelvic fractures the cystogram is first so that distal ureteral dye from the IVP will not mimic bladder extravasation. On the other hand, flank and rib injuries are more likely to have more proximal pathology, so the IVP is done first so no residual bladder dye will obscure the distal ureters. Should both investigations be indicated, it is wise to start with the cystogram.

29
Thermal Injury (Burns)

1. **B**, Page 575.

The presence of blistering without deeper damage makes this a 2nd degree burn. The most reliable sign of a full thickness burn is the presence of thrombosed blood vessels. Charring of the skin and subcutaneous tissues is considered 4th degree.

2. **E**, Pages 575, 576.

Burn shock is associated with all of these factors. Acute renal failure secondary to the profound hypovolemia is seen if adequate fluid resuscitation is not given.

3. **A**, Page 580.

All patients with major burns require hospitalization. Major burns include: in adults, 2nd degree with greater than 18% TBSA or 3rd degree with greater than 5% TBSA; in children 2nd degree with greater than 12% TBSA or 3rd degree with greater than 5%

TBSA; burns to airway, face, hands, perineum, or feet; presence of significant other disease, i.e., diabetes or severe cardiac disease; and associated smoke inhalation or any electrical burn.

4. **E**, Page 583.

The Neosporin isn't the removal factor but the ointment vehicle is. The ointment contains polyoxyethylene sorbitan, which will dissolve the tar and since it is water-soluble, will facilitate washing off the residue. Alternative agents are Tween 80 or Neosporin cream.

5. **A**, Pages 578, 579.

Moist air carries many times more heat than dry air. The upper airways are extremely efficient heat exchanges and can reduce the temperature of dry hot air from 280° to 50°C from the nose to the trachea and bronchi. Respiratory complications are the major cause of mortality in burn victims. The goal of therapy is to provide adequate ventilation, maintain a patent airway, and give maximal tissue oxygenation.

6. **D**, Page 580.

Early elevation of a burned extremity with active exercise may eliminate the need for an emergency escharotomy. All of the answers are appropriate indications for escharotomy, as well as decreasing pulse strength distal to the burn.

7. **C**, Page 580.

Metabolic acidosis (caused by inhibition of carbonic anhydrase) is a side effect of mafenide acetate therapy. However, mafenide acetate remains preferred over silver sulfadiazine for therapy of massively colonized burns because it has better penetration properties.

8. **D**, Page 580.

Gram-negative organisms are the most serious pathogens isolated from infected burns. These organisms usually are from the patient's own GI tract and not from external sources. The incidence of infection may be reduced by gentle hydrotherapy to remove dead tissue and topical antibacterial agents.

9. **B**, Page 579.

The half-life of carboxyhemoglobin is 5.5 hours in 21% FiO_2, 1.5 hours in 100% FiO_2, and 20 minutes in 3 atm hyperbaric oxygen. High-flow oxygen is the mainstay of therapy, but hyperbaric oxygenation is indicated for patients with markedly elevated carboxyhemoglobin levels and acidosis.

30
Inhalation Injuries

1. **E**, Pages 601, 603.

   This patient presents with a history consistent with combined toxic levels of carbon monoxide and hydrogen cyanide exposure. He is in need of aggressive airway maintenance and immediate antidotal therapy, which would include amyl nitrite and sodium thiosulfate. You would want to avoid using sodium nitrite because this may cause worsening of hypotension (and worsen acidosis) as well as induce a fatal methemoglobinemia, particularly in children. In addition, hyperbaric oxygen therapy is indicated to reduce half-life of carboxyhemoglobin as adjunctive therapy. Fifty percent of the general population lack the genetic trait to detect odor of bitter almonds.

2. **C**, Pages 601, 602.

   Profound lactic acidosis commonly accompanies cyanide poisoning and the calculated anion gap is frequently 25–30 mEq/L. Bicarbonate levels are usually diminished, and if the pH is uncompromised, the serum potassium levels will be elevated.

3. **D**, Page 598.

   Only in the face of new electrocardiogram changes or with severe carbon monoxide exposure are serial cardiac enzymes indicated.

4. **B**, Page 587.

   Although evolution of byproducts varies with each material, the yield of the product is dependent on one of these four "critical" (A, C, D, E) factors either singly or in combination.

5. **A**, Pages 598, 599.

   Patients whose symptoms clear after oxygen therapy in the emergency department can be discharged; however, it is imperative that a follow-up examination be performed at 3 weeks to identify any delayed neuropsychiatric deficits.

6. **B**, Page 587.

   Although all of the above are toxic products of combustion of PVCs, the anhydrous HCl loosely bound to soot aerosol is delivered deep to the lung parenchyma and following hydration, a severe chemical pneumonitis occurs, which may closely parallel that of adult respiratory distress syndrome.

7. **C**, Page 597.

   Calculated oxygen saturation may be normal even in the face of profound carbon monoxide exposure. Only measured oxyhemoglobin saturation is considered accurate.

8. **D**, Page 596.

   Partial saturation of hemoglobin with carbon monoxide will result in a tighter bond with the remaining oxygen shifting the oxyhemoglobin dissociation curve to the left. This impairment of oxygen unloading will worsen the hypoxic state.

9. **C**, Pages 599, 600.

   All of the above are indicated in significant carbon monoxide exposures. Aggressive management of cerebral edema is indicated with hyperventilation, barbiturates, and diuretics. Hyperbaric oxygen is also helpful with its resultant cerebral vasoconstriction.

31
Frostbite

1. **C**, Page 609.

   Chilblain is a superficial form of cold injury. It is more commonly seen in young women. It is also perennial, starting with the first cold weather and spontaneously remitting with warm weather. A delay in relaxation of spastic vessels in these individuals with excessively high vascular tone in the extremities is the pathologic basis of the disorder. Raynaud's disease, collagen vascular disease, and macroglobulinemia predispose. The resulting vasculitis and edema in the dermis results in itching, burning, and red patchy swelling of the skin.

2. **A**, Page 610.

   Immersion or trenchfoot is a nonfreezing cold injury. It is seen with exposure to cold and wetness, usually less than 50°F, for more than 10 to 12 hours. It classically occurs in three phases: the initial ischemic phase resulting from vasoconstriction, a hyperemic phase resulting from the vasodilation of rewarming, and finally a recovery period during which depigmentation may occur. Hypersensitivity and pain with weight-bearing may persist for years after recovery.

3. **E**, Page 611.

   Frostbite is rarely seen in healthy people who are adequately dressed. There are always other associated factors but the largest predisposing factor (50% of cases in a study of 163 injuries) was alcoholic intake or mental illness. Acute injury is the common predisposing factor. Race is reportedly associated with susceptibility to frostbite with a greater racial predisposition in blacks. Acclimatization seems to protect individuals from frostbite since persistent exposure to cold results in less vasospasm and augments heat protection.

4. **E**, Pages 612, 613.

   Frostnip is not a true frostbite, since there is no loss of tissue, if it is treated immediately. Blister formation is characteristic of superficial and deep frostbite.

5. **D**, Page 613.

In superficial frostbite the injured area is white, non-blanching, but remains soft and resilient to the touch. Hard, unyielding tissue is characteristic of deep frostbite. The skin takes on a waxy appearance and is anesthetic. Bullae will form within 1–24 hours. In deep frostbite bullae formation is either absent or takes weeks to develop along the lines of demarcation.

6. **B**, Page 613.

Rapid rewarming has been shown to decrease tissue loss more than slow rewarming. Never partially rewarm frostbitten tissue because refreezing or partial thawing increases tissue loss. The water should remain at a constant temperature range (104–108°F) and should not exceed 112°F since rewarming temperatures above this result in thermal tissue damage and at lower rewarming temperatures the maximal benefits are not achieved.

7. **C**, Page 614.

All patients with significant frostbite should be hospitalized and kept in protective isolation to minimize risk of infection. The injured soft tissue is allowed to amputate itself spontaneously before extirpation and debridement occurs. All blebs (blisters) are left intact and covered with sterile sheets, and no dressings or ointments are applied if they rupture. Daily whirlpool therapy is indicated to decrease infection and antibiotics are used only for deep infections. Smoking is contraindicated due to the vasoconstrictive effects of nicotine.

8. **A**, Pages 613–615.

Rapid rewarming with immersion of the frozen part in water (warmed to 104–108°F) has been experimentally and clinically proven to be the treatment of choice for frostbite. Low molecular weight dextran infusion to increase capillary blood flow has been suggested, but experimental evidence is conflicting. Sympathectomy has been controversial for years and remains so. Clinical trials have failed to show anticoagulants to be of benefit.

9. **D**, Pa~

potential long-term complications
udy suggests that as many as 82%
tivity, 73% have skin color chan-
erhidrosis, and 39% have con-
s suffering deep frostbite may
normalities due to damage of
ers.

32
Chemical Injuries to Skin

1. **B**, Page 617.

Acute injury may be deceptively mild but may be followed by extensive fluid loss and systemic toxicity. This response may take as long as 36 hours to develop.

2. **A**, Pages 617, 618.

Few specific antidotes are known for chemical skin injuries. Delaying institution of water lavage for as little as 3 minutes shows increased skin injury, while delays up to 15 minutes result in irreversible damage, depending on the chemical agent.

3. **E**, Page 618.

Self-explanatory.

4. **E**, Page 618.

Self-explanatory.

5. **D**, Pages 618–620.

6. **A**, Pages 618–620.

7. **F**, Pages 618–620.

8. **B**, Pages 618–620.

9. **E**, Pages 618–620.

PEG 300 and IMS allow better removal and dilution of phenol than water alone; glycerol is an acceptable substitute if PEG 300/IMS is unavailable. Mace and tear gas are treated with water lavage and will not produce chemical injury. Epoxy glue is easily removed by acetone except around the eyes and mucous membranes where acetone is too drying and vegetable oil should be used. Quick lime readily changes to calcium hydroxide on exposure to water and causes deeper injury. Phosphorus is treated with water lavage and copper sulfate aids in finding all remaining particles.

10. **B**, Page 619.

Ten percent calcium gluconate should be injected subcutaneously using a 26-gauge needle at a dose of about 0.5 cc/cm^2 of visible skin involvement or, if the skin is too painful, subcutaneous tissue, whichever is greater.

11. **E**, Page 619.

PEG 300 and 400 and glycerol are acceptable substitutes when swabbed on the phenol exposure area for 5–10 minutes. Cresol and carboxylic acid are phenol derivatives requiring treatment.

12. **D**, Page 619.

The application of 1% copper sulfate solution will form an insoluble black precipitate of copper phosphate that can then be debrided.

13. **A and E**, Page 619.

Sodium and potassium may ignite spontaneously; the others listed will burn if ignited.

14. **C**, Page 619.

Lavage with water is contraindicated because it will result in the production of the corresponding hydroxide and hydrogen, which is an intensely exothermic reaction that may produce a significant thermal injury. Calcium oxide can produce severe alkali burns. Treatment should be prompt usually before transport.

15. **D**, Page 620.

Vegetable oil will provide satisfactory removal. Acetone will dissolve glue but is too drying to use in eyes or mucous membranes.

33
Electrical Injuries

1. **B**, Pages 622, 623.

Human muscle tissue responds well to electrical currents at frequencies of 40–60 cp. Above 150 cp, tissue is less responsive and the current is less dangerous. Fatalities have been reported with voltages as low as 45 V. Amperage is most directly related to severity of injury. There have been reports of complete neurologic recovery after being struck by lightning and having no vital signs and fixed, dilated pupils. The dominant myocardial injury seen in lightning injury is asystole.

2. **E**, Page 625.

GI injury has been reported in 7–25% of conductive electrical injuries. Injuries include hemorrhagic necrosis of the intestines and gall bladder, esophageal ulceration, stress ulcers, pancreatitis, appendicitis, and intestinal perforation. All patients with GI complaints should be thoroughly evaluated and reevaluated since GI injuries may not be immediately apparent.

3. **C**, Pages 621, 622.

The greatest injury rate is seen from infancy to 4 years of age with an equal sex distribution. This reflects primarily electrical cord and outlet injuries. The incidence peaks again in the 20–50-year-old age group with a male predominance. This reflects primarily injuries occurring in the industrial work environment.

4. **D**, Page 622.

As little as 20 mA will produce tetanic contractions preventing voluntary release. Human muscle tissue responds well to frequencies between 40 and 150 cp. Unfortunately, 60 cp household current is that to which we are most frequently exposed. Above 150 cp, human tissue response is markedly decreased.

5. **E**, Page 623.

The greater the resistance, the larger the heat generated and thus the larger the entrance or exit wound. The smaller area of contact concentrates the current flow and generated heat to one area, resulting in a larger wound. Larger contact areas distribute the current flow over a larger area reducing the size.

6. **C**, Pages 623, 624.

Oral commissure burns usually occur in children less than 2 years of age and are most often caused by chewing on a lamp cord or sucking on the end of a line outline at household currents. Tongue and palatine injuries are infrequent.

7. **D**, Page 624.

The flexion crease burn results from current passing through approximated skin layers, resulting in a cutaneous arc. These burns have been termed "the hallmark of true conductive electrical injuries."

8. **B**, Page 625.

Alternating current will frequently induce ventricular fibrillation, while asystole is the predominant rhythm disturbance with direct current injuries such as lightning strikes.

9. **E**, Page 626.

Renal injury most commonly occurs when myoglobin released from massive muscle necrosis deposits in the renal tubules. Direct renal trauma and hypovolemia may also contribute to renal injury. Some authors believe renal injury may be reduced by aggressive fluid resuscitation, urine alkalinization, and osmotic diuretics.

10. **B**, Page 627.

Cataracts and thermal eye burns occur in 1–9% suffering electrical injuries. A history of entrance or exit wounds around the head is common in the development of cataracts, which may take 6 months to 1 year to become evident. Vascularization of the lens, which protects cataract development, may be evident on slit lamp exam 1–2 weeks after injury.

11. **D**, Page 628.

The use of burn formulas to estimate fluid requirements in electrical injuries should not be considered because they are likely to underestimate the severity of injury. The adequacy of circulatory volumes should be judged on urine output, which should be maintained at or above 1 ml/kg/hour with isotonic crystalloids.

12. **E**, Page 626.

Peripheral nerve injuries in an affected extremity was reported in 90% of all electrical injuries and may be permanent in 1–7%.

13. **A**, Page 622.

Electrical flash burns are simple thermal burns resulting from arcing. They are not conductive injuries because the body is not part of the electrical circuit. They may be 1st, 2nd, or 3rd degree, but characteristically have the appearance described above.

34
Lightning Injuries

1. **D**, Pages 632–634.

Because the duration of current flow with lightning injuries is so short, the amount of energy delivered is often much less than in a high-voltage electrical injury. The paucity of skin burns may also be explained by the short duration in that the energy delivered seldom has time to break down the skin and cause significant tissue damage. Although lightning is not technically a direct current, its oscillations are so rapid and its waveforms are so complex that one may think of it as a direct current for practical purposes, and as such it will tend to cause ventricular asystole rather than fibrillation.

2. **B**, Pages 633–635.

Deep muscle damage and myoglobinuria are rare. Over 50% of victims have at least one TM ruptured. Two-thirds of the seriously injured patients have vascular spasm and sympathetic nervous system instability. Burns, although infrequent, occur from clothing fires or formation of steam from sweat or rain. Confusion, loss of consciousness, and antegrade amnesia are universal.

3. **D**, Pages 634, 635.

Lightning seldom causes significant burns or tissue destruction. Therefore, there is no need for aggressive fluid therapy as required in other high-voltage electrical burns.

35
Radiation Injuries

1. **C**, Page 639.

Neutrons, as opposed to the other choices, are able to render a normal atom radioactive by being "captured." This explains persistent radioactivity following adequate cleansing.

2. **C**, Page 640.

He is displaying central nervous system effects soon after the exposure, therefore he has received at least 2000 rad.

3. **D**, Pages 640, 642.

Half of the people exposed to 350 rad will die.

4. **A**, Page 641.

Those systems with the most rapid cellular division rates will be most affected. Delayed death is usually due to infection in the face of leukopenia.

5. **B**, Page 638.

Alpha particles are emitted by plutonium and have the lowest penetration capability of the various particles.

6. **D**, Page 641.

Significant ongoing radiation exposure is possible if the skin and clothing are not fully decontaminated.

7. **A**, Page 641.

The most accurate prognostic indicator is the absolute lymphocyte count at 48 hours postexposure. If greater than 1200, the chances of a lethal exposure are small.

36
Near-Drowning

1. **C**, Page 645.

Drowning is the fourth most common cause of death and is second only to motor vehicle accidents in males 1–34 years of age and females 15–19 years of age. Children under 4 years of age account for 40% of all drownings. This underscores the need to safety-proof swimming pools, bathtubs, and aquatic recreational areas.

2. **C**, Page 645.

When death occurs minutes to days following initial recovery, this is termed *secondary drowning*. *Near-drowning* implies recovery has occurred following submersion. *Immersion syndrome* is sudden death after submersion in very cold water, probably resulting from dsyrhythmias induced by vagal stimulation.

3. **B**, Page 646.

Autopsy studies demonstrate that only 15% of those who die of drowning have aspirated enough fluid to cause life-threatening changes in electrolyte concentrations or blood volume. Although the differences between fresh water and sea water aspiration have been emphasized traditionally and demonstrated experimentally, most victims do not aspirate enough fluid to cause life-threatening changes.

4. **A**, Page 647.

Aspiration of sea-water may raise the concentration of all serum because fluid is drawn into the lungs and blood volume decreases. Fresh-water aspiration lowers serum electrolyte concentrations. However, potassium may be elevated due to red blood cell lysis.

5. **E**, Page 646.

Blood volume is contracted because of the osmotic effects of the sea water in the lungs.

6. **C**, Page 649.

Shock is uncommon, but when present it should be ascertained whether it is due to hypoxia, spinal cord injury, or hypovolemia.

7. **D**, Page 651.

Caution is required in discharging near-drowning victims from the emergency department due to the possibility of delayed pulmonary complications. Asymptomatic patients should be observed for at least 4–6 hours. Reliable patients with normal chest x-rays and arterial blood gases may then be discharged with specific instructions for follow-up.

8. **D**, Page 650.

Prophylactic antibiotics have not been shown to improve survival and should be reserved for those with clinical signs of infection. The use of steroids for treatment of pulmonary aspiration is controversial, but several outcome studies do not support their routine use. Positive pressure ventilation with PEEP or CPAP are indicated for patients with pulmonary insufficiency requiring intubation. A patient with clinically obvious pulmonary problems may still have a normal chest x-ray.

9. **D**, Pages 647, 648.

The mammalian diving reflex is present in infants and children but is diminished in adults. This may account for the higher salvage rates in children. The resulting hypothermia may have both beneficial and disastrous effects. In addition to imitating the diving reflex, hypothermia decreases metabolic demands and prevents or delays severe cerebral hypoxia. Hypothermia may, however, induce ventricular fibrillation and death. Successful resuscitation with neurologic recovery following submersion of up to 40 minutes has been reported. Furthermore, a severe hypothermic state may be indistinguishable from death. Aggressive core recovery is indicated.

37
Diving Injuries

1. **C**, Page 653.

Only nitrogen exerts toxic effects from increased partial pressure during sport diving.

2. **D**, Page 653.

Nitrogen narcosis, also known as "rapture of the deep," is caused by the nitrogen interfering with nerve conduction - like an anesthetic. Pulmonary overinflation is not associated with it.

3. **A**, Page 654.

Boyle's law states that as the pressure on a gas increases the volume changes inversely while temperature remains at a constant.

4. **D**, Pages 654, 655.

An antibiotic should be prescribed if a tympanic membrane rupture is present. A search of other squeeze syndromes should be prompted by the presentation above. A bloody nasal discharge could be associated with a middle-ear squeeze, but the headache should prompt one to also consider a sinus squeeze. The Frenzel maneuver is better than Valsalva's maneuver to prevent inner ear barotrauma, and hemotympanum dictates no further dives for 2–4 weeks.

5. **C**, Pages 656, 657.

The 20-year-old diver should have an expiratory view of the chest to rule out pneumothorax. The 30-year-old has Hamman's crunch. The 50-year-old is beyond the time limit noted for pulmonary overinflation syndrome. Another cause of his chest pain should be sought.

6. **B**, Pages 657, 658.

Dissolved gases come out of solution and form bubbles in the body when there is a decrease and tissues that are supersaturated begin to release nitrogen bubbles into the bloodstream and alveoli.

7. **D**, Pages 657, 658.

For unknown reasons older individuals have a higher incidence of DCS.

8. **C**, Pages 657, 659.

Although a thorough neurologic exam should be done, approximately 30% of those with Type I DCS have or will develop Type II DCS.

9. **B**, Pages 658, 659.

Symptoms of "chokes" can occur up to 12 hours after a dive and may persist for 12 to 48 hours.

10. **D**, Pages 658, 659.

11. **E**, Pages 658–660.

Although treatment should be started as soon as possible, patients should be transported for recompression therapy regardless of the time delay. Some patients may respond 10 to 14 days after the onset of symptoms.

38
Accidental Hypothermia

1. **B**, Page 663.
   As defined.
2. **A**, Page 664.
   The Babinski reflex is ongoing until it disappears at 26°C, followed soon after by the knee-jerk reflex.
3. **D**, Page 666.
   This is why the curled position to decrease the body surface area is so important.
4. **D**, Pages 667, 668.
   Increased thyroid hormone will aid in thermogenesis.
5. **E**, Page 669.
   All of the listed drugs predispose to hypothermia.
6. **C**, Page 670.
   A clue that blood gases are uncorrected is that a PaO_2 on room air is not physiologically possible. Partial pressures of O_2 and CO_2 increase with falling temperature while pH falls.
7. **A**, Page 670.
   For each degree Centigrade drop in temperature the pH should be corrected upward approximately .015.
   $$37 - 31 = 6$$
   $$6 \times .015 = .09$$
   $$.09 + 7.2 = 7.29$$
8. **B**, Page 672.
   Osborn waves appear between 25°C and 30°C and are a small positive deflection (avL, avF, and left precordial leads) at the junction of the QRS and the ST segment.
9. **D**, Page 673.
   A patient is not pronounced dead until he or she is warmed sufficiently without response. Numerous reports exist of neurologic recovery following long down times in the presence of hypothermia.
10. **D**, Page 674.
    This is the most effective field method for active rewarming
11. **C**, Pages 674, 678.
    Response to countershock is not usually seen until the core temperature is above 28°C.
12. **D**, Page 677.
    In mild hypothermia in an otherwise healthy individual, preventing further heat loss may correct the problem. Because humans are functionally unable to raise the core temperature when body temperature is less than 30°C, passive techniques are ineffective. In this range. Core temperature after drop may occur with this technique because cold blood from the periphery is shunted to the core due to peripheral vasodilation.

39
Heat Illness

1. **A**, Page 693.
   Active cooling is necessary at this temperature to maintain normothermia.
2. **D**, Page 693.
   Evaporation of sweat is the most effective mechanism because of the proportionately large heat of vaporization of water.
3. **B**, Page 695.
   Exercise or heat can decrease renal blood flow by 50%.
4. **D**, Pages 700, 703.
   Hypertonic solutions greatly aid in replacing lost electrolytes and protect against heat cramps.
5. **A**, Page 704.
   In order to make the diagnosis of heat exhaustion, it is necessary that mental function be unimpaired.
6. **E**, Pages 707, 708.
   The acute onset in the context of intense physical stress indicates exertional heat stroke as opposed to heat stroke, which comes on over days of heat exposure.
7. **C**, Page 710.
   Cold inhaled air is ineffective and ice water enemas can lead to water intoxication.
8. **B**, Pages 706, 707.
   The liver is extremely sensitive to heat stroke, which results in a decreased ability to clear lactate prolonging the metabolic acidosis. Myoglobinuria and renal failure are common due to muscle damage. Cardiac enzymes rise as well. The cerebellum is the most sensitive area of the brain.
9. **A**, Pages 706–708.
   The calcium is usually normal but can be drastically reduced in the presence of diffuse muscle damage. Phosphorous is decreased, supposedly due to heat-induced hyperventilation. Increased SGOT is due to hepatocyte damage and the PT is prolonged due to clotting factor abnormalities.

40
Orthopedic Injuries

1. **D**, Pages 718, 720.
   A fracture should be suspected if navicular (snuff box) tenderness is elicited despite a negative radiograph. Treatment involves application of a splint and follow-up radiographs if no improvement is seen 1 week later.

2. **C**, Page 733.
   The cast has been applied too tightly. A compartment syndrome is unlikely because the injury occurred 3 weeks previously. One must cut *both* the plaster cast as well as the inner padding to alleviate pressure. Fracture reduction is maintained by the application of the stockinette.

3. **C**, Pages 723–724.
   Greenstick fractures are a type of simple fracture. Dislocations should be radiographed before *and* after reduction. First-degree sprains exhibit *no* joint instability, and Salter IV fractures often cause growth arrest.

4. **B**, Pages 719–720.
   Reduction is best performed in the OR and is contraindicated until the wound has been irrigated and debrided. All other treatments are appropriate and mandatory.

5. **A**, Page ???.
   This radiograph depicts dorsal displacement of the distal radius. This question is intended to assist in distinguishing displacement from angulation. Compare text Figures 40–2 and 40–4.

41
Shoulder

1. **B**, Pages 736–739.
   Because of the proximity of the branchial plexus and especially the radial and axillary nerves, fractures of the humeral surgical neck most often result in neurovascular damage.

2. **C**, Page 738.
   Only three-part humeral fractures mandate open reduction and internal fixation (ORIF).

3. **A**, Pages 741–742.
   The patient's arm position is almost pathognomonic of an anterior shoulder dislocation. However, a prereduction radiograph should always be obtained.

4. **D**, Pages 744–746.
   Of all shoulder dislocations 2% are posterior, and the patient cannot perform external rotation or abduction. The subacromial position is the most common; however the axillary nerve is hardly ever involved.

5. **D**, Pages 741–746.
   Posterior dislocations are often missed on A-P radiographs. The glenoid fossa is often fractured and most posterior dislocations are subacromial. The Hill-Sachs deformity occurs mostly with anterior dislocations.

6. **A**, Page 747.
   Fractures of the body of the scapula are by far the most common. They usually heal rapidly and with little residual disability. They do result from high energy impact; therefore, the examining physician should rule out other injuries.

42
Humerus and Elbow

1. **B**, Pages 749–751.
   Nondisplaced elbow fractures are often not seen on routine elbow films. A sign indicative of an interarticular fracture is the "fat pad sign." Normally the fat pad lies posteriorly within the olecranon fossa. When the elbow joint is distended by an effusion or hemarthrosis, the posterior fat pad is displaced away from the cortex of the humerus, creating an area of radiolucency projecting posteriorly through the distal humerus on the lateral view. The anterior fat pad sign is a less sensitive indicator since it is frequently seen on normal x-ray films of the elbow.

2. **B**, Pages 749–752 (Fig. 42–2).
   In a fracture of the supracondylar area of the humerus, the distal fragment is displaced posteriorly and proximally. This allows the proximal fragment of bone to project into the antecubital fossa, compressing the brachial artery and median nerve.

3. **D**, Pages 752–753.
   Intercondylar fractures are rare and are generally seen in older adults, where the bones are more brittle. The injury in *A* is common in children but rare after age 20. Choice *B* is more common in children than adults, probably because the tensile strength of the collateral ligaments and the elbow joint capsule in children are greater than that of bone. Because both bones are tethered by the interosseous membrane, a dislocation of the radial head without an associated fracture is rare in adults.

4. **C**, Pages 757–759.
   The shaft of the humerus is a common site for metastatic disease. Radiographs of humeral fractures should be reviewed for evidence of metastatic disease.

43
Forearm

1. **A**, Page 764.
   Any patient with a fracture in the region of the elbow who has pain and altered sensation should be treated as if a compartment syndrome were developing.

2. **B**, Page 764.
Volkmann's ischemic contracture may result from the compartment syndrome described in Question 1.
3. **D**, Pages 761–764.
Radial-ulnar fractures are almost always displaced and usually require open reduction and internal fixation. Fractures of the radius usually can be treated by closed reduction. Proximal ulnar fractures are notorious for becoming displaced.
4. **B**, Page 772.
Perilunate dislocations are the most common carpal or fracture dislocation. Scaphoid fractures are the most common type of nondisplaced carpal fracture.
5. **C**, Page 771.
Dorsal chip fractures of the carpal bones most commonly involve the triquetrum.

44

Hand

1. **B**, Pages 776–777.
The lesion described is a "herpetic whitlow." These must be distinguished from a paronychia because herpetic whitlow is best treated nonsurgically in the manner described above. The diagnosis is made by both the appearance of the finger and by the presence of other characteristic lesions—such as blisters and ulcers—usually found in or around the mouth.
2. **B**, Pages 775–776.
The so-called "fish mouth incision" used to be one type of incision used for drainage of a felon. It is no longer advocated because it creates an unstable fingertip from severed septa.
3. **C**, Pages 775–778.
Patients with lymphangitis should be hospitalized, the hand and arm should be elevated and wrapped in a warm compressive dressing, and broad spectrum antibiotic coverage should be initiated until culture results are obtained.
4. **B**, Page 786–788.
This injury is an avulsion of the flexor digitorum profoundus tendon, usually caused by a forceful hyperextension of the DIP joint while the tendon is in maximum traction. The x ray films may or may not show an avulsed bony fragment. Occasionally the tendon retracts to the PIP joint or the level of the palm causing tenderness at that point. The diagnosis is made by demonstrating the inability of the patient to actively flex his DIP joint with the MP and PIP joints in full extension. Treatment is always operative.

5. **B**, Page 792.
Fractures of the metacarpal neck of the ring and little fingers with angulation of less than 10° may be immobilized without reduction, and angulation of 40° in older fractures (if clawing is not present) is acceptable. Any angulation in fractures of the second and third metacarpal necks must be reduced.

45

Cervical Hyperextension Injuries

1. **B**, Page 800.
The injury is not limited to ligamentous injury. It can also involve minor hematoma formation and muscle tears.
2. **A**, Pages 799, 800.
Hyperextension of the neck would not occur if the body is not accelerated relative to the head.
3. **B**, Pages 800, 801.
Subdural hematomas from torn bridging veins and retinal hemorrhages are pathologic changes seen in the shaken baby syndrome. An epidural hematoma would be unusual.
4. **D**, Page 801.
The history of shaking is usually not obtained until after objective evidence for abuse is obtained.
5. **C**, Page 802.
Retinal hemorrhages are seen on funduscopic examination.
6. **B**, Pages 805, 806.
7. **C**, Pages 805, 806.
8. **A**, Pages 805, 806.
9. **B**, Pages 806–808.
Nerve root irritation almost always radiates beyond the knee, often involving the foot. Others are self-explanatory.
10. **D**, Page 811.
Computed tomography is considered more accurate and more cost-effective than myelogram. The role of the magnetic resonance imaging has not been fully defined. Radionuclide imaging is useful only in localizing infectious and metastatic lesions

46
Pelvis and Thigh

1. **B**, Page 840.
   Avascular necrosis occurs most commonly after fractures of the neck of the femur. Tears of the posterior capsule such as those that occur during dislocations of the hip account for a significant number of these cases as well.
2. **C**, Page 836.
   The Ortolani click test should be performed as a routine part of every examination on all infants under 1 year of age to diagnose congenital hip dislocation. The hip is flexed 90° and the thigh is abducted. In infants with subluxation or dislocation, abduction is restricted and the involved hip is unable to be abducted as far as the opposite normal side, producing an audible click as the femoral head slips over the acetabular lip.
3. **D**, Pages 855–857.
   In some cases of iliopectineal bursitis, the physician may be able to palpate a mass lateral to the femoral vessels. This must be differentiated from a femoral hernia, psoas abscess, and synovitis of the joint.
4. **D**, Page 854.
   Myositis ossificans is a common condition in which extraarticular ossification occurs within a muscle or a group of muscles. It is most often seen in the thigh following a moderate or severe contusion and can usually be diagnosed 2 to 4 weeks following injury to the thigh. The patients are usually young, athletic individuals who have returned to active use of the quadriceps too early following injury to the thigh.
5. **C**, Pages 826–827.
   Posterior pelvic fractures are associated with more extensive hemorrhage than anterior pelvic fractures. The abdominal aorta descends to the left of the midline and divides at L4 into the common iliac arteries. At the level of the sacroiliac joints, the common iliac arteries divide, forming the external and internal iliac arteries. At this point these vessels (and the accompanying veins) are exposed to shearing forces when fractures occur in this area.
6. **D**, Pages 834–836.
   Tears of the posterior capsule such as those that occur during dislocations of the hip account for a significant number of cases of avascular necrosis of the femoral head.
7. **A**, Pages 833–834.
   Transient synovitis of the hip is a common, short-lived, nonspecific inflammation of the synovium of the hip. Often attributed to a mild traumatic episode or a low-grade febrile illness such as tonsillitis or otitis media.
8. **B**, Pages 832–833.
   Staphylococcus aureus in the most common organism causing septic arthritis of the hip. Other organisms that can cause this condition are *Streptococcus pyogenes* and *Haemophilus influenzae*.
9. **A**, Pages 833–834.
   Transient synovitis of the hip occurs most often in boys between the ages of 5 and 6. The onset of the condition is usually insidious, with the child complaining of pain in the hip that radiates down into the thigh and the knee. The temperature is usually normal to slightly elevated and is rarely high.
10. **B**, Pages 832–833.
    Septic arthritis is a disease of the young, and when the hip joint is affected age range is usually even lower: 70% of cases occur in patients 4 years old or younger. On examination the child has a high temperature, is irritable, has tenderness anteriorly in the groin and over the hip joint, and appears in a toxic state.

47
Proximal Femur and Femoral Shaft

1. **B**, Pages 839–841.
   Fracture of the superior aspect occurs with *anterior* dislocation. Impaction forces always are the cause of comminuted femoral head fractures, which often occur in conjunction with acetabulum fractures. Avascular necrosis is a common complication.
2. **A**, Pages 839–841.
   Often no history of trauma is obtained. The other statements are true.
3. **C**, Page 845.
   Application of a Thomas splint to a patient with a compound femur fracture with bone proturding is contraindicated because of the risk of osteomyelitis. All other choices are correct.
4. **D**, Pages 863–892.
   All are associated with distal femoral fractures. Additionally, damage to quadriceps apparatus is often seen.

5. **A**, Page 846.

Slipped capital femoral epiphysis occurs in children between the ages of 10 and 16 years. The patient may come to the emergency department with a history of minor trauma or strain several weeks to months before and symptoms continuing since this trivial episode. One should suspect the disorder in any adolescent who limps and complains of hip or knee pain associated with restriction of internal rotation of the hip.

6. **A**, Page 846.

These are the x-ray views that will demonstrate a slipped capital femoral epiphysis.

48
Knee and Lower Leg

1. **B**, Pages 874–876.

Partial disruptions of the quadriceps mechanism are treated by applying a cast with the knee in full extension. Complete tears are treated with early surgical repair.

2. **C**, Pages 881–882.

Osgood-Schlatter disease occurs in children, and symptoms have an insidious onset. It is often confused with superficial infrapatellar bursitis.

3. **A**, Pages 873–874.

The clinical situation described is that of a Baker's cyst, which is inflammation of the medial gastrocnemius bursa.

4. **A**, Pages 877–878.

Prepatellar bursitis secondary to trauma commonly becomes infected, as in this case. Fluid should be aspirated, and Gram's stain, culture, and white blood cell count should be done.

5. **A**, Page 877.

Chondromalacia patella is a disorder most commonly seen in young active females. The pain is poorly localized to the knee without any effusion or any history of trauma.

49
Ankle and Foot

1. **B**, Pages 897–900.

Patients with second degree sprains will have immediate pain whereas first and third degree sprains may be painless.

2. **A**, Page 923.

This is the classic description of tarsal tunnel syndrome. A positive Tinel's sign confirms diagnosis.

3. **C**, Pages 906–909.

Nondisplaced fractures are treated with padding and taping to adjacent uninjured toe—"dynamic splinting." Unstable displaced fractures often require open reduction and internal fixation.

50
Osteomyelitis

1. **E**, Page 936.

Both intravenous drug abusers, who are at risk for *Pseudomonas* osteomyelitis, and sickle cell amemia patients, who are at risk for *Salmonella* osteomyelitis, develop gram-negative osteomyelitis. Patients with chronic osteomyelitis usually have polymicrobial infections.

2. **A**, Pages 937–942.

Puncture wounds of the feet result in osteomyelitis 2% of the time by direct inoculation. The most common pathogen in *Pseudomonas*, which causes osteomyelitis in both children and adults, has been cultured from shoes. Cat bites often result in *Pasteurella multocida* osteomyelitis. Fresh water wounds are often contaminated by *Aeromonas hydrophilia*. A 3-year-old with hemotogenous osteomyelitis may have infection with *Staphylococcal*, group B *Streptococci*, or *Haemophilus influenzae*. Finally, diabetic foot osteomyelitis is often polymicrobial.

51
Foreign Bodies

1. **C**, Page 946.

After the removal of a corneal foreign body that leaves no rust ring, or for patients with a simple corneal abrasion, the therapy should include the instillation of an antimicrobial solution, one or two drops of a short-acting cycloplegic agent to relieve ciliary spasm, and an eye patch to be used for 24 hours. The patient should receive follow-up care by an ophthalmologist the following day. Immediate referral to an ophthalmologist is necessary if the emergency physician is unable to remove the foreign body, or if the foreign body has penetrated the globe.

2. **D**, Page 948.

All these methods may be used to remove a foreign body from the ear canal. One should examine the ear for evidence of tympanic membrane perforation before attempting irrigation of the ear canal.

3. **D**, Pages 951–952.

The symptoms depend on the size of the foreign body and how long is has been present.

4. **D**, Pages 951–955.

Patients who suffer complete airway obstruction secondary to aspiration are initially conscious and are recognized by their inability to speak. Stridor implies a partial airway obstruction. Loss of consciousness occurs in minutes if the obstruction is not relieved.

5. **B**, Pages 955–957.

Glucagon is successful in relaxing the esophagus enough to permit passage of esophageal foreign bodies in 37% of cases. Disk batteries should be removed immediately to prevent esophageal perforation. Disk batteries contain KOH in solution or various heavy metals. Those containing KOH can cause perforation while heavy metal intoxication may occur with the latter. Enzymatic degradation with papain has fallen into disfavor recently. While normal esophageal mucosa is resistant to papain, any defect in the esophagus may permit perforation with disastrous mediastinitis.

52
Animal Bites and Rabies

1. **B**, Pages 966–967.

Tetanus prophylaxis is indicated for all persons, even pregnant women. High risk wounds require only tetanus toxoid, even if more than 10 years have elapsed since the last immunization. Tetanus immune globulin is indicated only if the immunization history is unknown or if prior immunizations were inadequate.

2. **C**, Pages 968–969.

Involvement of the deeper structure of the hand requires hospitalization and parenteral antibiotics. Lacerations of the face may be closed primarily within 24 hours of injury. *Staphylococcus* species predominate in wound infections, hence penicillinase-resistant antibiotics are the drugs of choice. Local wound care is more important than antibiotic prophylaxis.

3. **C**, Pages 969–978.

Bites of cats, dogs, skunks, foxes, racoons, and bats account for most human and domestic animal cases of rabies. Bites of rabbits squirrels, hampsters, and rodents have never resulted in cases of human rabies and never call for antirabies prophylaxis.

4. **C**, Pages 969–978.

Immunization should be carried out only after exposure (i.e., bite) and should include both passive and active immunization. Hawaii has been consistently rabies-free. The presence of Negri bodies on microscopic exam is pathognomonic.

53
Venomous Animal Injuries

1. **C**, Pages 987–990.

All patients should receive skin testing with 0.02 ml of 1:100 solution by intracutaneous injection, regardless of their history. The other statements are true.

2. **A**, Pages 987–990.

Antivenin should never be injected around the wound or into a finger or toe. The other statements are true.

3. **A**, Pages 990–992.

Most fatalities are caused by allergic reactions to the sting. Bee and wasp venom can itself cause serious injury depending on the number of stings, the species of the insect, the size of the victim and the person's previous health, and the anatomic site of the sting. All of the other statements are true.

4. **C**, Pages 995–999.

Nematocysts should be fixed, if possible. Tetanus prophylaxis is indicated for all marine bites, as indicated by immunization history. At least as many deaths following envenomation are caused by drowning as are caused by toxic effects of the venom. Antivenin is available for stonefish (scorpionfish) envenomation only.

54
Soft-tissue Infections

1. **D**, Pages 1001–1003.

H. influenzae cellulitis has a number of unique features. It has a predilection for facial involvement, especially in patients younger than 5 years of age. Fever, leukocytosis, toxic appearance, and positive blood cultures are often seen.

2. **C**, Pages 1003–1004.

Acute rheumatic fever is never caused by impetigo; however, impetigo more often results in poststreptococcal glomerulonephritis than does streptococcal pharyngitis. Impetigo contagiosa may result in poststreptococcal glomerulonephritis, whereas bullous impetigo is caused by *S. aureus*.

3. **C**, Pages 1004–1008.

Most abscesses contain bacteria. However, approximately 5%, especially those associated with parenteral drug abuse, may be sterile. Hidradenitis suppuration is a disease consisting of chronic suppurative abscesses in the apocrine sweat glands. *S. aureus*, *Streptococcus viridans*, and anaerobes are usually found. Bartholin cysts are usually mixed aerobic and anaerobic infections, as are pilouidal and perirectal abscesses. Pilonidal cysts may yield *S. aureus*, whereas perirectal abscesses often yield *Bacteroides fragilis*.

55
Parasitology

1. **D**, Page 1023.
2. **F**, Page 1027.
3. **A**, Page 1013.
4. **B**, Page 1020.
5. **C**, Page 1021.
6. **G**, Page 1024.
7. **E**, Page 1025.
   Self-explanatory.
8. **A**, Pages 1013, 1015–1020.

The drug of choice for treatment is chloroquine phosphate. Mebendazole is used in the treatment of hookworm, whipworm, and roundworm. The other statements are true.

9. **B**, Pages 1021, 1023, 1024, 1027.
10. **D**, Pages 1021, 1023, 1024, 1027.
11. **A**, Pages 1021, 1023, 1024, 1027.
12. **E**, Pages 1021, 1023, 1024, 1027.
13. **F**, Pages 1021, 1023, 1024, 1027.
14. **C**, Pages 1021, 1023, 1024, 1027.

New onset of seizure activity can be the first indication of cysticercosis. In the southeastern United States hookworm infestation is classically recognized as a cause of iron deficiency anemia. The fish tapeworm *Diphyllobothrium latum* competes with the human host for absorption of vitamin B_{12}, which can lead to pernicious anemia. Onchocerciasis is a major cause of blindness in the world. Microfilariae migrate into the cornea, causing an allergic reaction with resultant corneal opacification. *Trypanosoma cruzi*, the cause

of Chagas' disease, invades the myocardium resulting in myocarditis. Conduction defects of various kinds are not uncommon. *Ascaris lumbricoides* (roundworm) can cause complete bowel obstruction due to its numbers and size.

15. **D**, Pages 1020, 1025, 1026, 1029.

Giardiasis is usually associated with the duodenal-jejunal mucosa. *Ascaris lumbricoides* can lead to malabsorption with steatorrhea as well as migrate into the biliary tree and cause ascending cholangitis. Suramin is used to treat African trypanosomiasis (sleeping sickness) while giardiasis is treated with quinacrine HCl or metronidazole. Rectal prolapse in young children can be caused by whipworm (trichuriasis). Giardiasis is one of the intestinal parasitic diseases referred to by the term *gay bowel syndrome* since it can be transmitted by the oral and anal sexual practices of male homosexuals.

16. **A**, Pages 1023, 1029, 1030.

Loa loa, a filarial infestation, is characterized by a migrating adult worm in the subcutaneous tissue; sometimes it can be excised when seen migrating through theocular subconjunctival tissues. The other statements are characteristic of trichinosis.

56
Common Ophthalmologic Problems

1. **E**, Pages 1033–1034.

Shallow anterior chambers predispose to acute angle closure glaucoma. Therefore, before dilating any pupil the examiner should shine a pen light transversely across the anterior chamber from the temporal side.

2. **D**, Pages 1045, 1047–1048.

Caustic burns of the eye and central retinal artery occlusion must both be treated immediately upon presentation.

3. **D**, Pages 1037, 1041, 1048–1049.

Hot metal may cauterize nerves as it penetrates and remain painless until ferrous oxide iritis develops 12 to 24 hours later. Lactate and corneal edema may leave the contact lens-injured cornea painless for 4 to 6 hours after removal of the lens. Ultraviolet exposure often is asymptomatic for 6 to 10 hours.

4. **A**, Page 1045.

Because of the need for immediate treatment, acuity is deferred in patients with caustic burns.

5. **B**, Page 1036.

Herpes zoster and true allergic conjunctivitis are the only indications for topical steroids. Steroids increase the patient's susceptibility to herpes simplex and fungal infections.

6. **A**, Page 1037.

Patches should not be worn for more than 12 hours and should not be changed by the patient, because they may improperly apply patch causing damage.

7. **D**, Page 1048.

In a young, otherwise healthy individual with a normal eye examination (except subjective acuity testing), sudden blindness is most often hysterical in nature.

8. **C**, Page 1046.

Ophthalmology consultation is required for corneal scrapings for culturing. Patching should not be done because it may enhance infection.

9. **C**, Page 1047.

Rust ring should be removed with a spud as soon as possible or in 24 to 48 hours after the surrounding cornea softens.

10. **A**, Page 1044.

Except for the lacerations listed in choices *B*, *C*, and *D*, lid lacerations are repaired as any facial laceration. Hematomas of the lid can be treated with ice packs.

11. **D**, Pages 1043–1044.

All choices suggest rupture of the globe, as does marked hemorrhagic chemosis.

57
Dental Emergencies

1. **A**, Pages 1057–1059.

Pain after extraction is common for 24 hours. Alveolar osteitis occurs 3 to 4 days postextraction and is characterized by sudden onset of excruciating pain. Alveolar osteitis (dry socket) occurs due to premature loss of blood clot with a localized infection of bone. Pericoronitis should not occur once the tooth is extracted. Osteomyelitis and gingival abscess occur later.

2. **F**, Page 1058.

Ludwig's angina is a bilateral boardlike swelling of the submental, sublingual, and submandibular spaces. The most serious immediate sequelae is airway obstruction. Antibiotics and surgical drainage are required.

3. **E**, Pages 1061–1065.

Ellis Class I and II fractures may be referred to a dentist. Ellis Class III fractures require endodontic therapy as soon as possible. Al veolar fractures re-

quire reduction and stabilization. Avulsion of a permanent tooth requires immediate reimplantation. A percentage point for successful reimplantation is lost for each minute that the tooth is outside of the oral cavity. After 2 hours reimplantation will not take.

58
Upper Respiratory Tract Infection

1. **D**, Page 1082.

Also associated are a severe sore throat, a low-grade fever, and dysarthria ("hot potato" voice). A fever over 103°F raises the suspicion of parapharyngeal extension and possible sepsis.

2. **D**, Page 1086.

Cellulitis of the floor of the mouth, Ludwig's angina, is rare but a true emergency. The rapid swelling and protrusion of the tongue makes the diagnosis obvious. Respiratory compromise can occur very quickly. It rarely requires surgery but broad spectrum antibiotics are necessary.

3. **E**, Page 1078.

All the suggested answers are true in favor of treating pharyngitis based on clinical suspicion: temperature greater than 101°F, tonsillar exudates, tender anterior cervical adenopathy, or known household exposure.

4. **E**, Page 1076.

Almost everyone has streptococcal pharyngitis at some time in his or her life. Previous strep does make a patient at increased risk of acute rheumatic fever but not for recurrent strep pharyngitis.

5. **E**, Pages 1077–1078.

There is no evidence that treatment prevents the type-specific antibody formation and decreases natural immunity. Treatment clearly prevents rheumatic fever but seems to have no effect on glomerulonephritis. People who have had acute rheumatic fever should be on long-term continuous antibiotic prophylaxis until at least age 20. If treated on clinical grounds, there is no reason to do a throat culture unless treatment of asymptomatic family members is planned.

6. **C**, Page 1076.

In children tonsillar exudates have not been found to correlate with streptococcal pharyngitis. All the other answers listed increase the likelihood of a positive strep culture.

7. **E**, Page 1079.

Infectious mononucleosis is usually a benign, if lengthy, disorder, but all of the listed answers are potentially fatal complications. Any patient with mononucleosis should avoid all contact sports.

8. **E**, Pages 1080–1081.

Treatment should be started on the clinical suspicion because mortality is directly related to delay in antitoxin administration.

9. **E**, Page 1073.

While the most common differential is between Group A streptococcus and viral etiologies, all of the listed pathogens must be considered in appropriate clinical settings.

10. **D**, Page 1086.

Soft tissue films of the neck would show an enlarged epiglottis confirming the diagnosis of acute epiglotitis in an adult. This disease is almost always missed on the initial presentation. Suggested clues are the patient's complaints out of proportion of physical findings and a muffled voice. A throat culture is of no help in a patient already on antibiotics. He has no exudates or cervical nodes to suggest infectious mononucleosis. His white count should be elevated, but this does not help make the diagnosis. This patient needs complete cultures and admission to the ICU with parenteral antibiotics.

11. **B**, Page 1086.

Ludwig's angina is a cellulitis of the floor of the mouth. It requires broad spectrum antibiotics and admission to the ICU to carefully monitor for airway obstruction. It may require surgical airway as intubation is often impossible due to swelling and destruction of landmarks. It rarely requires surgical decompression for the cellulitis itself.

12. **D**, Page 1082.

Isolated gonococcal pharyngitis is usually asymptomatic but can progress to disseminated gonococcemia. Most people with pharyngeal gonorrhea will also have genital involvement. It cannot be diagnosed with a Gram's stain because other gram-negatives also inhabit the pharynx. Spectinomycin is not effective treatment. Penicillin and tetracycline are recommended.

13. **C**, Page 1079.

Most patients with mononucleosis will develop a rash when given ampicillin. This is not an allergic reaction and these patients do not need to avoid ampicillin in the future. The rash of scarlet fever results in a generalized pinkish color with circumoral pallor that extends over the extremities. The rash of rheumatic fever does not begin until 3 weeks after a sore throat and consists of erythematous areas with clear centers and serpiginous margins.

14. **E**, Pages 1072–1073.

All of the pathogens listed can cause an acute pharyngitis with the above listed findings.

15. **D**, Page 1080.

Suspected cases of diphtheria require hospitalization, cardiac monitoring, and early use of penicillin and diphtheria antitoxin.

16. **C**, Page 1076.

Throat cultures, the mainstay of the diagnosis of streptococcal pharyngitis, have very high false negative and false positive rates. There is at least a 10% and probably higher false negative rate. Of even more importance, up to 50% of asymptomatic children may be carriers in lower socioeconomic groups in the winter months. A person truly has streptococcal pharyngitis and is at risk for subsequent rheumatic fever or glomerulonephritis only if there is a rise in antistreptococcal antibodies, which only occurs in 43% of patients with positive cultures.

17. **D**, Page 1084.

Most prevertebral space infections occur from direct extension of cervical osteomyelitis. The disease is often confused with a retropharyngeal infection, but the distinction is important since the etiology, pathogens, and treatment are all different.

18. **D**, Pages 1083–1085.

Patients with a retropharyngeal abscess may perfer the supine position and forced sitting may further compromise the airway. Soft tissue x-ray films of the neck are useful in the diagnosis of retropharyngeal abscess. Intubation may be quite difficult secondary to the swelling.

19. **D**, Page 1079.

Both infectious mononucleosis and streptococcus can be associated with low-grade or high fevers, and this does not differrentiate between the two. Mononucleosis is relatively more frequent among an older age group, typically college students, while streptococcus peaks around 12 to 13 years of age.

20. **B**, Page 1080.

While some patients die from respiratory obstruction caused by extension of the membrane, all infected patients will die as the result of exotoxins acting on the cardiac and peripheral nervous system unless early specific antitioxin is given. There is no evidence that antibiotics alter the course of the disease.

21. **B**, Page 1078.

Erythromycin is the drug of choice in a penicillin-sensitive patient. Tetracycline and sulfonamides are ineffective in eradicating pharyngeal streptococcus. Ampicillin is contraindicated in a penicillin-allergic patient.

22. **B**, Page 1077.

At least one-third of patients that develop acute rheumatic fever have no history of sore throat. Therefore, even with the best of care for pharyngitis, only two-thirds of cases of rheumatic fever would be eliminated. The fact that treatment even as long as 10 days after symptoms begin decreases subsequent rheumatic fever makes penicillin worthwhile even when *Streptococcus* is diagnosed late.

23. **C**, Page 1079.

Bullous myringitis is essentially pathognomonic for *Mycoplasma pneumoniae*. A chest x-ray film that looks much worse than the patient sounds clinically is characteristic of this entity.

24. **C**, Page 1086.

Epiglottitis is being increasingly recognized in the adult where its presentation is subtle. Like pharyngitis, dysphagia . is a prominent symptom, but adenopathy is uncommon. The patient may have a muffled voice and speak softly, but true hoarseness is rare. These patients usually have minimal pharyngitis and their pain is out of proportion to objective signs.

59
Sinusitis

1. **E**, Page 1092.

Anaerobes are more commonly associated with chronic sinusitis because of the increased pressure in the sinus that decreases blood supply and oxygen tension.

2. **D**, Page 1093.

The diagnosis of sinusitis is very difficult to make clinically. The classic history and physical findings correlate very poorly with culture-proven infection. However, complete opacification of the sinus to transillumination is felt to correlate well.

3. **D**, Page 1093.

There is no way to accurately culture the sinus in the emergency department. Treatment must be based on probable organisms. Nasal sprays should be used for only 3 days. After that a mucosal rebound can occur, which results in more severe congestion.

4. **C**, Page 1095.

Mucormycosis should be considered in a debilitated patient, especially a diabetic who may be acidotic. This patient has a typical presentation. Treatment is with antifungal agents. If antibiotics are ineffective, surgery may become necessary.

5. **C**, Page 1095.

Patients with cavernous sinus thrombosis have high fevers and appear quite toxic, often with altered mental status. High doses of antibiotics to cover *Staphylococcus*, gram-negative organisms, and anaerobes are the mainstay of therapy.

6. **C**, Page 1092.

All the listed answers are associated with both acute and chronic sinusitis but *S. pneumoniae* and *H. influenzae* are by far the most common causes of acute sinusitis. That's why ampicillin is the drug of choice.

7. **B**, Page 1093.

Nasal swabs do not reliably yield the causative agent in acute sinusitis and are even less accurate in chronic sinusitis.

8. **C**, Page 1092.

Rhinocerebral phycomycosis or mucormycosis is a fungal infection seen in the immune-compromised, classically the diabetic while in ketoacidosis. The disease can be rapidly fatal if not promptly recognized. Treatment includes surgical debridement and antifungal drugs.

60
Acute Bronchitis

1. **E**, Pages 1099–1100.

The tuberculin skin test or PPD usually becomes positive after 2 weeks of infection. Bronchitis is an extremely common disease, and it is the most common cause of hemoptysis, although in any given case of bronchitis hemoptysis is unusual.

2. **A**, Page 1098.

Amantadine is as effective as immunization in prophylaxis against influenza A and it also shortens the clinical course. It is not effective in non-A influenza types.

3. **B**, Page 1097.

Acute illness generally lasts 2–5 days and is followed by weakness and malaise that may persist up to 3–4 weeks. Viral pneumonia is quite common, especially in the elderly, but generally is not of clinical significance unless the patient is debilitated or at greater risk from other concomitant pathology.

4. **A**, Page 1098.

Both types of bronchitis may become chronic if unrecognized or untreated. The precipitating cause may be the same. Cortical steroids are most effective for allergic bronchitis. A great service to the patient with chronic recurrent bronchitis may be the identification of the allergic component. Asthmatic bronchitis can frequently be distinguished by the presence of eosinophils in unstained or weight-stained sputum.

5. **A**, Page 1099.

Pneumomediastinum is frequently associated with substernal chest pain, dysphagia, "crunching" heart sounds, or a cervical subcutaneous emphysema. It is easy to overlook radiographically unless a high index of suspicion is maintained and evidence is specifically sought.

6. **A**, Page 1099.

The absence of fever favors a bronchitic process rather than pneumonia, but the patient may have a normal temperature secondary to antipyretic drugs or general debilitation. An elevated respiratory rate may be a manifestation of fever, bronchospasm, or early respiratory failure or may be related to more benign causes such as anxiety or vigorous crying in a small child. An increased heart rate may be from a variety of causes and should be investigated if persistent.

7. **B**, Page 1100.

Indications for chest x-ray include unexplained fever, localized pulmonary findings on physical exam, increased respiratory rate out of proportion to physical findings, debilitated patients with chronic lung disease or immunosuppression, patients whose symptoms have become chronic (persisting for 2 or more weeks), asymmetric breath sounds, mediastinal crunch, hemoptysis, chest pain, or unresponsive bronchospasm.

8. **C**, Page 1100.

Fingings that can be expected are a normal study or slightly increased bronchopulmonary markings. Flattening of the diaphragm may indicate acute bronchospasm or COPD. Hilar adenopathy, usually unilateral, may suggest tuberculosis or neoplasm. Signs of complications of acute bronchitis include pneumomediastinum, pneumothorax, and pleural effusion.

9. **B**, Page 1100.

The most cost-effective expectorant is guiafenesin, which is readily available in most cough remedies. Iodine preparations and acetylcysteine carry either a high risk of allergic reaction or a high cost of delivery when aerosolized, which limits their usefulness.

10. **A**, Page 1097.

Purulent secretions are rarely seen with a purely viral infection. The most common pathogens in purulent bronchitis are *S. pneumoniae* and *H. influenzae*. Mild fever is the usual response of viral bronchitis in the adult.

61
Pneumonia

1. **A**, Page 1105.

This is the classic presentation for *S. pneumoniae*.

2. **E**, Page 1105.

S. aureus pneumonia has a higher incidence in IV drug abusers and is associated with pneumatoceles.

3. **D**, Page 1112.

In any individual where the etiologic organism's identification is critical or a reliable sputum must be obtained, transtracheal aspiration is the method of choice.

4. **B**, Page 1114.

Outpatient treatment with oral penicillin is acceptable provided the patient is compliant and is not immune-compromised.

5. **D**, Page 1105.

Although unusual organisms are much more likely in immune-compromised patients and all these agents must be considered, *S. pneumoniae* remains the single most common organism causing pneumonia in the healthy and debilitated alike. It accounts for 80% of cases of pneumonia requiring hospitalization.

6. **C**, Page 1106.

Unlike most epidemic diseases, Legionnaires' disease is much more common in the summer. A middle-aged smoker who has fever, severe shortness of breath but a nonproductive cough, especially if associated with diarrhea, should be suspected of having this disease.

7. **C**, Page 1110.

Most patients with mycoplasma will have positive cold agglutinins. They may also be positive in mononucleosis, influenza, or rubella. Cultures and Gram's stains are uniformly negative for this nonbacterial agent. Leukocytosis is unusual; most patients have fewer than 10,000 WBCs.

8. **C**, Page 1114.

Although tetracycline is listed as adequate treatment for *Mycoplasma* it is now considered a second line drug because of emerging resistance. Erythromycin has the added advantage of also being effective against *S. pneumoniae*. Together these two account for 90% of community-acquired pneumonias in otherwise healthy people.

9. **C**, Page 1114

Erythromycin initially given IV is the best agent for Legionnaires' disease. Rifampin should not be used alone because of rapid emergence of resistance. It does seem to be additive to erythromycin in clinical effectiveness.

10. **A**, Page 1114.
This patient has classic symptoms of pneumococcal pneumonia, which is the most common community acquired pneumonia even among the immune-suppressed. Erythromycin is as effective as penicillin and the drug of choice for the penicillin allergic. Tetracycline is increasingly ineffective against *Streptococcus pneumoniae*. The toxicity of chloramphenicol makes it unwarranted here. Ampicillin should not be used in a penicillin allergic patient. Cefoxitin, a second generation cephalosporin, is unnecessary shotgun therapy for this patient.

11. **C**, Page 1110.

12. **D**, Page 1110.

13. **A**, Page 1110.

14. **E**, Page 1110.

15. **E**, Page 1110.
A sputum Gram's stain is more reliable than a sputum culture, and accurate interpretation a must for every emergency physician. First, assure an inadequate specimen by looking for inflammatory cells. The presence of epithelial cells represents an inadequate specimen contaminated with oral flora. Leukocytes should appear gram-negative (pink), which help assure a properly prepared slide.

16. **B**, Pages 1105–1107.
There are times when early pneumonia can be difficult to diagnose. Pneumococcal pneumonia is one particular type that lacks physical or radiographic signs early in its course. Staphylococcal is a necrotizing infection that often shows abscess formation at any early stage. Legionnaires' disease, considered an opportunistic infection, can also be difficult to diagnose and should always be considered in the differential diagnosis of atypical summer pneumonias. Although respiratory failure may occur in viral pneumonia, its course is usually mild, self-limited, and without permanent sequellae.

17. **F**, Page 1116.
Hospitalization may be necessary for the patient to receive adequate therapy. Each case must be evaluated individually considering such factors as living circumstances, high morbidity pneumonias, high-risk patients, presence of sepsis, extensive pulmonary disease, and degree of respiratory impairment.

18. **C**, Page 1107.
Pneumocystis carinii in the immune-supressed host carries a very high risk of fatality. The disease can be rapidly progressing even in the face of a normal physical examination and/or radiographs. Early signs and symptoms are frequently out of proportion to radiographic findings. Signs and symptoms include fever, tachycardia, tachypnea, and nonproductive cough, hypoxia, and dyspnea.

19. **B**, Page 1112.

PTTA carries some risk of serious complications yet can be very helpful in obtaining an accurate etiologic diagnosis required for optimal management. PTTA is generally recommended in the following situations: (1) lower respiratory tract infection in the compromised host, (2) established infection after aspiration, (3) necrotizing pulmonary infection, (4) suspected anaerobic pulmonary infection, (5) hospital acquired infection, (6) suspected superinfection in established pulmonary infection, and (7) undiagnosed pulmonary disease when possibly infectious causes need to be ruled out.

62
Acute Bronchial Asthma

1. **E**, Page 1130.
One of the major benefits of theophylline appears to be improvement in diaphragmatic and other respiratory muscle function. With COPD, respiratory muscles can "fail" much like heart failure from prolonged overwork. Theophylline does stimulate cardiac contractility and promotes a mild diuresis, both of which may be of value in treating chronic obstructive pulmonary disease. Theophylline will cause nausea and vomiting in toxic doses from CNS stimulation, but it has no effect on gastric acid.

2. **D**, Page 1125.
The chest x-ray film in severe asthma may show an increased A-P diameter and flattening of the diaphragm secondary to air trapping. Infiltrates are not expected with primary bronchospasm, and their presence suggests a complication such as infection or aspiration. A patient with severe bronchospasm may not be moving enough air to wheeze and may have a silent chest. After treatment increases tidal volume, wheezing may become apparent for the first time. Likewise, arterial blood gases may deteriorate during treatment because of pulmonary vasodilatation of underventilated areas from sympathomimetic stimulation.

3. **E**, Pages 1129–1131.
A mist or oxygen tent, while useful for croup, should be avoided in acute asthma attacks. It produces no beneficial humidification of the lower respiratory tract and can hinder accurate observation of respiratory decompensation.

4. **E**, Pages 1128–1130.
In severe life-threatening asthma in children, an infusion of isoproterenol may be used. The infusion is started at 0.1 μg/kg/min and gradually increased with careful monitoring of pulse and blood pressure.

5. **B**, Page 1131.

There is a general consensus based on clinical experience that the early administration of steroids is perhaps the most important therapeutic measure to be taken in severe resistant asthma. An initial PEFR of less than 100 liters per minute with improvement of less than 60 liters per minute suggests aggressive therapy that includes the use of cortical steroids. Steroids should be used during treatment of a patient receiving long-term steroid therapy whose asthma is worsening. One reason for avoiding topical steroids during an acute attack is that these agents such as beclomethasone can precipitate bronchospasm during the acute attack.

6. **B**, Page 1132.

Anxiety is best reduced by relief of bronchospasm and emotional support, not sedatives and/or tranquilizers. There is no evidence that mucolitic agents cause significant improvement in acute asthma. Bacterial infections generally play an insignificant role in acute exacerbations of asthma; thus routine use is unwarranted. Although antihistamines are effective in allergic rhinitis, they are generally ineffective in acute asthma.

7. **C**, Page 1129.

Isoproterenol is one of the most potent adrenergic agents acting on beta receptors. Among its problems, however, are cardiac stimulation with dysrhythmias, including ventricular fibrillation, hypoxemia secondary to pulmonary vascular dilatation and intrapulmonary shunting, short duration of action, and psychological dependence on the hand-held, freeon-propelled nebulizers.

8. **A**, Page 1120.

Extrinsic asthma, those patients with a history of allergy, is characterized by a well-defined sensitivity to a specific inhaled allergen, personal or familial history of multiple allergic diseases, increased levels of IGE, and positive immediate skin test. The asthma characterized by a change in the FEV_1 brought on by exercise is known as exercise-induced asthma. Psychological factors can mediate changes in airway caliber, but the actual extent of participation of psychological factors in the induction or continuation of any acute attack is unknown.

9. **D**, Page 1125.

Frequently the pattern of arterial blood gases in the asthmatic is progressive from normal arterial blood gasses (4) to an initial hyperventilation that maintains oxygenation (1) to hyperventilation with decreasing oxygenation (3), to normalization of the PCO_2 as the patient begins to tire (5), to eventual acute respiratory failure (2).

10. **A**, Page 4.

A significant pulsus paradoxus greater than 10 Torr occurs in approximately one-third of acute asthmatic episodes. Its presence does signify severe airway obstruction but it can be absent in one-third to one-half of patients with severe obstruction. Frequently it disappears with minimal improvements in air flow through larger airways. Because of its variability, the presence of significant pulsus paradoxus cannot be used as a reliable indicator of the need for inpatient treatment.

11. **C**, Page 1125.

Some authorities recommend routine measurements of arterial blood gasses in acute asthma to stage severity; however, there frequently is a poor correlation between pulmonary function and PaO_2 or $PaCO_2$. It is true that extreme airway obstruction and fatigue may be associated with normalization and eventual elevation of the $PaCO_2$ and a corresponding worsening of hypoxia as the patient begins to tire. This may precede a sudden deterioration of the patient's status and therefore may be extremely helpful.

12. **B**, Page 1123.

Classic symptoms are cough, dyspnea, and wheezing. Cough probably secondary to subendothelial vagal stimulation may or may not be associated with sputum production. Dyspnea is present, although the exact mechanism is unknown. Hypoxia is not the cause. The wheezing that develops depends on velocity of air movement and the development of turbulence. It must be kept in mind, however, that some patients with asthma do not always wheeze but rather note intermittent shortness of breath and cough. Rales are generally not present in uncomplicated asthma.

13. **C**, Page 1123.

Patients too dyspneic to speak or with a disturbance of consciousness require immediate therapy, and history may have to wait. Some investigators have reported clear historical patterns in severe asthma. Others have not. Nevertheless, a brief history can serve as a guide to therapy. Knowing the duration and onset is helpful in that well-established asthma is usually more resistant to therapy. Uncovering a precipitating cause such as bee sting may prevent severe complications and serve as a guide to therapy. Knowing previous requirements for hospitalization is important in that these patients tend to develop similar future episodes. Present or previous requirements for systemic steroids often help identify patients with probable resistant bronchospasm.

14. **C**, Page 1126.

The predictive index scoring system looks at seven (7) categories. A score of 4 or higher is said to have a 96% accuracy in predicting need for hospitalization. Unfortunately, the index does not deal with the problem of relapse or incorporate assessments of response to therapy; therefore, its usefulness is open to question. This example, the patient with tachycardia, moderate wheezing, moderate dyspnea, and tachypnea, meets the criteria for admission.

15. **D**, Page 1134.

Calcium channel blockers have been found to do all of the following: (1) decrease airway smooth muscle sensitivity to contractile agonists, (2) reduce chemical mediator release from mast cells, and (3) inhibit exercise-induced bronchospasm, cold air- and antigen-induced airway narrowing.

16. **B**, Page 1130.

A therapeutic theophylline level is 10–20 μg/cc. For each 1 mg per kg given the serum level can be expected to increase by 2 μg/cc. Thus, a 200-mg loading dose would increase the patient's serum level to about 12. At higher serum levels side effects of nausea, vomiting, and arrhythmias can occur.

17. **C**, Page 1124.

Pulsus paradoxus is an exaggeration of the normal decrease in blood pressure with inspiration. A greater than 10 mm Hg difference is considered positive. If present, it indicates severe obstruction but may not be positive even in the presence of severe airflow. The value of the absolute level of pulsus paradoxus remains controversial.

18. **A**, Page 1130.

The loading dose of theophylline will be the same for each of the listed conditions, but maintenance doses should be reduced for all except smokers. Smokers have a more rapid metabolism of theophylline and maintenance doses should be increased.

19. **B**, Page 1133.

With pregnancy, one-third of asthmatics will improve, one-third will remain the same, and one-third will develop more severe disease. Terbutaline can be used during pregnancy but does inhibit uterine contractions and in fact is used as a tocolytic to stop labor in some centers. Aminophylline and steroids have no untoward effects on the fetus.

63

Chronic Obstructive Pulmonary Diseases

1. **A**, Page 1153.

This case represents iatrogenic blunting of the patient's hypoxic drive, which results in profoundly decreased ventilation with hypercapnia and acidosis. The Po_2 should be low because of the lack of ventilation and the CO_2 displacing O_2 from the alveoli.

2. **E**, Pages 1150–1152.

Patients with chronic bronchitis respond to their disease by increased cardiac output, not ventilation as do patients with emphysema. They do not respond to hypoxia or hypercarbia with increased ventilation, leading in turn to secondary polycythemia and cor pulmonale, which causes right-sided failure. At times, the right heart failure is incorrectly attributed to primary left heart failure.

3. **A**, Page 1160.

Water is the best expectorant. Many patients with asthma and COPD are dehydrated for a number of reasons, mainly respiratory losses. Careful hydration is an important, although often neglected, part of therapy.

4. **C**, Page 1155–1157.

This patient is obviously hypoxic, but probably is not severe enough to require immediate intubation. The patient's mental status is the best guide to the need for intubation. High-flow oxygen may blunt this "blue bloater's" respiratory drive and decrease minute ventilation and cause decompensation. A 5- to 10-minute trial of a Venturi mask at 24% is the best initial therapy. Terbutaline subcutaneously must be used with extreme caution in the elderly. Aerosolized bronchodilators are much preferred. Aminophylline is a mainstay of treatment but is not rapidly effective.

5. **B**, Page 1155.

Cor pulmonale is caused predominantly by vasospasm secondary to hypoxia. Improving oxygenation relieves the spasm and decreases pulmonary artery pressure. Aminophylline can improve cor pulmonale, but it is largely secondary to improved oxygenation. Nitroprusside is dangerous in these patients, because increased pulmonary shunting can cause further deterioration of systemic oxygenation. Propranolol is contraindicated in COPD patients because of increased bronchospasm. Furosemide further raises the hematocrit and so causes increased viscosity and cardiac work.

6. **D**, Page 1144.

Patients with COPD have altered host defenses for a variety of reasons and are at increased risk of infection. What would be a trivial URI to a normal person can be life-threatening to a borderline compensated COPD patient. Furthermore, infection may be difficult to diagnose in this population. They often have chronic coughs and their lungs are difficult to accurately auscultate.

7. **C**, Page 1147.

Cardiac output in patients with emphysema would be expected to be low. This is a major reason that these patients don't develop pulmonary hypertension in spite of widespread destruction of the pulmonary vascular bed. Alph-I antitrypsin deficiency is a well-described etiology of severe panacinar emphysema at an early age. Patients with emphysema are constantly fighting for breath and are much more symptomatic and limited in activity than the chronic bronchitic who will exist with a lower PO_2 and a higher PCO_2 and be relatively symptom-free. The loss of elastic recoil found in emphysematous patients accounts in large part for their air trapping and prolonged expiratory phase.

8. **B**, Page 1158.

Aminophylline has been a mainstay in the treatment of asthma. However, its role in COPD is less clear. Its benefits incude increasing diaphragmatic contractility, which makes it useful in COPD patients even without bronchospasm. Ventricular tachycardia and seizures are generally not seen in asthmatic patients before 40 $\mu g/ml$. However, more caution is advised for class D and E COPD patients. Aminophylline's ability to reduce fibrillation threshold is aggravated by hypoxia and hypocarbia. Because of the risk of cardiovascular toxicity, it is recommended that one should assist ventilation and be relatively sure that significant bronchospasm and subtherapeutic theophylline levels are present before aminophylline is used.

9. **C**, Page 1159.

The interrelationships between specific bacteria, the clinical course of acute and chronic bronchitis, sputum gram's stain and culture, and antiobiotic therapy are not clear. Numerous antibiotic regimens have been shown to shorten episodes of acute bronchitis. Broad-spectrum drugs have outperformed narrow-spectrum antibiotics. The choices generally include ampicillin or amoxicillin, tetracycline, cephalosporin, trimethoprim/sulfamethoxazole, and chloramphenicol.

10. **A**, Page 1155.

The most important therapeutic modality in the emergency department is ventilation since it is almost certain that oxygen administration without assisted ventilation to a patient in severe respiratory failure would result in less ventilation. Intubation to assist in adequate ventilation will often be necessary. Intubation, however, must be rapid and accurate.

11. **D**, Pages 1117–1118

Drug therapy in COPD is fraught with many complex problems. First, reactive airway disease and COPD is different from that in asthma, and therapy that works for one situation may or may not work in the other. Second, it is virtually impossible to determine if and

to what degree a given patient may have reactive airway disease. Third, even those patients without reactive airway disease may benefit from some actions of bronchodilators such as the increased diaphragmatic contractility with aminophylline. Fourth, there is great variability in patient's individual responses to specific bronchodilators. Fifth, even though objective benefits may not be noted, some patients describe subjective relief of dyspnea. In addition, some studies regarding the efficacy of drugs in COPD do not clearly define the type of COPD patient being studied.

12. **D**, Page 1153.

ACLS golden rule #1 states that for every 10 mm increase above 40, the pH will decrease by .08 units and for every 10 mm decrease in the PCO_2 below 40, the pH will increase by .08 units. The expected pH for a PCO_2 of 55 would be 7.28. The actual pH was 7.20, indicating some metabolic derangement in addition to the respiratory acidosis.

13. **D**, Page 1154.

The findings of criteria for right ventricular hypertrophy strongly suggest established cor pulmonale but the absence of such criteria does not rule it out. A vertical QRS axis of plus 90 or greater in a heavy-set person who normally would have a more transverse axis can be especially helpful. "P-pulmonale" strongly suggests COPD but may also be present with acute increases in right atrial pressure. Low QRS voltage clockwise rotation, and poor R-wave progression are interesting correlates of COPD but are both insensitive and nonspecific.

14. **B**, Pages 1146–1152.
15. **B**, Pages 1146–1152.
16. **B**, Pages 1146–1152.
17. **A**, Pages 1146–1152.
18. **A**, Pages 1146–1152.
19. **A**, Pages 1146–1152.
20. **A**, Pages 1146–1152.
21. **B**, Pages 1146–1152.
22. **D**, Pages 1146–1152.
23. **B**, Pages 1146–1152.

Pink puffers are characterized as dyspneic, frequently become cachectic with the work of breathing, and suffer from severe tissue hypoxia and air hunger, and yet may maintain relatively normal arterial blood gases in the early stages. The blue bloater is characterized by cardiac involvement recognized by a retrosternal heave of right ventricular failure, chronic hypoxemia, hypercarbia and polycythemia. It is often misdiagnosed as left ventricular failure. In spite of severe hypoxemia, the bronchitic patient probably has better tissue oxygenation than the pink puffer. Both can develop cor pulmonale, although it generally develops much earlier in the blue bloater.

24. **C**, Page 1146.

The two principle mechanisms of airway obstruction are bronchoconstriction and mucus plugging. The variable obstruction of small airways often leads to air trapping, hyperinflation, right-to-left shunting, and hypoxcmia. Bronchoconstriction is generally readily apparent whereas mucus plugging is less dramatic and more difficult to diagnose. Mucus plugs are found consistently in patients dying of asthma.

25. **C**, Page 1146.

Any change in the level of consciousness in a patient with COPD suggests the onset of severe acute respiratory failure and CO_2 narcosis. The number of words expresed at one time can give a rough measure of FEV_1. Gasping answers of 2–3 words is worrisome. Phrases are better, short sentences better still. High-pitched wheezes indicate more severe bronchospasm than lower-pitched wheezes but a "silent chest" indicates little air exchange and is most ominous. Many patients are their own best judge of the degree of airway obstruction.

26. **A**, Page 1144.

Once the emergency physician has assessed the type and severity of the three basic components of COPD, aggravating factors that precipitate the acute episode must be considered. These factors can be divided into disease-related, patient-rclatcd, and physician-related factors. The disease-related factors are further subdivided into acute, subacute, and chronic. The three major acute factors are pneumothorax, large pulmonary embolism, and lobar atelectasis. Pneumonia, pleural effusion, and small pulmonary emboli are but a few of the subacute precipitating factors.

27. **E**, Page 1145.

Inappropriate therapy can significantly impact a COPD patient. Many drugs may directly or indirectly produce bronchospasm, including aspirin, propranalol, reserpine, cholinergics, opiates, and all antirheumatic drugs with prostaglandin-inhibiting properties.

64

Pulmonary Embolus

1. **C**, Page 1165.

The most commonly cited symptoms, in order of decreasing frequency, are chest pain 88%, dyspnea 84%, and apprehension 59%.

2. **E**, Page 1166.

The most commonly found physical findings are tachypnea 92%, trachycardia 44%, and fever 43%.

3. **E**, Page 1168.

An EKG is a relatively nonspecific adjunct in diagnosing pulmonary emobolism, but it can be helpful if comparative EKGs show new changes. The "classic" $S_1Q_3T_3$ pattern can be a normal variant and is infrequently seen in pulmonary embolism. Thirteen percent of patients will have normal EKGs. Therefore, all of the answers are possible.

4. **A**, Page 1168.

Ventilation/perfusion scans are sensitive but not specific for pulmonary embolism because many other pulmonary disorders (such as in *C*) can interfere with interpretation. V/Q scans are more sensitive than pulmonary angiograms in detecting pulmonary embolism but less specific. If a multiview V/Q scan is totally normal, one can essentially rule out a pulmonary embolism.

5. **A**, Page 1168.

The most common fingings on a chest x-ray film are related to decreased volume and include an elevated diaphragm, parenchymal consolidation, and atelectasis. The other answers listed are all more specific for a pulmonary embolism but less common. A wedge-shaped pleural-based density is a "Hampton's hump." A unilateral dilated pulmonary artery with diminished segment perfusion distally (answers *D* and *E*) is Westermark's sign.

6. **D**, Page 1173.

Protamine is a specific antidote for heparin. It is given as 1 mg to neutralize 10 units of heparin up to 100 mg. Although heparin can cause a thrombocytopenia, it does not do so acutely and platelets will not help. Both fresh-frozen plasma and cryoprecipitate can cause a volume overload, as well as hepatitis, and are not indicated. A patient with active bleeding given this much heparin should have it reversed since it can be done quickly with little risk.

7. **A**, Page 1168.

A perfusion lung scan is more sensitive than even a pulmonary angiogram, which can miss multiple small emboli in vessels below 2 mm. A normal perfusion lung scan virtually excludes the possibility of a pulmonary emboli and more invasive tests are not needed. However, the procedure is limited by its lack of specificity. Five percent of normal volunteers will have an abnormal scan and virtually any pulmonary pathology, including completely reversible bronchospasm, will have an abnormal scan. The procedure is noninvasive and risk-free with no danger of anaphylaxis or arrhythmias as there is with pulmonary arteriography.

8. **E**, Page 1166.
   Malignancy and obesity may facilitate thrombogensis by one or more mechanisms. Prolonged immobilization of lower extremities may lead to stasis, thrombosis, and embolization. A history of drug abuse or other sources of infection should be considered as possible sites of septic embolization.

9. **B**, Page 1168.
   A normal young person has gradient of 5–15 mm Hg. Old patients and those with pulmonary pathology may normally have a gradient as high as 25–30 mm Hg. Pulmonary emboli increases the A-a gradient through intrapulmonary right-to-left shunting.

10. **C**, Pages 1165–1166.
    A history of cough, fever, chills, and sputum production preceding the onset of chest pain and dyspnea suggests pneumonia or pleurisy. Chest wall tenderness to palpation suggests muscular skeletal chest pain but is not inconsistent with a peripheral emboli irritating the intercostal nerves. The acute onset of dyspnea alone is not helpful in determing a diagnosis.

11. **E**, Page 1165.
    The majority of experimental and clinical evidence indicates that atelectasis is the major cause of hypoxemia with resultantly increased right-to-left shunt. The diffusion impairment in pulmonary vasculature does attribute but is not thought to be the major cause of hypoxemia. Pulmonary AV anastamoses are thought to open, thereby increasing the shunt. Pulmonary vasoconstriction is not thought to be a major factor.

12. **E**, Page 1168.
    A pleural-based rounded density with a convexity towards the hilum is an unusual but highly specific (Hampton's hump) radiographic feature of a pulmonary emobli. The other listed answers are all seen more often but are less specific.

13. **A**, Page 1167.
    The mean PAP is usually elevated when a degree of pulmonary arterial occlusion approaches 30%. There is also an elevation of the mean RAP when the extent of occlusion exceeds 35%. Jugular vein examination may reveal large A-waves. LVEDP may be normal or decreased but is not generally elevated as the result of an acute pulmonary emboli.

14. **D**, Page 1173.
    Most fatalities are secondary to a recurrence of embolism. When in doubt, heparin may prevent the second episode. Anticoagulation can be reversed with protamine if hemorrhagic complications develop. The unavailability of lung scan along with the strong likelihood of pulmonary emboli and absence of contraindications would favor heparin therapy. Age of the patient should not be a factor.

15. **A**, Pages 1165–1166.
    Predisposing factors include deep vein thrombosis, immobilization, congestive heart failure, chronic lung disease, peripheral vascular disease, malignancy, obesity, oral contraceptives, and previous history of embolism. Tachypnea was found in 92%, tachycardiac in only 44%, and fever over 38.5°C in 43%. A patient with dyspnea, fever, and infiltrates may well have a pulmonary embolus, not a pneumonia. (That's why we pay malpractice premiums.)

16. **D**, Pages 1172–1173.
    Heparin does very little to dissolve a clot once formed, whether in the pulmonary circulation or deep venous system. It works by preventing *propagation* of a clot and depends on the body's intrinsic system to dissolve the clots already present. Heparin has been shown to decrease some of the secondary actions of an embolism on the pulmonary vasculature but its main effect is on preventing further emboli.

65

Aspiration

1. **D**, Pages 1181–1182.
   Early intubation and mechanical ventilation have proved useful in reversing hypoxia and improving survival after aspiration. Several studies have stressed mechanical ventilation, even if oxygenation appears good. It appears to protect the pulmonary vascular system through an unknown mechanism. Both antibiotics and steroids appear to worsen the outcome of aspiration when used early in the course. Initially diuretics are also contraindicated, since these patients develop a relative hypovolemia from pooling of fluid in the lung.

2. **A**, Page 1178.
   Secondary bacterial infection is very common and may be hard to diagnose. These patients all have fever, leukocytosis, purulent sputum, and pulmonary infiltrates from their initial insult. Prophylactic antibiotics are not helpful. They merely alter the causative agent to a more resistant strain. Anaerobes from the oropharynx are the most common pathogens. Although gentamicin should be used in a hospital-acquired, secondary pneumonia, clindamycin would be a better choice than a cephalosporin. PEEP has no effect on the incidence of secondary infection.

3. **B**, Page 1178.

Most lung abscesses are secondary to aspiration of oropharyngeal flora. Anaerobes are 10 times as common as aerobes in the mouth and account for 88% of community-acquired lung abscesses. High-dose penicillin is the drug of choice, even though identified pathogens such as *Bacteroides fragilis* may be resistant to it.

4. **A**, Page 1180.

The earliest radiographic change seen with aspiration is atelectasis seen after the first hour. Of particular importance is the fact that infiltrates from aspiration alone do not progress beyond 36 hours. If there are progressive infiltrates beyond 2 days, a secondary infection must be considered.

5. **D**, Pages 1175–1176.

Paralyzing agents occasionally used to control patients during intubation place patient at great risk for aspiration because of all the listed factors. In general patients are at high risk if they have lost the reflex protection of their airways, lost control or coordination of the muscles involved in swallowing or regurgitation, or have structural defects in the gastrointestinal tract.

6. **B**, Page 1175.

Aspiration carries significant morbidity and mortality rates, as high as 70% even with the best treatment regimens. Difficulty and confusion concerning the diagnosis occur because the aspiration event is often silent. The prognosis of patients with aspiration is related to the character and volume of the aspirate.

7. **B**, Page 1176.

The presence of an N/G tube disrupts the competency of the upper and lower esophageal sphincters. This, in addition to the risk of inducing vomiting with a full stomach during the insertion process, may increase the risk of aspiration with use of N/G tube. Once the N/G tube is in place and functioning properly to keep the stomach empty, there is little risk of aspiration.

8. **D**, Page 1178.

The major factors that determine the progression of aspiration to pneumonitis are dental hygiene, general state of health, integrity of cough, as well as smoking habits. The cough and gag reflex along with pulmonary macrophagias, the mucociliary membrane, and intact immune system generally can handle aspiration of oropharyngeal secretions unless the innoculum of infective material is so large that the defense system is overwhelmed.

9. **D**, Page 1177.

In the first few minutes following water or saline aspiration, there is a rapid fall in PaO_2; this leads to a marked reduction in compliance, a decreased O_2 saturation, and an increased shunt. These are the result of a reflex airway closure and microatelectasis.

10. **C**, Page 1180.

Signs and symptoms occur in most patients within the first hour. A few patients will have a lag time up to 6 hours before the onset of symptoms. Apnea has been found immediately in as many as one-third of patients who aspirate. Initially, the chest x-ray shows no change but in 6–12 hours after the insult, development of infiltrates resembling pulmonary edema can be found.

11. **B**, Page 1179.

Initially the cardiac index is normal-to-high with a normal-to-low CVP. Within the first hours sequestration of fluid in the lungs causes massive pulmonary edema, and a fall in blood pressure will occur if hypovolemia is untreated. The combination of hypotension and pulmonary edema was once believed to represent cardiogenic shock. However, hemodynamic monitoring has shown there is no direct effect of aspiration on myocardial function.

12. **D**, Page 1182.

Prophylactic antibiotic use has not been shown to prevent infection and is associated with the onset of suprainfections and the development of resistant strains. Bacterial pneumonia occurs eventually in as many as 50% of patients with acid aspiration. Indications for antibiotics after an aspiration are: (1) new fever or higher fever, (2) new or expanding infiltrate more than 36 hours after aspiration, (3) increasing leukocytosis, (4) purulent sputum, (5) positive cultures, (6) consistent gram's stain, and (7) unexplained patient deterioration.

66

Thrombophlebitis

1. **A**, Page 1185.

Vessel wall injury, a hypercoagulable state, and venous stasis are the necessary factors in producing DVT, although the relative importance of each is unknown. Decreased factor X and elevated antithrombin III would both prevent clotting, not enhance it.

2. **E**, Page 1187.

When well-accepted clinical signs of DVT are considered individually or in any combination, there still is an unacceptable frequency of false-positives and false-negatives. Fifty percent of patients with these signs will have normal venograms, while 50% of patients will pedal edema but no signs will have DVT on venogram.

3. **A**, Pages 1188–1189.

Venography is the single most sensitive and specific test for diagnosing DVT. Doppler ultrasound takes considerable experience and even then has a large number of associated false-negatives. Impedance plethysomography has demonstrated an overall accuracy of 95% compared with venography, but there are false-positives associated with COPD and altered right-sided heart hemodynamics. ^{125}I-fibrinogen requires a 24-hour delay from injection until scanning can be done, as well as a high number of false-negatives in the thigh. Radionuclide phlebography will not identify isolated calf vein thrombi unless extensive disease is present.

4. **C**, Page 1192.

While it is true that DVT limited to the calf rarely causes clinically significant pulmonary emboli, they may cause subclinical pulmonary emboli. Twenty percent of them extend proximally to the popliteal area where there is a much greater chance of significant embolization. These patients should be fully anticoagulated with IV heparin.

5. **D**, Page 1186.

Antithrombin III is a circulating protein that inhibits the action of thrombin on fibrinogen. Heparin works by increasing circulating antithrombin III.

6. **E**, Pages 1187–1188.

Bruits are expected with arterial disease and are not associated with venous thrombosis. This diagnosis is impossible to make clinically and a high index of suspicion in appropriate clinical settings. Early laboratory consultation is mandatory.

67

Aortic Aneurysms

1. **E**, Pages 1202–1203.

Hypertension is the most common cause of a dissecting aneurysm. A patent ductus arteriosa overloads the pulmonary circulation but does not cause increased pressure along the aorta. These patients are not predisposed to developing dissection.

2. **C**, Page 1205.

While all of the listed answers can complicate dissection of a thoracic aneurysm, by far the most common is hypertension. It is important to treat not only the absolute blood pressure but also the rate of pressure development which determines the extension of the dissection. Classically trimethaphan is used; the combination of nitroprusside and propranalol can also be used.

3. **E**, Pages 1198–1199.

Abdominal aortic aneurysms can remain asymptomatic even when quite large; as many as 65% are found unexpectedly during routine physical examinatin or radiographs for other reasons. All of the other listed answers can be the initial presentation of an abdominal aortic aneurysm.

4. **E**, Page 1200.

For all of the reasons listed ultrasound and/or CT scanning has largely replaced aortography in the evaluation of abdominal aortic aneurysms. A false-negative examination is possible when only the functional lumen is identified and aortic wall calcification is absent.

5. **A**, Page 1199.

The physical examination has reported accuracy of 80–90% of detecting abdominal aortic aneurysms. This emphasizes the importance of careful palpation of the abdomen even when pathology is not suspected.

6. **B**, Page 1200.

It should be emphasized that it is the natural history of all aneurysms to rupture. In a patient younger than 65 who is a good surgical candidate any size aneurysm should be replaced. The cut-off for following expectantly an aneurysm in a poor surgical risk candidate seems to be 6 cm. All aneurysms of 6 cm should be surgically repaired.

68

Arteriovascular Diseases

1. **A**, Page 1214.

Raynaud's disease is caused by increased sympathetic stimulation. This results in the classic triple phasic response of pallor followed by cyanosis and finally redness. This most typically involves the hands and is induced by cold exposure and occasionally by emotional stress. Reserpine depletes the sympathetic nerves of catecholamines, allowing for local vasodilatation.

2. **A**, Page 1209.

The hallmark of acute arterial occlusion is pallor, pulselessness, paresthesias, paralysis, and pain. *B* and *D* are incorrect because ulcerations of the skin are signs of chronic arterial insufficiency and would not be associated with an acute event. *C* is incorrect because the hand should be pale, not flushed.

3. **D**, Page 1211.

The most common source of peripheral emboli is mural thrombi from a diseased heart. Approximately 50% of patients have atrial fibrillation. Valvular heart disease is also common.

4. **D**, Pages 1213–1214.

Although this is a good history for Raynaud's disease, several other conditions should be considered. Peripheral emboli, Raynaud's phenomenon, and thoracic outlet syndrome can give symptoms such as these, which is why an EKG, ANA and sedimentation rate, and Adson's maneuver, respectively, should be evaluated. Systemic hypoxia would not give the localized constellation of symptoms described, so ABGs are not useful.

5. **B**, Page 1220.

All of the answers are true causes of thoracic outlet syndrome except for *B*. The symptoms are produced when the shoulders are moved backward and downward, not anterior and cephalad. Compression in this case is caused by hypertrophy of the subclavian muscle, abnormalities of the first rib, and old clavicular fractures.

6. **B**, Page 1220.

The thoracic outlet syndrome is caused by pressure on the neurovascular bundle in the neck or thorax. The presenting symptoms are paresthesias, usually along the ulnar border of the forearm and hand. Sympathetic dystrophy can occur, which is confused with Raynaud's syndrome. All of the answers can cause thoracic outlet obstruction, but a cervical rib is the most common.

7. **A**, Page 1213.

While Raynaud's syndrome can be associated with any connective tissue disease, it is most commonly associated with sclerodema and the mixed connective tissue disease syndrome. Raynaud's syndrome is the initial presentation of sclerodema in 70% of cases.

8. **B**, Page 1224.

Even with good control of blood pressure, with progressive stenosis renal failure can occur. Surgery has been found to improve blood pressure in 89% of patients (it will completely cure it 55% of the time) and will improve renal function. The renal vein renin index is helpful for predicting responses to surgery, but the high incidence of bilateral disease may give a false-negative. Fibromuscular disease is seen most often in young women.

9. **E**, Page 1223.

A symptomatic bruit that can be found in 4% of those over age 50 is not necessarily an indication for arteriography. A noninvasive study such as a Doppler is done and then arteriography only if a high degree of obstruction is suggested.

10. **E**, Page 1217.

Buerger's disease is a vasculitis involving the *distal* small arteries seen most often in Jewish men who are smokers. It is not associated with ischemic heart disease, but frequently amputation of fingers and toes is necessary. There is no truly effective treatment, although preganglionic sympathectomy is advocated by some.

69

Infective Endocarditis and Acquired Valvular Heart Disease

1. **E**, Page 1236.

Many arrhythmias are associated with prolapse of mitral valve, supraventricular tachycardia and PVCs most often. However, third degree block is rare. The best way to diagnose a suspected case is with echocardiography.

2. **A**, Page 1233.

Alpha streptococcus or *S. viridans* is the most common cause of subacute bacterial endocarditis. The pathogen usually infects a valve damaged by rheumatic fever or congenital heart disease, most commonly the mitral valve followed by the aortic. *S. viridans* is very sensitive to penicillin.

3. **A**, Page 1238.

A loud S_1 is caused when the ventricles have relatively less volume at end diastole. As the ventricles fill with blood the mitral valve leaflets float upward into a more nearly closed position. Thus, with any lesion that causes volume overload of the ventricle, the valve is in a nearly closed position at the beginning of systole, and a soft S_1 is heard.

4. **A**, Pages 1237–1240.
5. **A**, Pages 1237–1240.
6. **C**, Pages 1237–1240.
7. **B**, Pages 1237–1240.
8. **D**, Pages 1237–1240.
9. **G**, Pages 1237–1240.

10. **E**, Pages 1237–1240.

The left atrial hypertension of mitral stenosis can progress to pulmonary hypertension and ultimately right heart failure. Atrial fibrillation frequently complicates valvular disorders and is most commonly found in mitral stenosis, mitral regurgitation, tricuspid stenosis, and tricuspid regurgitation. The cardinal symptoms of aortic stenosis are dyspnea on exertion, angina, and exertional syncope. Aortic stenosis can result in sudden death from dysrhythmias, and once symptoms are present early valve replacement is advocated. The characteristic murmur of mitral regurgitation is a grade 3–6 apical holosystolic murmur radiating to the axilla. Aortic regurgitation patients can be asymptomatic for years. The first complaints are generally dyspnea and fatigue. Chest pain and palpitations can also occur. Pulmonic valvular disease is associated with a parasternal lift, a widening split S-2, a systolic injection click, and a harsh systolic murmur loudest in the left second intercostal space and increasing with inspiration. Tricuspid stenosis causes prominent A waves in the jugular venous pulse and tricuspid regurgitation causes prominent C-V waves along with jugular venous distention.

11. **B**, Pages 1237–1238.

The best way to hear the sometimes subtle diastolic rumble of mitral stenosis is to have the patient exercise by doing several rapid sit-ups and then quickly lie down on the left side, while you listen over the apex with the bell of the stethoscope. Having the patient lean forward with hands tightly clasped during exhalation is the best position to hear the high-pitched murmur of aortic insufficiency along the left sternal border. Valsalva's maneuver will accentuate the murmur of IHSS and prolapse of the mitral valve while it diminishes all other murmurs.

12. **B**, Page 1233.

Virtually any organism appears capable of causing this infection, including gram-negative bacteria and *S. aureus*. Gram-positive cocci of the *streptococcus* species is the most common cause.

13. **C**, Page 1233.

Most commonly endocarditis affects the mitral valve with rheumatic valvular disease being the most common predisposing factor. Any lesion that involves turbulent blood flow can predispose to endocarditis. Common sources of transient bacteremia include dental procedures, GI or GU manipulations, and skin infections. Echocardiography is particularly helpful diagnostically by aiding in the visualization of vegetations, especially in a subacute process.

14. **C**, Pages 1235–1236.

Currently four (4) basic valve types are in use, each with different normal and abnormal sounds. In general, dampening of any sounds or the presence of a *new* murmur suggests dysfunction such as thrombosis, infection, or valvular degeneration. Sharp opening and closing sounds in the aortic ball cage valve are normal. Apical diastolic rumbles are present in two-thirds of the mitral tissue valves but not aortic tissue valves. Central occluder disk valves produce opening sounds. Both tilting disk valves and central occluder disk valves produce a high-pitched click-closing sound.

15. **C**, Page 1236.

Mitral valve prolapse, although the most common valvular abnormality, generally has the least clinical significance.

16. **D**, Page 1234.

Despite antibiotic therapy, up to 25% of patients die from this disease. Congestive heart failure is the most common cause of death followed by emboli to the brain. Mycotic aneurysms, coronary artery embolus, ruptured sinus of valsalva, and dysrhthmias are also significant contributors to morbidity and mortality. Causes of right-sided endocarditis have a high incidence of lung abscess or infarction.

17. **D**, Pages 1234–1235.

Currently the American Heart Association recommends a throat culture for individuals in the age group at risk for rheumatic fever (4–20 years of age). In older or younger patients, the culture should be done selectively. Positive cultures are treated with penicillin or erythromycin for penicillin-allergic patients.

18. **B**, Page 1233.

The hallmark of infective endocarditis is the nonspecificity of its clinical manifestations. Common complaints include fatigue, malaise, arthralgia, headache, weight loss, night sweats, and fever. Many patients also develop various neurologic complaints related to embolization ranging from focal defects to coma or meningitis.

19. **D**, Page 1234.

Most patients will develop a new heart murmur at some point during the course of their disease. Up to 95% have fever. Microvascular lesions such as petechia tend to occur in more subacute cases. Leukocystosis and an elevated sedimentation rate commonly occur, but the cornerstone of the diagnosis is positive blood cultures, which are present in up to 95% of patients.

20. **B**, Page 1234.

Migratory nondeforming polyarthritis, which is seen in 80% of cases, is the single most common manifestation of acute rheumatic fever. Carditis is next, seen in 40% of cases, and is usually manifested as murmurs of mitral or aortic regurgitation. The others are seen in 10–15% or less of cases. Besides the Jones criteria, supporting evidence of recent streptococcal infection (positive throat culture, increased ASO titer) is essential to the diagnosis of acute rheumatic fever.

21. **E**, Pages 1236–1237.

The EKG in patients with the click murmur syndrome is usually normal. Often, however, especially when the patient is symptomatic with chest pain, inverted T-waves in leads 2,3 and AVF are seen. This is felt to be due to ischemia of the papillary muscle.

22. **D**, Page 1238.

Palpation of the carotid upstroke and volume is the most sensitive indicator of the severity of aortic stenosis. It is unreliable, however, when a patient has combined aortic stenosis and aortic insufficiency. The length or intensity of the murmur do not correlate with the pressure gradient across the valve.

23. **E**, Page 1233.

Right-sided endocarditis is most likely to involve a normal valve and is seen most often in intravenous drug users. Nafcillin or oxacillin is the drug of choice.

24. **D**, Page 1238.

Mitral stenosis causes a pressure gradient between the left atrium and left ventricle, forcing the atrium to work harder and hypertrophy. Many patients do well even with increasing left atrial hypertrophy but suddenly decompensate when atrial fibrillation develops and the atrium no longer helps overcome the pressure gradient.

25. **E**, Page 1236.

In addition to these criteria, a pansystolic murmur with light systolic accentuation, multiple frequent premature ventricular contractions, and angiographic or echocardiographic severe mitral valve prolapse increases the risk of serious dysrhythmias. There is an increased risk of sudden death if many of these criteria are present and prophylactic treatment with beta blockers is indicated.

70

Hypertension

1. **A**, Page 1249.

Malignant hypertension is caused by fibrinoid necrosis of small arteries and is a medical emergency. It is always associated with papilledema and usually with a diastolic pressure greater than 130, although it can be as low as 110. Malignant hypertension can be associated with hypertensive encephalopathy, but either can exist without the other.

2. **E**, Page 1247.

Seizures are quite common during hypertensive encephalopathy, as are focal neurologic defects or coma. Many of these patients are first diagnosed as having intercerebral bleeding; however, the CT scan is negative. The encephalopathy is completely reversible if the blood pressure is controlled quickly. However, death can occur in a few hours if not treated promptly.

3. **A**, Page 1253.

Toxemia of pregnancy is associated with a 10–15% maternal mortality, most often from cerebral hemorrhage. Antihypertensive therapy with hydralazine should be initiated, and if seizures seem imminent (i.e., hyperactive reflexes) magnesium sulfate should be given promptly.

4. **E**, Page 1254.

Most aortic dissections are missed on their initial evaluation in the emergency department. Myocardial infarctions affect the same patient population of middle-aged hypertensive males and are much more common. A high degree of clinical suspicion is mandatory. The EKG is not helpful because ischemic changes are common with aortic dissections, and even an acute myocardial infarction may be caused by proximal dissection with compromise of coronary arteries.

5. **E**, Page 1247.

Angina is a relative contraindication to diazoxide because it may worsen the pain or precipitate an infarction from decreased perfusion of the myocardium. Diazoxide, when given, should be used with Lasix to counter its sodium-retaining properties.

6. **B**, Page 1250.

7. **A**, Page 1250.

8. **E**, Page 1250.

9. **C**, Page 1250.

10. **D**, Page 1250.

It is important for the emergency physician to be aware of the complications and side effects of drugs that patients may be taking. Minoxidil, a potent direct arteriolar vasodilator, is unique in causing a pericardial effusion. Aldomet frequently causes a positive Coombs test, which occasionally progresses to a hemolytic anemia. It can also cause liver damage. Hydralazine is associated with a positive antinuclear antibody that progreses to a lupus-like syndrome 10% of the time. Propranolol can exacerbate asthma and congestive heart failure, as well as precipitate hypoglycemia while masking the signs and symptoms. Furosemide can cause electrolyte disorders by its potassium-wasting properties, causing a metabolic alkalosis. In large doses it can also cause hearing loss.

11. **A**, Page 1246.

This patient has clonodine withdrawal, which often mimics a pheochromocytoma. Inderal can cause an increased blood pressure and other symptoms, but the sweating and tremor especially are not seen. Hyperthyroidism is not associated with sudden hypertension and is rare in middle-aged males as is a pheochromocytoma. Hydralazine does not cause symptoms on abrupt withdrawal.

12. **C**, Page 1256.

An *asymptomatic* patient with this level of blood pressure and no evidence of congestive heart failure or renal failure does not require urgent therapy or admission. Every patient should have a thorough physical examination with particular attention to the optic fundi and cardiovascular system. In the newly diagnosed patient, a chest X-ray and EKG should be obtained as should baseline electrolyte and renal studies, BUN, and urinalysis. Outpatient therapy should not be initiated by the emergency department, but patient education and prompt referral for follow-up is required.

13. **E**, Page 1247.

Nitroprusside has been evaluated in acute myocardial infarction as an aide to decrease infarction size. However, studies have not shown it to be effective. In some studies it actually seems to increase infarction size. It remains the agent of choice for rapidly controlling blood pressure in most clinical situations, eclampsia and dissecting aortic aneurysm being the main exceptions.

14. **A**, Pages 1244–1245.

Any young person with hypertension should have a careful search for a secondary cause of elevated blood pressure. Fibromuscular disease is the most common cause of elevated blood pressure in an otherwise healthy young woman. The diagnosis requires renal arteriograms but flank bruits offer a significant clue. Other findings with coarctation include a systolic murmur, heard best over the back, and delayed femoral pulses.

15. **A**, Page 1248.

Labetalol is a nonselective beta blocker with alpha 1 blocking properties. Postural hypertension can occur, so these patients should be treated in a supine position. Acute monitoring in an ICU setting as with nitroprusside is not required, however. It is contraindicated in pheochromocytomas as well as the other usual contraindications for beta blockers (congestive heart failure or COPD).

16. **A**, Page 1245.

This patient has a coarctation of the aorta. The notching of the ribs is due to increased collateral flow through the posterior intercostal arteries. The diagnosis is strongly suggested by a significant difference in blood pressure between the upper and lower extremities. Bobbing of the head can be seen with severe aortic regurgitation. Blue sclera are seen with osteogenesis imperfecta. An opening snap and diastolic rumble are found with mitral stenosis. An arm span greater than the patient's height suggests Marfan's syndrome, which can be associated with aortic insufficiency or aortic dissection.

17. **C**, Page 1249.

Hypertensive encephalopathy and malignant hypertension often coexist in the same patient and are both related to failure of autoregulatory mechanisms, but either can exist without the other. Malignant hypertension is rarely seen with a blood pressure of less than 130, but most people with pressures of this level do not develop malignant hypertension. Admission to the hospital with prompt control of blood pressure is necessary, but the agent used depends on the severity of the clinical syndrome. The underlying pathology is fibrinoid necrosis of small arterioles due to loss of autoregulation.

71

Dysrhythmias

1. **A**, Pages 1270–1273.

Quinidine is a very good drug for a patient who has been converted out of artrial fibrillation or flutter to a sinus rhythm, because it maintains the sinus rhythm. It is dangerous in atrial flutter, because it will increase conduction over the AV node and slow the flutter rate enough to allow for one-to-one conduction to occur with an increase in the ventricular response.

2. **A**, Page 1266.

Although all of the drugs can be used effectively, verapamil is now felt to be the drug of choice for SVT. From 5 to 10 mg given slowly IV will abort 90% of attacks.

3. **E**, Pages 1265–1267.

Verapamil is a calcium channel blocker with no effect on acetylcholine. Digitalis directly blocks the AV node as well as indirectly stimulating the vagal nerve, which increases conduction everywhere except the AV node. Edrophonium is a cholinesterase inhibitor that prevents the local breakdown of acetylcholine. Metaraminol and carotid massage increases vagal stimulation through local reflexes.

4. **C**, Page 1284.

As with any other tachyarrhythmia in an unstable patient, cardioversion is the most effective therapy. It carries no greater risk than in the normal population and may prove more effective because WPW is often resistant to standard drug therapy.

5. **D**, Page 1288.

Three of the most commonly used agents to slow rapid atrial fibrillation—digitalis, propranolol, and verapamil—are contraindicated in patients with WPW. While these drugs do decrease conduction over the AV node, they can also increase conduction over the bypass tract and increase the ventricular response. Bretylium has not been used for supraventricular arrhythmias, but its initial adrenergic release would be expected to increase the ventricular rate. Procainamide, which slows conduction over both the bypass tract and the AV node, is the drug of choice.

6. **B**, Page 1269.

The dysrhythmia described is atrial flutter with 2:1 conduction. Digitalization is the treatment of choice in stable patients. Quinidine is contraindicated in this case without prior digitalization because it enhances conduction through the AV node, causing 2:1 conduction to become 1:1 conduction. Cardioversion is reserved for unstable patients, lidocaine has very little effect on atrial dysrhythmias.

7. **B**, Page 1270.

Digitalis, verapamil, and propranolol are all drugs that may be used to slow the ventricular response in this particular dysrhythmia, which is atrial fibrillation. Cardioversion should be reserved for unstable patients.

8. **D**, Page 1272.

PVCs have a QRS that is 0.12 second in duration or greater, not 0.10 second.

9. **D**, Page 1274.

The dysrhythmia is now ventricular tachycardia. All of the answers may be appropriate management except for digitalis. Digitalis has no place in the treatment of arrhythmias of ventricular origin.

10. **C**, Page 1280.

Acute Mobitz type II block, even in a stable patient, requires a pacemaker. Atropine or Isuprel can be used while preparing the equipment; however, it can be associated with a decreased ventricular response, even though the sinus and AV nodal rates are increased. Likewise, lidocaine can increase the degree of block and should be avoided until a pacemaker can assure an adequate ventricular rate.

11. **C**, Page 1266.

Because the combined effect of IV beta blockers and calcium channel blockers can result in severe bradycardia, the two should not be used together, especially when given intravenously. Verapamil should also be avoided in patients with heart block, cardiomyopathy, or the sick sinus syndrome.

12. **D**, Page 1283.

The sick sinus syndrome is caused by a degenerative process involving the sinus and AV node. It is rarely caused by ischemic heart disease. These patients experience dizziness or syncope and may have an associated thromboembolic stroke. The therapy is a pacemaker, then adding suppressive antiarrhythmics as needed to control any tachyarrhythmias. It is often refractory to atropine, but if pushed to the full dose of 2 mg will usually respond.

13. **B**, Page 1268.

PAT with block is caused by digitalis over 80% of the time. However, the most common digitalis-induced arrhythmia is PVC. PAT with block is sometimes misdiagnosed as atrial fibrillation and treated with more digoxin.

14. **B**, Page 1272.

A PVC does not affect sinus node function. Therefore, while one sinus beat will be blocked at the AV node by the PVC, the next beat will occur exactly where expected in the cycle—two P-wave intervals from the last sinus beat. A PAC that originates in the atrium causes the sinus node to reset, so the next normal beat after a PAC is closer than expected to the aberrant beat.

15. **C**, Page 1284.

WPW is characterized by the short PR interval and delta waves or slurred upstroke of the R wave, best seen here in leads 2 and 3. This syndrome can mimic acute infarction, ventricular hypertrophy, or conduction delays, which is why it is so important to correctly identify the short PR interval and delta waves.

16. **B**, Page 1280.

This represents a second degree heart block with some of the sinus beats not conducting through to the ventricles. The gradual prolongation of the PR interval resulting in a dropped beat characterizes a Wenckebach or Mobitz type I second degree AV block.

17. **B**, Page 1272.

Multifocal atrial tachycardia is characterized by a somewhat irregular rhythm associated with different configurations of P waves and a varying PR interval. The definite P waves distinguish this arrhythmia from atrial fibrillation, which it can degenerate into.

18. **D**, Page 1274.

The patient with 6 PVCs in 24 hours is probably not at any greater risk than any other patient with an acute myocardial infarction. Bigeminy, multifocal PVCs, and R on T phenomena probably do confer a greater risk to the patient but the significance is unclear. Repetitive runs of PVCs have been clearly shown to predispose these patients to sudden death. These patients should be considered for long-term antiarrhythmic therapy.

19. **E**, Page 1264.

Once a dysrhythmia is identified, the clinical significance must be determined prior to the initiation of treatment. All EKG rhythms must be correlated with the patient's clinical status. When patients are unstable by any of these criteria, attempts to convert the acute dysrhythmia must be initiated immediately.

20. **F**, Page 1265.

This diagnosis should be reserved for regular tachyarrhythmias when the mechanism cannot be ascertained. Approximately 70% of SVTs are junctional in origin. The remainder are atrial tachyarrhythmias or atrial flutter in which the flutter wave cannot be identified.

21. **D**, Pages 1265–1266.

The preferred vagal maneuvers would be carotid massage and valsalva's maneuver. Eyeball pressure, although sometimes effective, has been associated with retinal detachment. Pulling on the tongue and the diver's reflex (holding the breath and placing the face in ice water) are also sometimes effective but uncomfortable for the patient. Valsalva's maneuver and carotid massage are the preferred vagal mechanisms and should be repeated if ineffective initially after pharmococolic therapy.

22. **C**, Page 1274.

Torsades de Pointes is morphologically distinct from other ventricular tachycardias. Its recognition is important in that the treatment differs slightly from other causes of ventricular tachycardia or ventricular fibrillation. If sustained, this is a life-threatening condition and ventricular cardioversion is indicated. If not immediately life-threatening, distinction needs to be made between the pause-dependent and adrenergic-dependent long Q-T syndromes. The pause-dependent type usually begins with a pause followed by an ectopic beat occurring on the U wave and can be treated with beta-adrenergic agonist. The adrenergic-dependent type occurring at times of increased rate, may be aggravated by beta agonist and is treated with beta blockers or calcium antagonist.

23. **C**, Page 1278.

AIVR occurs most often during the course of a myocardial infarction. Although this rhythm looks like slow ventricular tachycardia, it does not have the malignant potential of premature ventricular contractions for degenerating into ventricular fibrillation. No treatment is necessary.

24. **D**, Page 1261.

The relative refractory period is important because during this time an abnormal action potential or ectopic rhythm can be generated. During phase 3, a greater than normal stimulus is required to initiate a beat; therefore, it is relatively refractory. The absolute refractory period during the initial stage of the action potential is completely refractory to any new action potential generation. The so-called super normal period actually occurs during the relative refractory period at a time when a smaller than normal stimulus can generate a new impulse. This period correlates with the down slope of the T wave.

25. **D**, Page 1261.

The specialized atrial tissues that conduct impulses slightly faster than normal are Wenckebach's bundle, Thorel's bundle, and Bachmann's bundle. The bundle of Kent is an accessory pathway found in the Wolff-Parkinson-White syndrome.

26. **A**, Page 1277.

Ventricular parasystole is a rhythm originating from a slow single focus in the ventricle competing with the underlying rhythm. The rate is usually 40–60 beats per minute. The characteristic EKG features include a changing coupling interval, frequent fusion beats, and a constant interectopic interval. This rhythm does not have the potential for deterioration to a life-threatening rhythm, even though R on T phenomena can occur. Treatment is of underlying cardiac failure frequently associated with ventricular parasystole.

27. **A**, Page 1283.

The sick sinus syndrome is caused by disease involving the sinoatrial node and is characterized by sinus bradycardia, sinus arrest, and sinus block. Concomitant irritability of the atrium results in atrial tachycardia, Paroxysmal atrial tachycardia, or atrial fibrillation. A-V conduction is usually well-preserved. The syndrome often presents with rapid swings from slow to rapid rhythms known as the tachybrady syndrome.

28. **A**, Page 1272.

Multifocal apical tachycardia is seen most in hypoxic patients with COPD. It is very difficult to treat and most authorities recommend treating only the underlying COPD. It often alternates with atrial fibrillation.

29. **C**, Pages 1259–1261.

The summation of all the depolarizations of the ventricle make up the QRS complex, while the repolarization of the ventricle is reflected by the T wave. Thus, the Q-T interval is equal to the action potential duration. The P wave is the summation of all the atriomyocardial depolarizations.

30. **B**, Page 1280.

A-V dissociation occurs when the ventricular rate is controlled by a junctional or idioventricular site that is dissociated from the sinus rhythm. Regular PP intervals and RR intervals are observed, representing atrial and ventricular rates functioning independently of each other. This can be the result of endstage atrial ventricular block or an overriding accelerated junctional or ventricular pacing site

31. **D**, Page 1259.

In myocardial working cells, fast channels allow the influx of sodium during phase zero (0) of the action potention. Sodium, calcium, and potassium are returned to their previous position by an energy-dependent electrolyte pump. In pacemaker cells there is a spontaneous loss of internal negativity allowing threshold potential to be reached, and a spontaneous action potential thus occurs. The steeper the slope of phase 4 depolarization causes both greater automaticity and a faster rate of spontaneous depolarization.

32. **D**, Pages 1261, 1263.

Enhanced automaticity affects phase 4 of the action potential by either changing the rate of automaticity in normal conducting tissue or allowing for certain areas to suddenly develop unusually increased automaticity. Reentry is a common cause of many tachyarrhythmias. It results when there is a difference in the refractoriness in two areas of tissue, causing an area of unidirectional block. Trigger automaticity is a third recently proposed mechanism related to a transient instability of the cell membrane after depolarization. Increased excitability may be caused by ischemia or electrolyte imbalance but is not a major mechanism for arrythmia genesis.

72
Congestive Heart Failure

1. **B**, Page 1293.

The earliest sign of left-sided failure is related to the increased left atrial pressure. This initially causes an upward redistribution of pulmonary blood flow to the upper lobes, followed by interstitial edema and finally alveolar edema.

2. **D**, Page 1294.

Morphine is the mainstay of the treatment of congestive heart failure in both the child and the adult. It decreases both preload and afterload, diminishes anxiety, and increases cardiac contractility. In appropriate doses of 0.1 to 0.2 mg/kg, it has no more respiratory depression than in adults.

3. **E**, Page 1298.

Unlike verapamil, nifedipine has very little effect on the AV node and is not useful for controlling the ventricular rate in supraventricular tachycardia or atrial fibrillation. It is the most potent vasodilator, and therefore the most likely to cause hypotension. Verapamil has the most effect on the AV node conductivity and is the most likely of calcium channel blockers to result in bradyarrhythmias. Diltiazem is primarily a vasodilator but is less likely than nifedipine to cause hypotension or than verapamil to cause bradyarrhythmias.

4. **E**, Page 1299.

Digitalis is contraindicated in acute myocardial infarctions unless they have a supraventricular tachyarrhythmia. In cases of acute myocardial infarction, digitalis can decrease left ventricular function. Most people would agree with prophylactic lidocaine in a definite infarction even without PVC's. O_2 is an important part of therapy and should not be withheld because this patient has COPD. Initial low flow and an early check on blood gases are indicated. This patient has been on nitrates before and they should be continued during her current acute event. Withdrawal of the nitrates may precipitate vascular spasm and worsen ischemia.

5. **B**, Page 1293.

A myxomatous mitral valve is a common congenital anomaly that will account for an asymptomatic murmur. Under stress, the chordae tendineae can rupture and precipitate sudden acute mitral insufficiency and congestive heart failure. The sea-gull-type murmur is typical for this. An acute myocardial infarction should not be associated with a murmur this loud unless papillary muscle rupture is present, which is quite rare.

6. **C**, Page 1295.

Furosemide causes increased calcium excretion in the urine, unlike thiazide diuretics, which decrease calcium excretion.

7. **E**, Page 1293.

All of these entities can precipitate pulmonary edema as well as being masked by predominant signs and symptoms of pulmonary edema. Every patient that presents with pulmonary edema must undergo a diligent search for the precipitating event.

8. **D**, Page 1291.

Although all the listed disorders can produce congestive heart failure, the most common cause is hypertension, which is completely preventible with appropriate therapy.

9. **C**, Page 1299.

PVCs are the most common arrhythmia associated with Digitalis. However, they are also seen in many other clinical conditions, so they rarely suggest Digitalis toxicity. PAT with block is the most pathognomonic arrhythmia of Digitalis toxicity, but it is rarely seen.

10. **D**, Page 1299.

Digitalis works by binding to the myocardial cell ATP pump and increasing the intracellular sodium content. All of the answers listed diminish the sensitivity to Digitalis except for hypokalemia, which significantly increases it.

11. **C**, Page 1377.

Nitroglycerin results in dilatation of the capacitance vessels leading to a reduction in left ventricular size and wall stress and thus a decrease in MVO_2. Concurrent acceleration of heart rate does cause increase in MVO_2. The net result, however, is a decreased MVO_2.

12. **E**, Page 1294.

The ideal approach would be to have a Swan-Ganz catheter in place so that pulmonary capillary wedge measurements would tell you if you needed to increase or decrease preload, and systemic vascular resistance measurements could tell if afterload reduction was needed. If the patient is hypovolemic because of vigorous diuresis, a fluid challenge may be necessary. Dopamine would be relatively ineffective without adequate vascular volume but may be needed along with nitroglycerin and/or nitride to maximally unload the left ventricle.

13. **C**, Page 1294.

Pulmonary edema with a normal heart size may indicate constrictive pericarditis, massive myocardial infarction, noncardiogenic pulmonary edema, and mitral stenosis but not mitral regurgitation.

14. **A**, Page 1291.

The Frank-Starling mechanism refers to the increased force of contraction that results from increasing end-diastolic volume and resting muscle length. Ionotropic state or velocity of contraction of cardiac muscle can be enhanced via increased circulating catecholamines and adrenergic drugs, or digitalis. In a failing heart, increasing heart rate has a greater effect on cardiac output than on the normal heart. These three mechanisms are all effective on a short-term basis. On a longer-term basis, hypertrophy of cardiac chambers may assist in compensating for increasing demand.

15. **B**, Pages 1297–1298.

Hydralazine is a direct arterial dilator. Captopril, an angiotensin-converting enzyme inhibitor has both potent preload and afterload reducing properties. Nifedipine, a calcium channel blocker, has a predominant effect on afterload. Prazosin is an alpha-adrenergic blocker causing marked venodilatation and mild arterial dilatation.

16. **A**, Page 1298.

One advantage of dobutamine over dopamine is its ability to decrease afterload without tachycardia. There is some debate about whether dobutamine is less arrythmogenic; however, most experts feel that this is true. Dobutamine does not selectively increase renal blood flow as dopamine does in low doses. The single best indication for Digitalis is uncontrolled atrial fibrillation and congestive heart failure. Recent studies have shown that patients with sinus rhythm and chronic stable congestive heart failure can have Digitalis withdrawn without causing clinical deterioration. Amrinone is a noncatecholamine, recently introduced as an ionotropic agent.

17. **C**, Page 1293.

Pulmonary edema occurs first interstitially. Kerley described A, B, and C lines. A lines are straight nonbranching lines in the upper lung fields. The B lines are horizontal nonbranching lines at the periphery of the lower lung fields. C lines are nonbranching short lines in a reticular or honeycomb pattern in the lower lung fields. The B lines are the most easily recognized and most clinically useful.

18. **E**, Pages 1294, 1377.

Morphine is a valuable drug, both for its analgesic and hemodynamic effects. Morphine can dilate arteries, thereby decreasing systemic vascular resistance and improving coronary blood flow. It increases venous capacitance, thereby decreasing preload by effectively unloading the ventricle, and the stroke-work index is improved or increased.

19. **D**, Page 1297.

Venodilators decrease filling pressure or preload but do not affect afterload. Arterial dilators decrease systemic vascular resistance but do not affect preload. Most vasodilators have mixed effects with one or the other predominating. There are some vasodilators whose primary effect is afterload reduction such as nifedipine.

20. **E**, Pages 1292, 1293.

Dyspnea is a sensitive nonspecific symptom in congestive heart failure. Paroxysmal nocturnal dyspnea occurs in both congestive heart failure and exacerbations of chronic lung disease. The patient's appearance and neck vein examination are useless indicators of congestive heart failure since they may not only be misleading but are associated with several other disease states. The S_3 gallop is a specific indicator of a failing ventricle in the adult patient.

21. **C**, Page 1293.

The EKG and blood chemistry may help identify the precipitating cause of congestive heart failure but are not the most helpful to confirm the diagnosis. Arterial blood gases are useful to determine the impact of congestive heart failure on oxygenation and acid base balance, but again do not help with the differential diagnosis. The chest x-ray is most valuable in that with early failure redistribution of blood flow is seen, progressing to Kerley A, B, or C lines, indistinct pulmonary vessels, pleural effusions, interstitial edema, and "butterfly shaped" infiltrates in the hilar areas.

73
Cardiogenic Shock

1. **E**, Pages 1307–1308.

   A Swan-Ganz does not interfere with pulmonary blood flow or gas exchange and thus won't interfere with a match of ventilation and perfusion. All the other complications listed can occur and must be watched for closely. The balloon should never be left inflated, and the catheter is advanced only until a wedge tracing is first obtained.

2. **D**, Page 1307.

   The sudden onset of congestive heart failure after a myocardial infarction, especially when associated with a new murmur, suggests some structural alteration. Rupture of the papillary muscle or the ventricular septum is the most common. Papillary muscle rupture is more common with an inferior myocardial infarction and a murmur at the apex that radiates to the axilla.

3. **C**, Page 1309.

   This patient is hypotensive with a normal wedge pressure. A fluid challenge is what he needs, not vasopressors, which would increase blood pressure, but at the expense of myocardial oxygenation which is already compromised. The ventricles work most effectively with a wedge pressure of approximately 20. Fluids should be given until the wedge pressure reaches at least that level. Pressors should then be considered if the patient remains hypotensive.

4. **C**, Page 1307–1308.

   A patient with hypotension after an acute infarction should have invasive monitoring of ventricular function. If the wedge pressure is low, fluids should be given until it is in the 18 to 20 range. After that, pressor agents can be used to maintain a satisfactory blood pressure. In this patient who has no signs of failure, volume challenge should be used before resorting to dopamine if a Swan-Ganz is not readily available.

5. **B**, Page 1303.

   The central venous pressure only reflects the hemodynamics of the right ventricle. There may be a significant elevation in left ventricular end diastolic pressure without any change on the central venous pressure. This is why a pulmonary artery catheter is so important.

6. **B**, Page 1309.

   A pulmonary capillary wedge pressure of less than 15 torr indicates hypovolemia, but careful rehydration must be titrated to pulmonary capillary wedge pressure and pulmonary assessment, not blood pressure. Normal capillary wedge pressure is 8–12 Torr but in cardiogenic shock a higher filling pressure up to 18 Torr may be needed to maintain adequate cardiac output. If pulmonary congestion occurs, fluid administration should be discontinued and pharmacologic intervention (such as dopamine) should be considered.

7. **C**, Page 1310.

   There is no clear-cut preference of pharmacologic agents used in the treatment of cardiogenic shock. Each drug carries its particular advantages and disadvantages. Dopamine is still the most commonly used drug, but mortality of cardiogenic shock remains high despite its widespread use.

8. **B**, Page 1304.

   Cardiogenic shock commonly occurs when 40% or more of the ventricular mass has been damaged. When both right and left ventricular muscle have been damaged, there is also greater risk of the onset of cardiogenic shock. Cardiogenic shock carries a variable mortality, however. A left ventricular end diastolic pressure (LVEDP) of greater than 29 Torr carries a 100% mortality. However, a cardiac index of less than 2 l/min/m^2 with an LVEDP of less than 15 Torr carries a much better prognosis.

9. **E**, Page 1306.

   A number of noncardiac factors take on greater significance in the management of cardiogenic shock. Although slight volume loss does not profoundly alter cardiac output in a normally functioning myocardium, even slight alterations in this setting can profoundly affect cardiac output. Tachycardia may not allow sufficient time for ventricular filling and thereby limit stroke volume in addition to increasing myocardial oxygen demand. Myocardial contractility may be further depressed by the presence of acidosis. If metabolic derangements persist, vessel walls are themselves damaged and the shock state is worsened. The vasodilators may adversely affect vascular resistance, preventing the maintenance of perfusion pressure and the delivery of oxygen to myocardial cells. All of these factors take on greater significance in a patient with cardiogenic shock.

10. **A**, Page 1308.

    Although controversy exists regarding the appropriateness of Swan-Ganz catheterization in the emergency department, there are some clear indications for its use. Manipulation of hemodynamic variables is the cornerstone of management of cardiogenic shock and clinical data can be highly misleading. Therefore, pulmonary artery pressure monitoring is very helpful. A possible exception is hypovolemia that is corrected by fluid challenge. Invasive monitoring is not indicated unless hypotension is unresponsive to volume challenge.

11. **A**, Page 1303.

All of the described signs and symptoms may be present in cardiogenic shock. The features that distinguish cardiogenic shock from other types of shock are the presence of an increased left ventricular filling pressure as reflected by an elevated pulmonary capillary wedge pressure of greater than 16 Torr and a decreased cardiac output that becomes worse with IV fluids.

74

Ischemic Heart Disease

1. **D**, Page 1368.

In 66% of patients with sudden death, there is no associated infarction, although all have severe atherosclerotic disease. Paradoxically, for survivors of sudden death the prognosis is better when associated with an infarction. This is thought to be because a continuously ischemic area can continue to produce arrhythmias, whereas a dead area will become electrically silent after an infarction.

2. **E**, Page 1375.

Anterior myocardial infarctions are generally associated with a worse prognosis once the patient reaches the hospital. It is more likely to be associated with infarct extension, aneurysm formation, ventricular thrombi, and cardiogenic shock. However, early arrhythmias precipitating sudden death are seen with equal frequency in both.

3. **E**, Pages 1372–1375.

Coronary artery spasm is classically seen with Prinzmetal's variant angina, but it is increasingly associated with all types of coronary artery disease. The most common feature is spasm associated with a fixed stenotic lesion that can cause any of the disorders listed.

4. **B**, Page 1336.

Digitalis causes a downward sloping of the ST segment but not ST segment elevation. All of the other conditions can be confused with an acute myocardial infarction.

5. **C**, Page 1358.

The clinical course of acute myocardial infarction, transmural or subendocardial, is essentially the same. Ventricular ectopy, hypotension, and pericarditis occur with equal frequency in both. The electrocardiogram has not proved a good differentiator of transmural from non-transmural infarctions when anatomic studies are correlated. Recently it has been appreciated that subendocardial infarctions have a higher incidence of late arrhythmias after discharge from the hospital.

6. **B**, Page 1329.

Most murmurs decreased during Valsalva's maneuver because of the decreased blood returned to both the right and left ventricles. IHSS and prolapse of the mitral valve are exceptions in which increased intensity occurs. Valsalva's maneuvers can terminate a reentrant tachyarrhythmia by its parasympathetic stimulation, but it is dangerous in acute coronary ischemia because it reduces coronary blood flow.

7. **E**, Page 1355.

Pericarditis is frequently confused with myocardial ischemia because of the ST and T wave changes associated with it. However, it does not cause Q waves. Left ventricular hypertrophy can cause Q waves in V_1 through V_4. IHSS can cause Q waves anteriorly and inferiorly or posterior laterally. WPW can cause Q waves most often in the inferior leads. A left-sided pneumothorax can mimic an anterior myocardial infarction; however, the electrocardiogram will normalize if taken in an upright position.

8. **E**, Page 1363.

Left bundle branch block both mimics and masks acute myocardial infarctions. It is usually associated with a significant cardiac disease ischemia, hypertrophy, valvular disorder, or cardiomyopathy. Rarely is it seen in congenital heart disease.

9. **A**, Page 1367.

Both false negatives due to small infarctions and improper sampling and false positives due to chest trauma, cardioversion, or hypothermia can be seen with cardiac enzymes. Most importantly, they have little use in the emergency department. Patients with myocardial ischemia without infarction and therefore no rise in cardiac enzymes are still at high risk for sudden death and should be admitted and monitored.

10. **A**, Page 1328.

A tachycardia with wide complexes can be due to ventricular tachycardia supraventricular tachycardia with aberrancy. There are various ECG criteria to distinguish the two, but the physical exam can also be helpful. Cannon A waves are seen in the jugular vein when the atria contract against a closed ventricle. With ventricular tachycardia there is a dissociation between the atrial activity and the ventricles. At times the atria contract against a closed tricuspid valve resulting in intermittent cannon A waves. With supraventricular tachycardia the relationship between the atria and ventricles is preserved. However, a patient with an underlying atrial fibrillation will not have intermittent cannon A waves.

11. **A**, Page 1333.

Acute elevation of the R wave is a transient phenomenon lasting only a few minutes. It is recorded within seconds of the ligation of a coronary artery and can be seen with spasm as well as total thrombotic occlusion.

12. **B**, Page 1372.

Variant angina is due to spasm of a coronary artery. The arteries can be normal, but often spasm occurs in the region of a fixed atherosclerotic obstruction. It is associated with serious arrhythmias, AV block, ventricular fibrillation, and ventricular tachycardia. The calcium channel blockers are effective therapy in most cases. The EKGs show ST segment elevation during an episode of pain, which reverts as the spasm subsides and pain ceases.

13. **C**, Page 1373.

Angina due to ischemia at a distance from the infarct zone is associated with a 44% 1-month mortality and 72% overall mortality, significantly worse than the 15% mortality at 1 month and 33% overall mortality when the ischemia was in the area of the infarction. Ischemia at a distance angiographically represents a total occlusion of one vessel (the infarction area) and another severely narrowed vessel supplying the area of new ischemia.

14. **B**, Page 1359.

The right coronary artery supplies both the right ventricle and inferior portion of the left ventricle. Anterior myocardial infarctions, although usually more extensive, are not associated with a right ventricular infarction. Right ventricular infarctions usually present as right-sided congestive heart failure with jugular venous distention and peripheral edema with relatively clear lung fields. The treatment is to increase fluids to ensure adequate peripheral perfusion, not to give diuretics.

15. **B**, Pages 1339–1342.

All of these features suggest pericarditis rather than ischemia but the best differential is the P-R deviation. The T waves of pericarditis typically do not invert until after the ST segment has returned to base line, unlike ischemia where both occur together.

16. **E**, Pages 1346-1350.

Most authorities recommend a prophylactic pacemaker in all the listed conditions, regardless of location of the infarction. Also, lidocaine must be used with great caution here for fear of precipitating complete heart block.

17. **D**, Page 1346.

Right or left bundle branch block is not necessarily a reason for admitting a patient in the absence of other findings. It is important to carefully evaluate the patient and arrange for appropriate follow-up. Right bundle branch block and left anterior hemiblock are forms of bilateral bundle branch block, and a temporary pacemaker should be inserted if an acute infarction is suspected.

18. **E**, Page 1380.

Right ventricular infarction may be suggested in association with an elevated jugular venous pressure and EKG evidence of inferior wall myocardial infarction without congestive heart failure. The emergency department management is aggressive fluid resuscitation. Invasive monitoring is essential once the patient is admitted.

19. **D**, Pages 1329–1331.

The classic EKG changes of an acute transmural infarction are ST segment elevation that evolves with the development of pathologic Q waves. ST segment elevation, pathologic Q waves, ST segment depression, and T wave inversion are all suggestive of myocardial pathology but may be caused by such things as ventricular aneurysm, coronary artery spasm, old infarction, misplacement of leads, or electrolyte disturbances, to name but a few. There is no single EKG criteria that can accurately diagnose an acute myocardial infarction alone.

20. **A**, Page 1333.

Although rarely seen in the emergency department, the earliest EKG manifestation of acute myocardial ischemia is a marked increase in R wave voltage. Giant R waves are best seen in precordial leads and are usually accompanied by some ST segment elevation. Prominent T waves, hyperacute ST segment elevation, and Q waves all may accompany various phases of the acute myocardial infarction and are the expected EKG changes seen in the emergency department.

21. **B**, Page 1316.

The lessons learned from the institution of Coronary Care Units are many, including: (1) ischemic heart disease patients have the highest risk of developing ventricular fibrillation before the onset of symptoms; (2) electrical instability is the most common cause of cardiac arrest; (3) continuous monitoring is required for immediate detection of electrical instability; (4) the aggressive containment of lethal or potentially lethal rhythm disturbances is highly feasible; and (5) the authority to act quickly and decisively can be effectively delegated to specifically trained nurses.

22. **D**, Page 1318.

The ischemic condition involves more than disruption of the delivery of oxygen to the heart. It also involves disruption of 2 other key functions: the delivery of metabolic substrates to the heart and the removal of deleterious metabolic end products. All of these factors play a role in the progression of ischemia to cell death.

23. **B**, Page 1318.

Myocardial ischemia is more than oxygen deprivation alone, as illustrated by comparing a patient who has sustained an acute myocardial infarction and a patient who has hypoxemia as a consequence of congenital heart disease. Both patients have reduced oxygen delivery to the heart, but the patient with the acute myocardial infarction has the added problem of reduced coronary blood flow. In this example of congenital heart disease, hypoxemia is present without myocardial ischemia.

24. **D**, Page 1315.

Decline in mortality related to ischemic heart disease between 1968 and 1976 is 20.7%. The reason for this decline is unknown but probably has been influenced by many factors, including lifestyle changes, improved medical care, emergency medical services, and coronary artery bypass surgery.

25. **C**, Page 1319.

Myocardial ischemia may be precipitated by several mechanisms, including: (1) normal coronary artery perfusion with sudden acceleration of myocardial demand, (2) normal demand and suddenly decreased coronary perfusion, or (3) a mixture of stable decreased coronary perfusion and sudden acceleration of demand. This patient, judging by his medications, probably has coronary artery disease controlled with beta blockers, diuretics, and nitrates. The increased demand of mowing his lawn probably exceeded his myocardial reserved precipitating ischemia.

26. **D**, Page 1319.

All of the factors play a part in determining MVO_2. MVO_2 will be augmented by hypertension or by failure and subsequent dilatation of the left ventricle. Conversely MVO_2 will be diminished by decreasing arterial blood pressure, reducing left ventricular size, or improving left ventricular function.

27. **C**, Page 1378.

Each hospital must establish its own criteria for the use of thrombolytics, addressing such issues as age of the patient, length of time following the onset of symptoms, EKG criteria, and contraindications. The capacity of doing emergency cardiac catheterization is not necessary unless intracoronary thrombolytics are used.

28. **B**, Page 1379.

Because clinical findings do not always correlate with the correct measurements of hemodynamic status, a rational approach must be developed. This begins with an assessment of cardiac output through blood pressure, heart rate, urine output, and mental status. Left ventricular filling pressure is assessed through careful cardiopulmonary exam (listening for S_3 and rales and chest x-ray). Based on this assessment, the patients can be placed in one of four groups. First, those with no evidence of hypoperfusion or pulmonary congestion. Second, those with decreased cardiac output without pulmonary congestion (who are clinically hypovolemic and merit a cautious fluid challenge with regular reassessment). Third, those with evidence of pulmonary congestion and an adequate cardiac output. These patients usually do not require invasive monitoring and respond well to agents that decrease preloads. Fourth, those with a decreased cardiac output and pulmonary congestion do require hemodynamic monitoring for optimal therapy.

29. **D**, Page 1355.

Hypothermia produces a distinctive elevation of the J point known as the J wave or Osborn wave. The heart rate is generally slow even in the presence of atrial fibrillation. The Q-T interval is invariably prolonged. These changes are often present when the rectal temperature descends to 32°C or below.

30. **A**, Page 1355.

Failure to find a new Q wave in the presence of an old one does not exclude acute myocardial infarction. The other statements are all true and exemplify the difficulty in either determining the presence of acute myocardial infarction or excluding an old infarction. General conclusions supported by recent studies correlating Q waves with necrosis are as follows: (1) the EKG is relatively good in identifying an old myocardial infarction; (2) the EKG is fair in locating an infarction if it is a single event; and (3) the EKG is poor in reflecting the extent of infarction.

31. **D**, Page 1336.

The following are causes of prominent T waves resembling acute myocardial ischemia and need to be considered in the differential diagnosis: (1) acute myocardial infarction, (2) benign early repolarization, (3) left bundle branch block, (4) left ventricular hypertrophy, (5) IHSS, (6) hyperkalemia, (7) subarachnoid hemorrhage, and (8) acute hemopericardium. The hyperacute T wave does not have a high degree of sensitivity in the diagnosis of acute myocardial ischemia.

32. **A**, Page 1339.

Although a common emergency department problem, much confusion still surrounds the accurate diagnosis of BER. BER is generally found most often in V_3 through V_6 but may be exhibited only in the limb leads or all of the precordial leads. ST segment elevation of BER is usually not associated with reciprocal changes, but these can occur. Although a distinct notched J point has been considered pathognomonic of BER, this sign is often absent and conversely can be exhibited in some leads by genuine ischemic current of entry. BER can only effectively be excluded when ST segment contour is convexed upward or the ST segment elevation exceeds 5 mm.

33. **D**, Page 1360.

Many conditions are known to produce pseudoinfarction patterns, including all of the depolarization and repolarization abnormalities associated with ischemic heart disease. Not only can they obscure a significant process, but they can mimic an acute infarct both by EKG criteria and clinical signs and symptoms.

34. **B**, Page 1363.

Bifascicular blocks carry considerable risks of developing complete AV disassociation. Although sudden death is usually secondary to ventricular fibrillation, it can be related to the onset of complete heart block. The most common types are complete left bundle branch block and right bundle branch block with left anterior fascicular block. Any symptomatic patient with bifascicular block warrants admission to the Intensive Care Unit and consideration for pacemaker.

35. **B**, Pages 1369–1378.

Ventricular tachyarrhythmias are significant problems in bundle branch block and complete heart block. When Isoprel is infused, PVCs can indicate either too much or not enough of the drug. Lidocaine can be extremely hazardous in this setting and may promote terminal asystole. Patients with this combination of heart block and PVCs should be treated as patients sustaining major trauma in terms of prompt evacuation to the hospital since only a combination of a pacemaker and pharmacologic control of the dysrhythmias is truly life-sustaining.

36. **B**, Page 1377.

Nitroglycerin has been a cornerstone in the drug management of ischemic heart disease for many years. Its actions include a venous and arterial vasodilatation (venous more than arterial) decreasing preload and afterload, direct vasodilatation especially in the epicardial collateral vessels, increased cardiac blood flow and oxygen supply, and direct relief of coronary vasospasm. Reflex increase in heart rate and hypotension may be seen secondary to vasodilatation.

75

Nontraumatic Acute Abdominal Pain

1. **C**, Page 1391.

Pain referred to the top of the shoulder secondary to diaphragmatic irritation is called Kehr's sign. It is a very helpful finding because it signals a significant intraabdominal disease. Cholecystitis is typically referred to the lower edge of the scapula.

2. **E**, Page 1389.

Over 40% of people with acute abdominal pain will not be diagnosed in the emergency department. All other causes listed account for less than 10% each. The emergency physician's job is not necessarily to make a specific diagnosis; rather it is to recognize life-threatening disease and be able to initiate proper work-up and referral.

3. **E**, Pages 1397–1400.

Many extraabdominal disorders initially produce abdominal pain. All of the disorders listed may go undiagnosed while a thorough gastrointestinal work-up is undertaken.

4. **E**, Pages 1392, 1398.

Pneumonia is a frequent cause of abdominal pain often associated with abdominal distention and vomiting in a child. The physical findings of rales or consolidation are easily missed in an uncooperative child. Chest x-ray films should be part of the evaluation of any child with unexplained abdominal pain.

5. **E**, Page 1397.

Ultrasound is felt to be "the" test of choice in the evaluation of all the conditions listed except pancreatitis. It is useful to detect pancreatic pseudocyst, a complication of chronic pancreatitis, but is usually nonspecific in the evaluation of acute pancreatitis.

6. **A**, Page 1392.

Diarrhea and constipation are reported with equal frequency in 15% of patients with appendicitis. Abdominal pain that clearly precedes nausea and vomiting is a significant clue to a surgical abdomen. Nausea and vomiting usually precede or coincide with the onset of pain in gastroenteritis. Fifty-six percent of patients with acute appendicitis have a temperature of less than 100°F. Fortunately, 96% have some abnormality in their WBC count.

7. **B**, Page 1390.

While the exact etiology of abdominal pain is usually not found in younger patients, acute cholecystitis has been found in 26% of patients over age 70 who present to the emergency department. Thirty-three percent of those in a younger age group will.

8. **B**, Page 1397.

Plain films of the abdomen have a notoriously low yield and have been found to influence patient management in only 10–13% of cases. All of the listed findings increase the chances of a radiographic abnormality, but high-pitched increased bowel sounds will have a positive x-ray 57% of the time, more than the other listed answers combined.

76
Upper Gastrointestinal Tract Disorders

1. **D**, Page 1427.

   As with any cause of acute blood loss, the hematocrit does not accurately reflect the full extent of volume depletion. Reticulocytosis is expected since the marrow increases production of red blood cells to replace those lost. Bleeding disorders are especially common in the patient with liver disease but are adequately evaluated with a combined PT, PTT, and platelet count. GI bleeding of digestion is associated with an elevated BUN because of digestion of red blood cells. However, creatinine should be normal.

2. **B**, Page 1418.

   Esophageal reflux is caused by an incompetent lower esophageal sphincter. Treatment is aimed at increasing sphincter tone and diminishing the effects of reflux. Elevation of the head of the bed uses gravity to diminish reflux. Antacids both increase sphincter tone and diminish the noxious effect of reflux material, as does cimetidine. Smoking, alcohol, and caffeine all decrease lower esophageal sphincter tone and increase the incidence of reflux. Anticholinergic agents, which may be useful for esophageal spasm, decrease the sphincter tone and lead to increased reflux.

3. **A**, Page 1424.

   Duodenal ulcers account for 25% to 40% of all causes of gastrointestinal bleeding. Erosive gastritis is the second most frequent cause, occurring in 12% to 37% of the cases, depending on the population studied.

4. **B**, Page 1420.

   Any change from a regular pattern of pain is suggestive of a penetrating ulcer, but the most characteristic sign is pain radiating to the back. Peritoneal irritation and diminished bowel sounds are seen with perforated ulcer and contamination of the peritoneal cavity, but not necessarily with a penetrating ulcer.

5. **A**, Pages 1416–1417.

   Esophageal spasm can mimic cardiac pain, especially its propensity for relief by nitroglycerin. Helpful differentiating features include the associated dysphagia and pain at rest. Because it can be associated with a normal endoscopy, manometry is a better diagnostic aid.

6. **A**, Page 1418.

   Boerhaave's syndrome is a tear of the esophagus permitting contrast material to leak out into the mediastinum. While a chest film may be highly suggestive, showing mediastinal air and a left pleural effusion, the gastrograffin swallow is almost always diagnostic.

7. **E**, Pages 1414–1415.

   The differentiation between cardiac and esophageal pain is often impossible. However, a careful history can help. Dysphagia, although rare, points strongly to an esophageal etiology as does relief of symptoms with antacids. Pain waking the patient from sleep is not helpful and can be from either source. Relief of pain with nitroglycerin, although suggesting a coronary etiology, can be seen with esophageal spasm. Water-brash, regurgitation into the back of the throat, is found in 48% of the patients with reflux.

8. **E**, Pages 1424–1425.

   Any patient presenting with a GI bleed requires confirmation of the bleeding with N/G and stool aspirate and hemocult test. (False positives can occur with vitamin C ingestion.) Urgent endoscopy is usually required after stabilization in order to confirm the bleeding site.

9. **C**, Pages 1418–1420.

   The superior mesenteric artery syndrome is caused by partial obstruction of the duodenum as the SMA runs over it in the retroperitoneal space. The classic presentation is midepigastric abdominal pain precipitated by eating, which helps to differentiate it from peptic ulcer disease, which is usually relieved by eating.

10. **D**, Page 1407.

    Vomiting involves primarily loss of the acid hydrogen chloride produced by the stomach. This results in a metabolic alkalosis. The kidney attempts to compensate for this by excreting potassium in place of hydrogen in the urine, resulting in hypokalemia.

11. **E**, Pages 1425–1429.

    The laceration found with the Mallory-Weiss syndrome typically occurs in the cardioesophageal region of the stomach just below the gastroesophageal junction. It occurs most often in alcoholic men after violent retching. It will usually abate spontaneously without requiring surgery and without recurrence.

12. **D**, Page 1424.

    All of the answers listed except the antacid aluminum hydroxide can cause black stools. The hemocult test can distinguish them from true melena secondary to GI bleeding.

13. **E**, Page 1420.

    Penetration of an ulcer as opposed to perforation with contamination of the peritoneum is seen in up to 25% of patients with peptic ulcer disease. It usually responds to intensive medical management but can be associated with all of the complications listed except abscess formation, which is very rare. Sudden erosion into a vessel can lead to massive life-threatening hemorrhage. The pancreas is the most common site for penetration of an ulcer, but the associated pancreatitis is usually mild. Persistent weight loss and intractible pain are indications for surgical repair.

14. **A**, Pages 1418–1420.
15. **C**, Pages 1418–1420.
16. **B**, Pages 1418–1420.
17. **A**, Pages 1418–1420.
18. **D**, Pages 1418–1420.

Gastric ulcers and duodenal ulcers are not the same pathophysiologic event, one occurring in the stomach instead of the duodenum. Gastric ulcers are due to a primary deficiency of the gastric mucosa, which allows a back diffusion of hydrogen ions from the stomach. Thus, the gastric pH is often low. Duodenal ulcers have normal mucosal defenses that are overwhelmed by greatly increased acidity, often because of rapid gastric emptying that results in unbuffered gastric acid reaching the duodenum. Ten percent of gastric ulcers prove to be malignant and can be associated with a firm supraclavicular (Virchow's) lymph node. The treatment is the same for both with the exception that anticholinergics should not be used with a gastric ulcer. Medical management is usually effective for both. Duodenal ulcers are clinically common four times as often as gastric ulcers, but on autopsy there is an equal incidence of each.

19. **C**, Page 1420.

Perforation of a peptic ulcer is associated with diminished or absent bowel sounds in over 90% of cases. Although usually associated with severe pain, an acute perforation may be associated with temporary relief of pain. The stools are invariably guaiac positive but rarely grossly so. Vomiting often occurs once or twice, but persistent vomiting is rare. The hallmark of this disease is diffuse abdominal guarding usually associated with direct and rebound tenderness from contamination of the peritoneum.

20. **B**, Page 1429.

Peripheral vasopressin is generally as effective as intraarterial effusion for esophageal varices. It does cause coronary artery vasoconstriction as well as decreasing cardiac output. Mortality with emergency portacaval shunt is 25–50%. The most common complication of a Sengstaken-Blackemore tube is pulmonary aspiration. When using the Sengstaken-Blackemore tube, an N/G tube should be taped alongside, ending in the esophagus to permit suction of the esophagus and decrease aspiration.

21. **A**, Page 1423.

Magnesium-containing antacids tend to cause diarrhea, while aluminum-containing antacids are constipating. Thus, antacids can be chosen to minimize the particular patient's more predominant complaints. The most effective antacid regimen is to give 100 meq. 1 and 3 hours after meals and at bedtime. Administered properly, antacids are as effective as the H2 blocker cimetidine and rantidine.

22. **D**, Page 1406.

Gastric outlet obstruction occurs in about 5% of patients with peptic ulcer disease, most of whom have had symptoms for over 10 years. Vomiting is the most common presenting complaint, usually of undigested food without bile. Aggressive medical management is usually attempted but most patients will require surgery. Anticholinergics are contraindicated because they decrease GI motility and may worsen a partial obstruction.

23. **C**, Page 1423.

Cimetidine has a large number of infrequent side effects including impotence, gynceomastia, leukopenia and confusion. Cimetidine diminishes hepatic blood flow and can cause elevated levels of many drugs including coumadin, benzodiazepines, lidocaine, propanolol, theophylline, and dilantin. None of the above has been associated with rantidine, which has the added advantage of BID dosage (a recent report suggested a single dose of 300 mg each day is as effective as 150 mg BID). In appropriate doses both result in equally effective gastric acid suppression.

77
Disorders of the Liver, Biliary Tract, and Pancreas

1. **D**, Page 1441.

This is a typical presentation of hepatic encephalopathy. Lactulose and neomycin are the agents of choice. However, neomycin is never given IV. It is used orally or rectally to decrease bowel flora. Paracentesis is a diagnostic procedure and this patient has no indication of bacterial peritonitis. Transfusion and Lasix may both worsen the encephalitis by increasing the protein, on one hand, and decreasing potassium on the other.

2. **B**, Page 1433.

Anti-HBsAg implies immunity to hepatitis B. Patients with this serologic marker do not require prophylaxis after exposure, nor do they require active immunization.

3. **B**, Page 1450.

This patient has emphysematous cholecystitis. Air can be seen in the gallbladder and its wall. This patient requires urgent cholecystectomy—not more tests.

4. **A**, Page 1456.

Pancreatic carcinoma is increasing in incidence and is now the fourth leading cause of cancer deaths. The diagnosis is difficult to make, but pancreatic ultrasound or a CT scan are the best initial tests. ERCP can confirm initial clinical impressions. Fasting blood sugar and CEA level are not helpful initially but both can be used to follow the progress of the disease.

5. **A**, Pages 1433–1449.
6. **D**, Pages 1433–1449.
7. **B**, Pages 1433–1449.
8. **C**, Pages 1433–1449.

Hepatic disease associated with jaundice can usually be differentiated by the biochemical and clinical profiles. Acute viral hepatitis is associated with a tender, sometimes enlarged liver, an ALT elevated more than SGOT, and a normal alkaline phosphatase. Alcoholic liver disease can closely mimic viral hepatitis, but the SGOT is usually elevated higher than the ALT. An elevated alkaline phosphatase suggests an obstructive process as would be expected with cholecystitis. Chronic active hepatitis can produce a clinical picture similar to acute hepatitis; it often has associated autoimmune phenomena such as elevated immunoglobulins.

9. **E**, Page 1437.

This patient has Gilbert's syndrome, which is a deficiency of the clearance of bilirubin from the circulation. This results in an elevated unconjugated (indirect) bilirubin with a normal or decreased direct bilirubin. A hemolytic anemia could cause such a picture, but a normal CBC and reticulocyte count excludes this.

10. **D**, Page 1449.

All of the tests listed can accurately access the anatomy but only the Hida scan (a nuclear medicine scan) can detect function of the gallbladder. Nonvisualization of the gallbladder with visualization of the liver and common duct is diagnostic of gallbladder disease, acute or chronic.

11. **A**, Page 1444.

Pancreatitis is often caused by gallstones but not the other way around. Obesity and estrogen use will increase the amount of cholesterol excreted in the bowel. Ileal resection will decrease the absorption of bile acids that are necessary to solubilize cholesterol. Hemolytic anemias have increased bilirubin excretion into the bile and lead to pigmented stones.

12. **E**, Page 1454.

All of the listed answers except amylase correlate with a poor prognosis. Other findings that reflect a poor prognosis include age over 55 and an SGOT over 250 IU/dl.

13. **E**, Page 1441.

Increased blood pressure can be associated with an encephalopathy that in many ways will mimic hepatic encephalopathy, but one does not cause the other. Hepatic encephalopathy is due to a failure of the liver to metabolize nitrogenous substances absorbed from the intestine. The exact biochemical pathogenesis remains elusive; however, certain clinical conditions are well described as worsening encephalopathy, notably those listed, which are all correctable.

14. **D**, Page 1441.

The only functional abnormality with a liver abscess is an elevated alkaline phosphatase. Both transaminase and bilirubin are only mildly elevated, if at all, and jaundice is rare.

15. **B**, Page 1452.

Alcohol and biliary tract disease are by far the leading cause of pancreatitis. There are many other causes, including those noted, but not hypothyroidism.

16. **E**, Page 1452.

Many intraabdominal disorders can cause an elevated amylase, often those in the differential of pancreatitis. An elevated amylase does signify a significant disease process but used alone is nonspecific as to etiology.

17. **C**, Page 1434.

This patient may well have hepatitis B but the particular blood sample was taken at a point in its course after HBsAg had diminished and before anti-HBsAg had risen to detectable levels. To rule out this window phase, and anti-HBc is usually used. If all three are negative it can be concluded that the patient does not have hepatitis B. The HBsAg always rises before clinical symptoms; thus in an icteric patient the sample could not have been drawn too early.

18. **D**, Page 1435.

Non-A, Non-B hepatitis is by far the most common cause of posttransfusion hepatitis now that there are effective screens for hepatitis B. However, episodic causes not associated with transfusion can occur. Non-A, Non-B hepatitis is typically milder than hepatitis B but can result in all of its complications.

19. **E**, Page 1437.

Immune serum globulin is not useful in treating acute hepatitis. It is used in prophylaxis of those exposed but who have not yet developed clinical disease. Hyperimmune globulin is used for known parenteral exposure to hepatitis B if the patient does not have anti-HBsAg. Immune globulin is recommended for non-A, non-B hepatitis, but proof of its usefulness is lacking.

20. **E**, Page 1438.

All of these agents can cause hepatic injury. A careful drug history is imperative in anyone presenting with jaundice.

21. **B**, Page 1439.

Alcoholic hepatitis is directly related to the amount of ethanol consumed. It will progress to cirrhosis in over 50% of those who continue to drink and a smaller percentage of those who abstain completely. Malnutrition does increase the risk of alcoholic hepatitis and subsequent cirrhosis but both can occur in the well-nourished alcoholic.

22. **A**, Pages 1433–1437.
23. **C**, Pages 1433–1437.
24. **B**, Pages 1433–1437.
25. **A**, Pages 1433–1437.
26. **D**, Pages 1433–1437.
    Hepatitis A is transmitted via a fecal-oral route with an incubation period of 6 days to 4 weeks. Most cases are not associated with jaundice; therefore most people don't realize they have hepatitis. By the age of 50 over 50% of the population have serologic evidence of previous disease. It can progress to fulminate hepatic failure and death, although not nearly as often as other forms of hepatitis. A carrier state does not develop. Hepatitis B is now most often transmitted sexually with an incubation period of 6 weeks to 6 months. Anicteric hepatitis can develop, but clinical jaundice is more common. A carrier state, chronic active, or chronic persistent hepatitis can all occur. Laennec's cirrhosis is the diffuse fine scarring associated with Mallory bodies seen in alcoholic liver disease.

27. **D**, Page 1436.
    All of the listed causes can lead to temporary elevation of transaminase levels except for respiratory failure. Severe right-sided heart failure, constrictive pericarditis, or inflammatory bowel disease can all progress to eventual cirrhosis.

28. **C**, Page 1434.
    The delta agent is a virus that requires hepatitis B in order to replicate. It only occurs in cases of acute or chronic hepatitis B and implies a worse prognosis.

78
Disorders of the Small Intestine

1. **C**, Pages 1469–1470.
   Selective arteriography is the best therapeutic modality. It can establish the diagnosis, and with infusion of vasodilators can correct the defect and avoid surgery on an unstable patient. Most people, however, do require operative intervention. Preliminary symptoms occur in 40% of the people. An unexplained lactic acidosis in a patient without hypotension should suggest this diagnosis.

2. **C**, Page 1474.
   Intussusception is a disease of the young child; 70% occur in the first year and 80% to 90% by age 2. About 90% of pediatric cases are idiopathic and believed to be secondary to lymphoid tissue at the ileocecal valve, whereas 90% of cases in adults are caused by local lesions, tumor, or a Meckel's diverticulum.

3. **A**, Page 1469.

Bilateral adnexal tenderness with pain on cervical motion has been reported with equal frequency in patients with appendicitis and those found to have PID at surgery. All of the other factors can help to suggest PID as opposed to appendicitis.

4. **E**, Page 1468.
   Fecaliths are relatively rare, occurring in only 5–10% of cases of appendicitis, but when present in an appropriate clinical setting, they are virtually diagnostic of appendicitis. The other features are all associated with appendicitis but are not pathognomonic.

5. **A**, Page 1460.
   Pain and vomiting with a history of prior abdominal surgery is a classic finding of small bowel obstruction. The bowel sounds should be increased early, while decreased bowel sounds will be seen later in the course. Most cases of small bowel obstruction have distention but no peritoneal signs until infarction occurs. Alcohol is not associated with small bowel obstructions.

6. **D**, Page 1472.
   There are numerous extra intestinal manifestations of regional enteritis that may at times dominate the clinical picture. Included are arthritis, particularly ankylosing spondylitis, erythema nodosum and pyoderma gangrenosa, and iritis.

7. **E**, Page 1472.
   There are myriad extra gastrointestinal complications of regional enteritis. Hydronephrosis can be caused by the obstruction of the ureters by an inflammatory mass. Megoblastic anemia is caused by vitamin B_{12} malabsorption because of disease of the terminal ileum.

8. **C**, Pages 1464–1465.
   Early in its course a bowel obstruction is associated with increased bowel sounds. As intraluminal pressure increases, they may diminish and even cease altogether. An ileus has absent bowel sounds from the beginning. It is often difficult to distinguish between the two and some entities can cause both, e.g., abdominal abscess or regional enteritis.

9. **D**, Page 1463.
   The most typical metabolic cause of ileus is hypokalemia. All of the others listed are well-recognized. An ileus must be watched for in an appropriate clinical setting.

10. **A**, Page 1459.
    Postoperative adhesions are the most common cause of small bowel obstruction in the United States. Hernias are second.

11. **C**, Page 1464.
    The omentum in children often does not reach into the right lower quadrant and help seal off a perforated appendix into a localized abscess; they are more likely to develop generalized peritonitis after appendiceal rupture.

12. **D,** Page 1472.

Most cases of regional enteritis involve both the colon and small bowel, although it can be limited to either area alone. The skip areas can help differentiate it from ulcerative colitis, with which it has many features in common. Involved bowel typically affects all layers, which is why the incidence of fistula formation is so high.

13. **A,** Pages 1469–1471.

Nonocclusive mesenteric infarction accounts for 30–50% of cases of mesenteric vascular disease, with primary embolic and thrombosis accounting for the rest. Diagnosis requires angiography, which must be done early, often on the basis of clinical suspicion with little physical evidence.

79
General Disorders of the Large Intestine

1. **A,** Page 1489.

Anal lesions, hemorrhoids, and anal fissures are the most common cause of rectal bleeding when all patient populations are considered. As the patient ages, the incidence of more serious disorders increases, especially carcinoma. Every patient with bright red rectal bleeding should have anoscopy and/or sigmoidoscopy performed.

2. **D,** Page 1491.

Adhesions, although the most common cause of small bowel obstruction, almost never produce obstruction of the colon. The most common cause of colonic obstruction by far is carcinoma, followed by volvulus, diverticular disease, and inflammatory bowel disease.

3. **C,** Pages 1484–1486.

Kaopectate does increase the incidence of formed stools. However, it has no effect on the frequency or water content of the stools and increases the total salt loss. The patient should be encouraged to drink fluids containing glucose, because they are easily absorbed. Milk should be avoided because of a transient lactase deficiency. Antimotility agents such as Imodium or Lomotil should be avoided if there are any signs of an invasive diarrhea. Pepto-Bismol has been shown to both prevent traveler's diarrhea and improve symptoms of nonspecific diarrhea.

4. **B,** Page 1489.

Juvenile polyps are the most common cause of rectal bleeding in children. They are usually single, have no malignancy potential, and have a peak incidence around age 5. Their initial symptom is painless rectal bleeding.

5. **E,** Page 1486.

The patient who presents with constipation must have potential metabolic causes considered. Diabetes usually causes diarrhea via an autonomic neuropathy, but it can be associated with constipation. Renal failure is associated with a chronic diarrhea.

6. **C,** Page 1482.

A toxin-mediated gastroenteritis is usually associated with a lack of true abdominal tenderness and fever and does have less peripheral leukocytosis. However, the best test to differentiate between the two is the presence or absence of fecal leukocytes seen on a Wright's stain.

7. **E,** Page 1490.

Although carcinoma is the most common cause of lower GI bleeding in adults, diverticular disease accounts for 65% of severe bleeding. It usually comes on suddenly and painlessly. It rarely requires surgery but often requires transfusions.

8. **A,** Pages 1489–1490.
9. **C,** Pages 1489–1490.
10. **D,** Pages 1489–1490.
11. **E,** Pages 1489–1490.

The number of diseases producing rectal bleeding are relatively small but can vary from a harmless anal fissure to a life-threatening hemorrhage from diverticulitis. Carcinoma usually has guaiac-positive stools long before other symptoms of pain or weight loss develop. Ulcerative colitis usually has its onset in the second decade with bloody diarrhea as well as multiple other extra gastrointestinal symptoms. Polyps usually present with painless bright red blood, often intermittently. Some have a potential for malignant degeneration and thus should be correctly identified and excised. Hemorrhoids are typified by bleeding that coats the stools or occurs after defecation; it may be painless or associated with irritation and puritis.

80
Acute Gastroenteritis and Colon Disorders

1. **C,** Pages 1518–1519.

This is a typical presentation of a sigmoid volvulus. The patient has no signs of impending strangulation, and initial nonsurgical management is desirable. Rectal tube decompression is successful 90% of the time. Later, elective resection can be considered.

2. **A**, Pages 1510–1512.

Grossly bloody stools are the hallmark of ulcerative colitis but are uncommon in granulomatous colitis. Otherwise, the symptoms are similar with elevated sedimentation rates when the disease is active. Both diseases can have peripheral arthritis as well as colonic ulcerations. Fistulas are much more common with granulomatous colitis.

3. **A**, Page 1498.

Antibiotics do not shorten the clinical course of salmonella and do increase the period of excretion of salmonella in the stools. This is believed to be due to the alteration of normal bowel flora that compete with and inhibit salmonella. Antibiotics are only indicated for bacteremia, in which case chloramphenicol is the initial agent of choice.

4. **D**, Page 1496.

TMP-SX is as effective as ampicillin and is preferred for the treatment of shigella. Amoxicillin is not effective even for those organisms sensitive to ampicillin. Antibiotics clearly do shorten the clinical course and should be initiated as soon as the diagnosis is made.

5. **D**, Page 1511.

Toxic megacolon is found in cases of inflammatory bowel disease, most often ulcerative colitis. The patient presents with high fever and increasing abdominal distention often following a barium study. Many of these patients require emergency colectomy.

6. **E**, Page 1509.

The best way to diagnose *Entobiasis* (pin worms) is with the scotch tape test. The tape is applied to the perianal area at night and examined under the microscope. If done for 3 days, it is 99% diagnostic.

7. **C**, Page 1503.

Antibiotics (trimethoprim sulfa or doxycycline) are effective for both prophylaxis and treatment. The duration of illness and severity of symptoms can be shortened with prompt treatment. Now most authorities do not recommend antibiotic prophylaxis but suggest starting them at the first sign of diarrhea.

8. **A**, Page 1506.

Peripheral esophinilia is rare with amebic dysentery, unlike other protozoal infections. This disease is on the increase, especially among homosexuals. Many people suggest a serologic test for *Entamoeba* before starting steroids for newly diagnosed ulcerative colitis.

9. **C**, Page 1505.

This patient has antibiotic-associated enterocolitis. This is due to a toxin produced by *Clostridium difficile*, which has overgrown in the bowel from the suppression of normal flora. Oral vancomycin is the therapy of choice.

10. **B**, Page 1509.

Mebendazole should be repeated 2 weeks after the first dose because unhatched ovum are resistant to the first dose. Even with effective treatment, it often tends to be recurrent.

11. **C**, Page 1508.

Giardiasis should be strongly considered in any patient with diarrhea after a backpacking trip in remote areas. While the cyst can usually be found in the stools, in acute cases with chronic disease duodenal aspirate is the best diagnostic method.

12. **E**, Page 1509.

Clindamycin is the most common antibiotic to cause serious enterocolitis, but all of the others have been reported to do so. The enterocolitis is due to overgrowth of a clostridial organism that produces a local toxin. It is treated with oral vancomycin.

13. **A**, Page 1499.

Increasing *Yersinia enterocolitica* is found to cause mesenteric adenitis, which can exactly mimic appendicitis. It can also mimic regional enteritis. However, most cases are mild diarrheal illnesses. Diagnosis is by stool culture, which unfortunately takes a long time to grow.

14. **B**, Page 1511.

Sigmoidoscopy with biopsy is the best way to diagnose ulcerative colitis. Several infectious processes can mimic it and must be ruled out. A barium enema can be useful to evaluate the extent of disease, but it is contraindicated if toxic megacolon is suspected. Examination of the stools will show red blood cells and white blood cells that are nonspecific. A gallium scan is occasionally useful if an intra-abdominal abscess is suspected.

15. **C**, Page 1503.

Scombrotoxin is produced by bacteria acting on certain dark fish meats, especially that of the Hawaiian tuna, mahi-mahi. They have histamine-like properties and the clinical manifestations are those of histamine release, facial swelling, palpitations, abdominal cramps, etc. Symptoms are promptly relieved with parenteral antihistamines.

16. **B**, Page 1501.

Clostridium perfringens grow on meat or poultry products. After ingestion they sporulate in the gut and release enterotoxins as a byproduct of their metabolism. Symptoms begin 6–12 hours after ingestion with abdominal cramps and diarrhea as the dominant symptoms. It rarely lasts over 24 hours. Stools are negative for red blood cells and white blood cells.

17. **D**, Page 1500.

Vibrio parahemolyticus is the only vibria species that produces disease through direct tissue invasion. It causes an intense inflammatory response in the intestinal mucosa. Stools contain both white blood cells and red blood cells.

18. **D**, Page 1511.
All of the listed infectious diseases can mimic ulcerative colitis both clinically and morphologically. Further treating amebiasis with steroids can exacerbate the disease. Stool cultures, examination for ova and parasites, and serology for amebiasis should be done on all newly diagnosed ulcerative colitis patients.

19. **A**, Page 1516.
Most patients with diverticula are asymptomatic. Thirty to forty percent will develop symptoms at some time including pain, bleeding, and inflammation. Diverticular disease is unique to Western cultures with our highly refined diets that lack fiber. This causes a chronic increase in intraluminal pressure that results in 50% of the population developing diverticuli in old age.

20. **C**, Page 1499.
Erythromycin is the best agent for *Campylobacter*. It produces a rapid clinical and bacterologic cure and prevents the frequent relapses. *Campylobacter* is increasingly recognized as a cause of gastroenteritis and in many places is the most common cause of an invasive diarrhea.

81
Disorders of the Anorectum

1. **A**, Page 1527.
External hemorrhoids resolve spontaneously after 4 to 5 days. Surgical incision is indicated for patient comfort.

2. **E**, Pages 1529–1530.
Both ischiorectal and supralevator abscesses require drainage within the operating room. Perianal abscesses and submucosal abscesses can be definitively treated in the emergency room, although both are likely to reoccur. Pilonidal abscesses can be initially drained in the emergency department, but later definitive surgical excision is needed.

3. **D**, Page 1532.
Proctalgia fugax is a disease of unknown cause that is very painful but of short duration. The symptoms tend to be intermittent and cannot be reproduced by digital rectal exam.

4. **B**, Page 1528.
The most common initial manifestation of internal hemorrhoids is painless bright red bleeding usually with defecation. External hemorrhoids usually present

with acute painful thrombosis and are not typically associated with bleeding. Painful bright red bleeding is most often due to an anal fissure.

82
Genitourinary Disease

1. **D**, Page 1555.
Trimethoprim-sulfamethoxazole is effective against the predominant organism causing prostatitis and is concentrated in the prostatic fluid. It is considered the drug of choice for this disease. Massage of the acutely inflamed prostate induces bacteremia and should be avoided. If urinary retention develops, a suprapubic catheter is safer and more comfortable. The urine culture will usually yield the responsible organism.

2. **D**, Page 1568.
The patient without signs of obstruction or infection does not require admission or antibiotics. Urologic consultation should be obtained for follow-up and stone analysis, but it need not be immediate.

3. **E**, Page 1568.
While all of these patients should be admitted, the true emergency is a stone with evidence of infection (fever, chills, significant pyuria). Sepsis and renal damage represent a significant risk, and immediate operative intervention is indicated.

4. **B**, Pages 1564–1567.
The narrowest part of the ureter is at the ureterovesicular junction just as the ureter enters the bladder. Therefore, careful attention to this area should be given when examining x-ray films.

5. **E**, Page 1559.
Torsion of the testicle is a true emergency requiring detorsion before 6 to 12 hours if testicular function is to be preserved. Almost half of patients will report a history of a similar pain which resolved spontaneously, believed to be caused by partial torsion. Relief of pain on elevation of the scrotum (Prehn's sign) is classically associated with epididymitis but has been found to be of little value in distinguishing between these two entities.

6. **C**, Page 1445.
Untreated bacteriuria even without clinical pyelonephritis is associated with an increased incidence of prematurity and fetal wasteage. During pregnancy the ureters dilate and peristalsis is decreased, making it easier for a lower urinary tract infection to spread upward to involve the kidneys.

7. **D**, Page 1546.

A not unusual occurrence is the development of post-IVP acute renal failure, which may prove fatal in a patient with diabetes, multiple myeloma, or other causes of renal disease. If an IVP is necessary, making sure that the patient is adequately hydrated will significantly decrease the risk of this complication. Sepsis, although a cause of renal failure, is not associated with a greater risk following IVP.

8. **A**, Page 1562.

The degree of hematuria from microscopic to gross bears no relationship to the seriousness of the etiology. Therefore, any degree of hematuria requires an expeditious, complete work-up.

9. **C**, Page 1562.

A bladder tumor usually presents with painless hematuria as its only sign. Stones usually have some pain while cystitis causes frequency, dysuria, etc. Renal carcinoma seldom causes gross hematuria, while prostatic hypertrophy is rare in this age group. Benign prostatic hypertrophy is the most common cause of gross hematuria in men over age 60.

10. **A**, Page 1560.

Urinary retention is not due to a problem with the kidneys or ureters, which is all that is accurately accessed with an IVP. It is not necessary unless there are signs of infection with systemic toxicity. As with prerenal azotemia, the BUN to creatinine ratio may be elevated beyond the normal 10–5, possibly because of reabsorption of excreted BUN. Sudden relief of a long-standing obstruction has been associated with a significant diuresis requiring careful fluid and electrolyte management for as long as 1 week. If a catheter cannot be readily placed, most urologists would prefer the emergency physician to proceed with a suprapubic tap rather than possibly doing more damage with filiforms and followers.

11. **E**, Page 1549.

Most women with acute cystitis will respond quickly and completely with a single dose of amoxicillin or trimethoprim-sulfamethoxazole. In fact, some authors suggest that the response to a single-dose therapy is the most practical way to distinguish upper from lower urinary tract infections. However, none of the above-mentioned patients are candidates for a single-dose treatment.

12. **D**, Page 1551.

All boys and any patient with suspicion of obstruction somewhere in the urogenital tract should have urologic referral. However, an uncomplicated urinary tract infection in an otherwise healthy girl can be managed by referral to a primary care physician for reevaluation in 2 weeks.

13. **A**, Page 1540.

During the first 3 months of life, 75% of babies with urinary tract infections will be males. Thereafter, the male:female ratio steadily decreases, favoring the female 1:50 during the reproductive years. In a geriatric population due to the incidence of prostatic hypertrophy, the ratio of males to remales is equal.

14. **A**, Page 1552.

Ampicillin is the agent of choice for proteus urinary tract infections. Proteus is a frequent pathogen is young boys. It should be considered in patients with pyuria and bacteriuria who have an alkaline pH because of its urea-splitting enzyme.

15. **B**, Page 1556.

Epididymitis rarely requires operative intervention. Appropriate antibiotics, elevation, and analgesia are usually curative. It is felt to be a sexually transmitted disease, particularly in the young population with *Chlamydia* and *Neisseria gonorrhea* being the most common organisms isolated.

16. **A**, Page 1556.

With increasing use of newer diagnostic modalities, *Chlamydia*, which does not grow on routine culture, is increasingly recognized in number of infections, including epididymitis. It is now felt to account for two-thirds of all cases of epididymitis in young men.

17. **A**, Page 1559.

Occasionally a testicle can be manually detorsed with resumption of blood flow. This should be viewed as a temporary maneuver and definitive surgery should be arranged. The defect is bilateral; therefore, both testicles should be repaired at surgery. Doppler studies and isotopic scans can be effective in demonstrating lack of blood flow, but a normal study does not preclude torsion. A reactive hydrocele can occur and be mistaken for a tumor.

18. **E**, Page 1565.

Primary hyperoxaluria is a rare, often lethal disorder that appears in childhood. Uric acid stones are radiolucent and would not show up on an x-ray. Renal tubular acidosis could not be present because of the low urinary pH. Magnesium-amonium-phosphate stones are found in urine infected with *Klebsiella* and require an alkaline pH. Idiopathatic hypercalcuria is usually due to increased absorption of calcium from the gut. It is a major cause of stones and can be treated with large fluid intake, decreased dietary calcium, and at times thiazide diuretics.

83
Abdominal and Pelvic Pain

1. **E**, Page 1576.

Appendicitis during pregnancy is often difficult to diagnosis. The appendix rides higher and higher in the abdomen as it is pushed upward by the enlarging uterus. Round ligament strain and uterine contractions are not often associated with nausea and vomiting this late in a pregnancy. It can be very difficult to separate pyelonephritis or ovarian torsion from acute appendicitis.

2. **E**, Page 1577.
The presentation of pyelonephritis is identical to that in the nonpregnant patient. Patients initially have frequency and dysuria followed by back pain, fever, and costovertebral angle tenderness. Admission is warranted to ensure high levels of antibiotics. Tetracycline is contraindicated both because of fetal teeth staining and toxicity to the maternal liver.

3. **B**, Page 1576.
Pregnant women are the same risk as the nonpregnant population for developing appendicitis. Symptoms, however, are often confusing. There is a normal leukocytosis with pregnancy, but a left shift should suggest an inflammatory process. The enlarged uterus inhibits the formation of an abscess after appendiceal rupture and makes generalized peritonitis more likely.

4. **E**, Page 1578.
Many women are afraid of birth control pills because of their potential complications. It should be pointed out to them that unprotected intercourse with its risk of pregnancy is of greater potential harm. Before starting birth control pills, pregnancy must be effectively ruled out because of the high risk of fetal abnormalities. Women on birth control pills should have their blood pressure checked and be warned about this potential complication.

5. **A**, Page 1577.
IUDs are effective contraceptives with less than 4 pregnancies per 100 women. However, birth control pills are much more effective with pregnancy between .7 and 2.5 per 100 women per year.

6. **D**, Page 1576.
The premenstrual tension syndrome is thought to be due largely to a decrease in neurotransmitters, especially dopamine. Pyridoxine is a cofactor in the synthesis of dopamine, which has been found effective to treat PMS. Naprosyn is useful for dysmenorrhea but not PMS. Progesteronal agents may actually make symptoms worse. Some women with fluid retention will be helped with mild diuretics, but pyridoxine remains the first line of therapy.

7. **D**, Page 1575.
Follicular cysts occur during mid-cycle and rupture with the release of an egg. Rupture of a follicular cyst is the cause of mittelschmerz syndrome; other types of ovarian cysts can cause dysmenorrhea.

8. **A**, Page 1574.

Mittelschmerz is the intermenstrual lower abdominal pain some women have 2 weeks before their menses. It is a completely benign disorder related to ovulation. Oral contraceptives suppress ovulation and therefore "cure" mittelschmerz. Intrauterine processes are not involved; therefore a D&C has no effect, nor is the patient at risk for endometritis. A slight amount of vaginal bleeding can occur due to the sudden decline in estrogen levels.

84
Complications of Pregnancy

1. **A**, Page 1586.
This patient has preeclampsia with most of the classic manifestations. Hydralazine is the drug of choice because it directly reverses the primary pathophysiologic lesion of vasospasm. It increases cardiac output and causes a reflex tachycardia. The drug is given in 5 mg boluses every 5 to 10 minutes until a total of 20 mg is reached. The other agents listed are not recommended because they adversely affect and fetus.

2. **A**, Page 1586.
Magnesium sulfate is used for its anticonvulsive effects and has minimal effects on blood pressure. The main complication is respiratory depression, which is seen after deep tendon reflexes are lost. The specific antagonist is IV calcium 1 gm.

3. **A**, Pages 1584–1585.
4. **B**, Pages 1584–1585.
5. **B**, Pages 1584–1585.
6. **D**, Pages 1584–1585.
The two common causes of third trimester bleeding are placenta previa and abrupto placenta. A pelvic examination is contraindicated (either with speculum or bimanual) because of the possibility of puncturing the placenta and greatly increasing the bleeding. An abrupto is a tearing away of the placenta from its implantation site. It is slightly more common than placenta previa. An abrupto typically presents with painful dark vaginal bleeding. There may be concealed blood loss as blood accumulates in the uterus. Baseline clotting studies should be drawn as soon as the diagnosis is suspected. Placenta previa occurs when the placenta implants low on the uterine wall covering the cervical os. These patients typically present with painless bright red vaginal bleeding. Diagnosis can be confirmed by pelvic ultrasound.

7. **C**, Page 1582.

Hydatidiform moles usually have greatly elevated levels of HCG, which often first suggest this diagnosis. The diagnosis is confirmed by ultrasound with evacuation of the uterus, the required treatment.

8. **A**, Page 1586.

By far the most common cause of delayed postpartum hemorrhage is retained products of conception. The treatment is curretage. This complication can cause both infection and clotting abnormalities as well as delayed bleeding.

9. **E**, Page 1585.

The most common cause of early postpartum hemorrhage is uterine atony. Intravenous oxytocin and uterine massage are used initially. If they fail to control bleeding, a curettage is performed for removal of possible retained products of conception. Of course blood loss needs to be replaced.

10. **C**, Pages 1587–1588.

Postpartum pituitary insufficiency (Sheehan's syndrome) is seen only after postpartum hemorrhage or infection. The other listed conditions can complicate a normal pregnancy.

11. **C**, Page 1587.

Amniotic fluid embolus is a rare, often fatal complication. It often causes diffuse intervascular coagulation as well as acute cor pulmonale.

12. **B**, Page 1586.

Toxemia of pregnancy is much more common during the first pregnancy among older primagravidas. All of the other statements are true. It can be associated with many initial complaints, including weight gain, headache, visual disturbances, or epigastric pain.

13. **A**, Page 1583.

Hypofibrinogenemia is a potential problem if the products of conception are retained for more than 3 weeks. All patients in the emergency department with a missed abortion should have a CBC and coagulation studies including fibrinogen level.

14. **E**, Page 1585.

Uterine rupture is a rare cause of hemorrhage in late pregnancy. It is associated with prior surgery or blunt abdominal trauma. Most of the hemorrhage is intraabdominal, which causes peritoneal irritation and lack of external bleeding. Fetal mortality is 50%, but urgent delivery, usually by section, is mandatory.

85
Ectopic Pregnancy

1. **C**, Page 1594.

All of the answers are relatively more common with a threatened abortion than C. If there is an anemia out of proportion to the vaginal blood loss, this suggests an intraabdominal source and thus makes an ectopic pregnancy more likely.

2. **E**, Page 1599.

A dry tap—the failure to obtain fluid—is considered nondiagnostic. Straw-colored aspirate is normal and effectively excludes a ruptured ectopic, but an intact ectopic pregnancy is still possible. Vascular blood can be differentiated from free peritoneal blood by the fact that fibrinogen precipitates along the peritoneum and blood aspirated from there will not clot. A hematocrit over 20% favors an ectopic, while one below 10% suggests another cause of intrauterine bleeding such as a corpus luteum cyst.

3. **E**, Page 1594.

Forty percent of women with ectopic pregnancies are misdiagnosed at their initial visit. Common missed diagnoses include pelvic inflammatory disease, threatened abortion, ovarian cyst, and appendicitis. Every woman of child-bearing age and abdominal or gynecologic complaints must have an ectopic considered. An ectopic pregnancy is the most frequent cause of nonapparent vascular collapse in this age group.

4. **A**, Page 1594.

While all of the answers are classically found in ectopic pregnancy, all of them except fullness of the cul-de-sac are found frequently with other conditions. Fullness of the cul-de-sac is due to significant bleeding or rarely to pus. The most frequent cause of significant intraabdominal bleeding in the woman during child-bearing years is an ectopic pregnancy.

5. **C**, Page 1601.

All of the answers are relatively more common with a threatened abortion except C. If there is an anemia out of proportion to the vaginal blood loss, this suggests an intraabdominal source and thus makes an ectopic pregnancy more likely.

6. **E**, Page 1595.

An adnexal mass is found in less than 50% overall of cases of ectopic pregnancy. Therefore, the diagnosis must be considered even it its absence. Abdominal pain is the most frequent sign, followed by amenorrhea.

7. **B**, Page 1592.

Prior history of a therapeutic abortion does not predispose a woman to have an increased incidence of ectopic pregnancies in the future. All of the other answers are associated with an increased incidence of ectopic pregnancy through mechanical interference of egg passage in the case of salpingitis, tubal ligation, and pelvic adhesions. IUDs are associated with an increased incidence of ectopic pregnancy through a mechanism that is not well understood.

8. **C**, Page 1593.
IUD users are not at greater risk than other women during the first 2 years of IUD insertion. After that they have a risk 3 times that of control subjects, which extends even after the IUD is removed. Birth control pills are the only method that suppresses ovulation and has a very low risk of ectopic pregnancy, but they can be associated with amenorrhea and ovarian cyst, which can mimic an ectopic.

9. **C**, Page 1597.
The whole molecule HCG assay interacts with lutenizing hormone, which can cause a high incidence of false positives. The beta-specific HCG is the most sensitive and specific. The more specific the test, the lower the incidence of false positives; the more sensitive the test, the lower the incidence of false negatives. A gestational sac should be detected by ultrasound when an HCG level of greater than 6,000 is present. If not, this is strong evidence of an ectopic gestation.

10. **A**, Page 1591.
The incidence of ectopic pregnancy has increased from 4.5 to 10.5 in the 10 years from 1970–1980. Possible reasons include an increased use of IUDs and increased antibiotics to treat salpingitis, which may leave the tubes damaged but not completely occluded as may have occurred in the past. The most common predisposing factor is previous infection.

86
Vaginal Bleeding

1. **A**, Page 1607.
Fewer than 1% of uterine leiomyomas undergo malignant degeneration. Therefore, unless they are causing symptoms they are not an indication for hysterectomy, especially since they often regress after menopause when estrogen stimulation wanes.

2. **E**, Page 1607.
Fibroids occur in 20% of women over age 35. They are usually asymptomatic but can be associated with all of the symptoms listed except *E*. The vaginal bleeding of uterine myomas is usually prolonged, excessive menses. While submucosal myomas can cause intermenstrual bleeding, other causes must first be ruled out.

3. **D**, Page 1607.
Cervical polyps are common and benign with little malignant potential. They can cause intermenstrual bleeding, often aggravated by contact during intercourse. Diagnosis is by direct visual inspection during a speculum exam.

4. **E**, Page 1605.
Passing clots suggests heavy bleeding, which does not remain in the uterus long enough to undergo fibrogenolysis. This should always be considered abnormal.

5. **D**, Page 1609.
Anovulatory cycles cause continuous stimulation of the endometrium by unopposed estrogen. There is no corpus luteum formed and thus no progesterone secretion. The result is endometrial hyperplasia. The endometrium will build up for several months with amenorrhea. Then when the endometrium has outstripped its blood supply, vaginal bleeding will ensue, which often mimics a threatened abortion. Treatment with progesteronal agents will cause in initial decrease in bleeding followed by increased bleeding as the hyperplastic endometrium sluffs.

6. **A**, Page 1609.
Oral contraceptives can cause abnormal bleeding via two mechanisms: breakthrough bleeding caused by endometrial hyperplasia or withdrawal bleeding from noncompliant usage. Temporary treatment of breakthrough bleeding is to double the normal dose of oral contraceptives.

87
Genital Infections

1. **B**, Page 1615.
Lymphogranuloma venereum is caused by a chlamydial organism. It is diagnosed by the Frei test and responds to both tetracycline and sulfa drugs. Chancroid is caused by the bacterium *Hemophilus ducreyi*, a gram-negative bacillus. Granuloma inguinale is a sexually transmitted disease caused by the bacteria *Donovania granulomatis*. Condylomata accuminata are caused by the papova-virus.

2. **D**, Pages 1617–1618.
3. **B**, Pages 1617–1618.
4. **A** or **B**, Pages 1617–1618.

5. **C**, Pages 1617–1618.

Vaginitis is a common complaint seen in every emergency department. Monilial vaginitis is easily diagnosed by the "cottage cheese" discharge that adheres to the vaginal mucosa, and it is treated with local antifungal agents. Trichomoniasis is associated with a frothy, foul-smelling discharge. It is easily confirmed when motile trichomonads are seen on a wet mount. The sexual partner as well as the patient should be treated with metronidazole. A nonspecific discharge with "clue" cells on the wet mount is seen with *Hemophilus vaginalis* vaginitis. Clue cells are vaginal epithelial cells coated with bacteria, which give them a stippled appearance. Herpes genitalis produces clear vesicles on the cervix and vaginal wall, which degenerate to form the characteristic ulcers. A smear will yield multinucleated giant cells.

6. **C**, Page 1617.

7. **C**, Page 1617.

8. **C**, Page 1617.

9. **A**, Page 1617.

10. **C**, Page 1617.

N. gonorrhea and *Chlamydia* often coexist in the same host. They can both cause pelvic inflammatory disease, as well as the acute urethral syndrome. Tetracycline cures both, whereas penicillin, ampicillin, or spectinomycin treats only gonorrhea. Both are commonly asymptomatic, which emphasizes the need to treat all contacts, symptomatic or not. Both can result in sterility in the male as well as the female.

11. **E**, Page 1613.

Even an asymptomatic person with no evidence of disease should be treated if known exposure to gonorrhea has occurred. He may still have the disease and transmit it to others even if Gram's stain and cultures are negative. In this case when the patient doesn't know what he was exposed to, tetracycline is the most reasonable choice since it covers both gonorrhea and *Chlamydia*.

12. **A**, Page 1614.

Topical Acyclovir is not as effective as oral medication, which significantly decreases the duration and severity of signs and symptoms. It is also effective for recurrent herpes simplex infections while topical ointment is not. Neonatal infection with herpes has a 50% mortality and therefore babies of infected mothers should be delivered by cesarean section. Women with herpes are predisposed to cervical cancer. The importance of a yearly Pap smear should be emphasized to these patients. Most fever blisters are caused by herpes simplex type I. However, 10% are caused by HSV-2.

13. **D**, Page 1620.

Toxic shock syndrome is believed to be caused by an exotoxin released during a vaginal infection with staphylococci. Antibiotics have not been shown to affect the course of the disease but may prevent recurrences. The underlying pathology is capillary leakage, and early vigorous fluids are by far the most important part of therapy.

14. **A**, Page 1613.

Erythromycin and penicillins are considered safe in pregnancy. Tetracycline can retard fetal long-bone growth and cause staining of the teeth. Sulfa compounds compete with bilirubin binding sites on albumin and can cause neonatal hyperbilirubinemia. Metronidazole and trimethoprim can cause fetal malformations.

15. **A**, Page 1618.

A vaginal foreign body can cause a foul-smelling discharge that can mimic an infection. Bits of toilet paper and pin worm are the most common offending agents in the pediatric age group.

16. **D**, Page 1616.

Condyloma acuminatum is a viral lesion and as such does not respond to antibiotics. It will usually respond to local podophyllin treatment, although several applications may be necessary.

17. **A**, Page 1618.

Monilial vulva vaginitis is the most commonly seen vaginal infection, accounting for approximately 50% of all cases. It is particularly common among diabetic women, among women on oral contraceptives, and especially after the use of broad-spectrum antibiotics, most commonly tetracycline.

18. **E**, Page 1615.

All of these regimens for treating gonorrhea are effective for exposure to syphylis except spectinomycin. These regimens are not effective for seropositive syphilis, however.

19. **D**, Page 1617.

Initially it was believed that while women were commonly asymptomatic, all men with gonorrhea would develop symptoms. However, it is now recognized that up to 10% of men may have culture-proven gonorrhea and remain completely asymptomatic. This emphasizes the need for close follow-up and treatment of all sexual contacts of both men and women.

20. **E**, Page 1615.

The hallmark of primary syphilis is a painless hard ulcer, the chancre. Most other causes of genital ulcers are painful. It is important to realize that at this stage, the serologic tests are often still negative. While the rash of secondary syphilis may not extend to the palms or soles, anyone who presents with such a rash should have syphilis considered (the other possibilities are Rocky Mountain spotted fever, atypical measles, and erythema multiforme).

21. **C**, Page 1619.

Most cases of PID will have an elevated white blood cell count and sedimentation rate, which is a point to help differentiate it from appendicitis where the sedimentation rate is usually lower. With increasing use of laparoscopy, the high incidence of both false positive and false negative diagnoses by clinical means is becoming appreciated.

22. **B**, Page 1618.

Uncontrolled diabetes is often associated with vaginal candidiasis. The other common cause is antibiotic suppression of normal vaginal flora, seen most often with tetracycline.

88
Anemia

1. **C**, Page 1632.

Any process associated with increased production of red blood cells will have an elevated reticulocyte count. Sickle cell disease, hemolytic anemias, and hemorrhage all involve rapid red blood cell turnover and, therefore, stimulate the marrow to increase red blood cell production. Polycythemia vera has as its basic pathologic mechanism an inappropriate stimulation of all marrow lines to increase production of red blood cells, white blood cells, and platelets. The basic defect in aplastic anemia is marrow unresponsiveness and always has a low reticulocyte count.

2. **A**, Page 1628.

A macrocytic blood picture is typical of all of these except thalassemia. Thalassemia is a disorder of synthesis of the globin chain of hemoglobin. Because of the inability to produce adequate amounts of the hemoglobin molecule, the individual cells are small and have a lower hemoglobin concentration than expected.

3. **B**, Page 1629.

In iron deficiency anemia, iron-binding capacity increases as an adaptive measure to hold on to iron. This is the best way to differentiate iron deficiency from the anemia of chronic disease in which the serum iron and iron-binding capacity are both decreases.

4. **A**, Page 1637.

Most patients with vasoocclusive crisis are somewhat dehydrated, largely because of urinary concentrating difficulties. Volume replacement, usually with 5% dextrose and half-normal saline, is an important part of therapy. While there is a real risk of narcotic addiction, adequate analgesia usually with parenteral narcotics is an important aspect of treatment. Oxygen may be of benefit for hypoxic patients and may help to prevent the acute sickling. Folic acid is important

because of the rapid turnover of red blood cells.

5. **D**, Page 1642.

Chronic myelogenous leukemia is usually associated with a white blood cell count over 50,000 but with a remarkably normal differential. Chronic lymphocytic lymphoma is much more common among adults. Splenomegaly is common. Paroxysmal nocturnal hemoglobinuria, and chronic myelogenous leukemia are the main pathologic conditions associated with a decreased leukocyte alkaline phosphatase. While platelets may occasionally be increased, almost all patients are anemic.

6. **B**, Page 1642.

The peripheral smear with CML usually has increased basophils and eosinophils while a leukomoid reaction does not, but the two can look exactly alike. Chronic myelogenous leukemia is associated with a decrease in leukocytic alkaline phosphatase, while the leukomoid reaction typically has an increased leukocyte alkaline phosphatase.

7. **E**, Pages 1640–1641.

Lymphocytes are divided into T, B, or null cells by antibodies found on their cell surface. Although each cell type has a distinctive function, they are morphologically identical. Exercise, stress, and epinephrine all increase the white blood count by decreasing the marginal pool, which is composed of mature polymorphonuclear leukocytes.

8. **E**, Page 1636.

All of the answers are frequent complications of sickle cell disease. Painless hematuria and a decreased urinary concentrating ability are frequently seen in sickle cell trait.

9. **D**, Page 1637.

In spite of advances in antibiotics, infectious processes remain the leading cause of death in sickle cell patients. These patients do have an increased risk of death from all of the other answers except hemorrhage. The patients have many disorders of their immune system, including autoinfarction of the spleen, decreased antibody production, and decreased leukocyte function.

10. **B**, Page 1637.

Patients with sickle cell disease have multiple disorders of their immune system and are particularly susceptible to encapsulated organisms. For reasons that are unclear, *Salmonella* is the leading cause of osteomyelitis among these children.

11. **C**, Page 1635.

Paroxysmal nocturnal hemoglobinuria is a rare intrinsic membrane disorder affecting red blood cells, white blood cells, and platelets. It is an acquired disorder due to an increased sensitivity to compliment. It manifests itself as an intrinsic hemolytic anemia with occasional decreased platelets and leukopenia.

12. **A**, Page 1631.

So-called hypersegmented polymorphoneutrophils are thought to be diagnostic of megaloblastic anemia, seen with B_{12} or folate deficiency. They can help differentiate a macrocytic anemia such as that seen in thyroid deficiency or liver failure from true megaloblastic anemia.

13. **C**, Page 1630.

Red blood cell basophilic stippling is seen in only 2 disorders: thalassemia and lead poisoning. It is vital that the emergency physician recognize this not uncommon problem of indigent children. Sickle cell disease may have Howell-Jolly bodies on their peripheral smear, which reflects defective splenic function. B_{12} and folate deficiency are associated with a macrocytic anemia. Aplastic anemia has normal red blood cell morphology.

14. **C**, Page 1630.

Twenty percent of patients with sideroblastic anemia will respond to large doses of vitamin B_6. Iron is contraindicated because iron overload is a major cause of death.

15. **B**, Page 1623.

Erythropoietin is the hormone made in the kidney and possibly activated in the liver that stimulates the bone marrow to produce red blood cells. Decreased erythropoietin is the major cause of anemia of renal disease. It is elevated in most other types of anemia as a response to tissue hypoxia.

16. **D**, Page 1634.

Haptoglobin binds to free hemoglobin in the serum and would be expected to be low in patients with intravascular hemolysis. A decreased haptoglobin is an early finding in hemolytic anemia. After the haptoglobin is depleted, this circulating free hemoglobin can damage the kidneys.

7. **C**, Page 1642.

Chronic myelogenous leukemia can terminate in a blastic crisis with increased production of immature granulocytes and decreased response to treatment. The most common cause of death in patients with CLL is infection. Many of these patients have various autoimmune disorders, commonly a Coombs' positive hemolytic anemia. Treatment is directed at complications, lymphadenopathy, decreased platelets, anemia, etc, and many patients with only an elevated leukocyte count can go for years without treatment.

89
Coagulation Disorders

1. **B**, Page 1653.

TTP is a disorder of unknown cause and is usually lethal. The diagnostic pentad includes thrombocytopenia, fever, microangiopathic hemolytic anemia, renal failure, and fluctuating neurologic symptoms. Coagulation studies are usually normal.

2. **A**, Page 1659.

In the typical case of DIC, all of the abnormalities listed are found. However, each of the tests can be abnormal from other factors. Fibrinogen degradation products are elevated because of increased activity of both thrombin and plasmin. Elevated fibrinogen degradation products are seen only in DIC and primary fibrinolysis.

3. **C**, Page 1649.

Thrombocytopenia is almost always an acquired disorder secondary to drugs, infections, or autoimmune mechanisms. Platelets are not involved in either the intrinsic or extrinsic clotting pathways, and therefore, both PT and PTT are normal. The bleeding time is the only clotting study that is abnormal with isolated thrombocytopenia. Aspirin causes a functional abnormality of the platelets, but no decrease in numbers. Clinically, epistaxis, gingival bleeding, and petechiae are seen. Hemarthrosis is a more common complication of clotting factor abnormalities such as hemophilia.

4. **C**, Page 1654.

Coumadin is a vitamin K antagonist and suppresses factors II, VII, IX, and X. Antihemophiliac factor VIII therefore would not help. Intravenous vitamin K_1 corrects the clotting defect but takes 6 to 12 hours. Fresh-frozen plasma has all of the necessary clotting factors and is the therapy of choice when rapid reversal of anticoagulation is indicated. Fresh whole blood has all of the required clotting factors but would necessitate a large volume load. Stored whole blood does not have all of the clotting factors.

5. **D**, Page 1649.

The bleeding time is a test of platelet number and function as well as vascular integrity. Aspirin inhibits platelet function, and patients with ITP have inadequate numbers of platelets. Vitamin C is necessary for capillary integrity, and steroids decrease the perivascular supporting tissue, both resulting in prolonged bleeding time. Heparin can cause a thrombocytopenia, but unless this complication is present the bleeding time is normal in patients treated with heparin or coumarin.

6. **D**, Page 1651.

Autoimmune disorders are often associated with thrombocytopenia from a variety of mechanisms. All of the other answers are associated with an increased platelet count. Reactive thrombocytosis is considered benign. Primary thrombocytosis is associated with both bleeding and thrombosis and requires a complete hematologic investigation.

7. **D**, Page 1658.

Both von Willebrand's disease and classic hemophilia share a decreased level of factor VIII activity. In addition, von Willebrand's has low levels of factor VIII antigen and a special factor VIII von Willebrand's factor, which is necessary for platelet adhesion. Therefore, both have a prolonged PTT, but only von Willebrand's has a prolonged bleeding time, which reflects its associated platelet defect. Hemophilia is transmitted as a sex-linked recessive trait, whereas von Willebrand's disease is transmitted as an autosomal dominant gene.

8. **B**, Page 1657.

Hemophiliacs can have a significant intracranial bleeding after seemingly minor head trauma. Hemophiliacs with any degree of head trauma should be treated with factor VIII and observed closely.

9. **E**, Page 1657.

The bleeding in hemophilia is often delayed, sometimes over 24 hours. Early treatment with factor replacement after injury, especially head trauma, even without evidence of bleeding at the time, is strongly recommended.

10. **C**, Page 1661.

The treatment for any form of symptomatic polycythemia is phlebotomy with normal saline replacement. Initially 500 cc of whole blood is removed; the procedure can be repeated as needed to lower the hematocrit to 60%.

11. **E**, Page 1660.

Polycythemia vera is a disorder that involves all cell lines and has increased red blood cells, white blood cells, and platelets. It also has an elevated leukocyte alkaline phosphatase and serum B_{12} level. Most secondary polycythemias are due to tissue hypoxia and thus a decreased PaO_2 is expected. The bone marrow picture would be the same with both disorders.

12. **E**, Page 1657.

von Willebrand's disease is transmitted as an autosomal dominant trait. Like classic hemophilia it has an elevated PTT but a normal PT. It is associated with a defect in platelet formation, but the number of platelets are normal. An unexplained finding is that a single dose of factor VIII replacement stimulates a progressive increase in factor VIII activity lasting 12–40 hours (the half-life of factor VIII is 8 hours). Even though it has defects involving both platelets and the

clotting sequence, it usually runs a milder course than hemophilia A.

13. **C**, Page 1652.

Splenomegaly can be associated with thrombocytopenia due to sequestration. However, the basic pathologic event in ITP is antibody-mediated platelet destruction, and splenomegaly is not expected. Platelet transfusions are a stimulus to further antibody production and thus should be avoided. Steroids have been found to help in adults but not children in whom the disease is usually self-limited. Posttransfusion thrombocytopenia is mediated by an antiplatelet antibody to the PLA-1 antigen. It can lead to significant bleeding requiring transfusion and thus further antigenic stimulation.

90
Oncologic Emergencies

1. **D**, Page 1677.

Sixty-eight percent of epidural compressions occur in the thoracic spine. Plain films show evidence of tumor in the vertebral body in 90% of patients with vertebral metastasis, the most common cause of epidural compression. Radiation therapy is the usual treatment but high-dose steroids should be started first to reduce cord edema.

2. **C**, Page 1666.

Pseudomonas aeruginosa is still a major pathogen and only this combination offers two drugs that are synergistic against it. Some recommend adding nafcillin as a third drug. If anaerobes are suspected, then clindamycin is a good choice.

3. **D**, Page 1672.

While any electrolyte abnormality can be found in a cancer patient, hypercalcemia is the most common, affecting 20% of cancer patients. Concomitant hypokalemia is found in 50% of those with hypercalcemia.

4. **B**, Page 1669.

The acute tumor lysis syndrome is seen with rapid destruction of tumor cells. Hyperuricemia occurs from breakdown of nucleic acids. Hyperkalemia, the most serious threat, occurs from massive cell lysis. Hyperphosphatemia occurs because of protein breakdown. Hypocalcemia occurs secondary to hyperphosphatemia.

5. **B**, Page 1667.

Keeping the head of the bed elevated can help slow the development of cerebral edema. Radiation therapy is the mainstay of treatment. Steroids have not been found to be useful but diuretics used carefully can provide temporary symptomatic relief. Because of the dual risk of increased bleeding due to increased venous pressure and decreased blood delivery to the tissues, all IVs should be started in the lower extremities.

6. **B**, Page 1670.

Hyperviscosity syndrome is due to sludging of flow through the microcirculation. The definitive treatment is plasmapheresis or leukopheresis. While waiting for that, a phlebotomy may reduce viscosity temporarily. Diuresis would be expected to increase viscosity. Allopurinol, Dilantin, or hydroxyurea may be used to treat a complication, but have no effect on viscosity.

7. **E**, Page 1670.

The hypocalcemia of the acute tumor lysis syndrome is secondary to increased phosphate. Excessive calcium can cause widespread precipitation of CA^{++} PO^{4+++} throughout the body. All of the other listed answers are important in managing the acute tumor lysis syndrome.

8. **E**, Pages 1665–1666.

Because of impaired ability to mount a classic inflammatory response, even the most thorough physical examination will often not identify a specific site of infection. Fifty percent of septic patients lack any distinctive physical findings.

9. **C**, Page 1666.

A lumbar puncture in the emergency department is indicated only when the patient's symptoms point to a CNS etiology (altered mental status, headache, stiff neck, etc). All of the other selections should be done *before* starting antibiotics.

10. **E**, Page 1678.

CNS infections are always vexing, more so in the oncology patient. Meningismus, one of the cardinal signs, is often absent. The mainstay of diagnosis is the lumbar puncture, but this is no help in a diagnosis of cerebral abscess (30% of CNS infections in oncology patients) and may be dangerous if there is elevated intracranial pressure. Furthermore, in the neutropenic patient, there may be no cells found in the CSF, even with meningitis.

91

Arthritis

1. **E**, Page 1697.

Reiter's syndrome is a triad consisting of non-gonococcal urethritis, polyarthritis, and conjunctivitis. The conjunctivitis is seen in only 30% of patients. Several types of skin lesions are seen, usually on the feet or penis. Most acute attacks respond well to nonsteroidal antiinflammatory drugs such as indomethacin.

2. **C**, Page 1695.

Gonococcal arthritis is by far the most common cause of septic arthritis among otherwise healthy young people. It is twice as frequent in women, probably because they are more likely to harbor an asymptomatic primary infection. It typically produces migratory arthralgias and tenosynovitis of the wrists. It then settles in one or more joints with a septic effusion. The typical skin lesions are present only 50% of the time. Gram's stains are unlikely to show the gram-negative diplococci. There is typically a rapid response to penicillin and if there is not, other diagnoses should be entertained. Frequent aspirations are recommended both to remove pus and relieve pain. Any patient with a septic joint should be started on antibiotics immediately to prevent destruction of the joint. The drug can be changed later when culture results are available.

3. **B**, Page 1695.

Patients with gonococcal arthritis that does not involve any weight-bearing joints do not universally require admission. The organism is very sensitive to penicillin and most get a response within 12 hours. All the other examples require admission for close monitoring of rheumatic fever and SLE and for parenteral therapy in septic arthritis and osteomyelitis.

4. **B**, Page 1689.

Normal synovial fluid has a white blood cell count of less than 2,000 cells, mostly mononuclear. It will form a string at least 3 cm long due to the presence of hyaluronate, which is also responsible for the positive mucent clot of normal fluid. With inflammation the hyaluronate is broken down, resulting in decreased viscosity with a poor string sign and a poor mucent clot. Uric acid crystals are negatively birefringent but calcium pyrophosphage crystals are positively birefringent. A high lactic acid should suggest infection with a nongonococcal agent.

5. **A**, Page 1699.

The development of vasculitis is a medical emergency. If not promptly treated with systemic steroids, irreversible neuropathy can occur.

6. **C**, Page 1699.

Felty's syndrome (rheumatoid arthritis with splenomegaly and leukopenia) is a late complication of rheumatoid arthritis. It is associated with a strongly positive rheumatoid factor. Dry eyes and dry mouth make up Sjögren's syndrome.

7. **D**, Page 1685.

Hydrochlorothiazide can cause an elevated uric acid and can precipitate gouty arthritis, but is not associated with lupus. All of the other listed agents can induce an antinuclear antibody reaction (50% of patients on procainamide) and less often clinical systemic lupus erythematosis.

8. **B**, Page 1700.

Migratory nondeforming polyarthritis is the single most common manifestation of acute rheumatic fever seen in 80% of cases. Carditis is next, seen in 50% of cases, and is usually manifested as murmurs of mitral or aortic regurgitation. The others are seen in 10% or less of cases. Besides the Jones criteria, supporting evidence of recent streptococcal infection (positive throat culture, increased ASO titer) is essential to the diagnosis of acute rheumatic fever.

9. **A**, Page 1693.

Allopurinol is useful for the long-term treatment of hyperuricemia. In the acute attack a rapid reduction in uric acid levels can cause a flare-up. Indomethacin and phenylbutazone are equally effective and probably the drug of choice for an acute attack of gout. Colchicine, orally or IV, is effective and also provides diagnostic information (only gout or pseudogout are relieved with colchicine). ACTH is effective but not often used because of the superiority of other agents.

10. **B**, Page 1693.

Pseudogout shares many features with gout. It is caused by crystals deposited in the joint and is treated with antiinflammatory agents or colchicine. Unlike gout, the knee is by far the most commonly involved joint.

11. **C**, Page 1695.

Only 2% of patients with psoriasis develop arthritis but of those who do, 90% will have pitting of the nails. This can help differentiate the acute arthritis from gout or rheumatoid arthritis, with which psoriasis can also be associated.

92
Dermatologic Problems

1. **C**, Page 1725.

Impetigo is a streptococcal infection that can result in poststreptococcal glomerulonephritis but not rheumatic fever. Penicillin is necessary for effective treatment of the skin lesions, but it does not prevent glomerulonephritis.

2. **C**, Page 1723.

Varicella is responsible for epidemic outbreaks of chickenpox usually in children 5 to 8 years old. Infection then remains dormant is the dorsal root ganglia until years later when it is reactivited as shingles. Viruses can be cultured from the vesicles of shingles, and chickenpox can be acquired from exposure. Rarely, exposure to chickenpox can result in shingles. Direct contact with shingles has not been reported to cause new cases of shingles.

3. **A**, Page 1712.

Measles is a highly contagious viral exanthem. However, it is not contagious beyond the fifth day of the rash or about the eighth day of illness.

4. **E**, Page 1706.

Epinephrine is the therapy of choice for all anaphylactic reactions. It reverses the bronchospasm, raises the blood pressure, and inhibits the mediators of anaphylaxis. In the hypotensive patient subcutaneous absorption is unreliable. Although IV epinephrine can cause myocardial damage especially to ischemic tissue, this patient's hypotension and hypoxia from bronchospasm represent a greater threat to life. Small boluses repeated frequently are less likely to present deleterious cardiac effects.

5. **B**, Page 1713.

Roseola is characterized by a highly febrile child (temperature 39°C to 41°C) who appears well and has few physical findings. The fever lasts 3 to 4 days and then breaks with the onset of rash, which clears over the next 1 to 2 days.

6. **C**, Page 1715.

This patient has a typical *Rhus* contact dermatitis from poison ivy or poison oak. While there may be a mild secondary infection, systemic antibiotics are not necessary in this afebrile nontoxic boy. Likewise, systemic steroids are not warranted for a small localized reaction without constitutional effects. Calamine lotion has no proven value. Topical steroids are often useful but are not retained on the skin well while there is significant oozing. They are more helpful in the subacute stage of erythema and pruritus without active weeping. Burow's solution is the therapy of choice for this patient, because it reduces swelling and itching and provides a local antibiotic effect.

7. **D**, Page 1721.

Most cases of erythema nodosum are idiopathic and no etiology is found. A thorough history and physical examination are necessary and most recommend a chest x-ray or PPD. But in an otherwise asymptomatic patient no further work-up is needed.

8. **C**, Page 1721.

Erythema nodosum is an inflammatory reaction consisting of erythematous nodules usually on the anterior tibia. All of the answers are associated with erythema nodosa but most cases remain idiopathic. Oral contraceptives are the leading cause of drug-induced cases.

9. **A**, Page 1709.

There are two distinct types of toxic epidermal necrolysis that are readily differentiated with a skin biopsy. The staphylococcal scalded skin syndrome affects young children and has a generally benign course without large fluid loss. Nonstaphylococcal toxic epidermal necrolysis has a high mortality associated with large fluid deficits. Steroids are indicated in this case. The cause is unknown but may appear secondary to penicillin or sulfonamides.

10. **B**, Pages 1703–1704.

Tinea capitus is fungal infection of the scalp caused by species of *Trichophyton* or *Microsporum*. Unlike Tinea corpus or pedis it requires oral griseofulvin usually for 3 to 6 weeks until there is complete clearing of the lesion. All the other statements are true.

11. **C**, Pages 1724–1725.

Most authorities suggest systemic steroids in doses of 40–80 mg of prednisone per day for the elderly. This group is more likely to develop postherpetic neuralgia. While steroids do not decrease the intensity of the pain, they do shorten the duration, which can be as long as 1 year. Topical steroids are used for ocular involvement of herpes zoster (unlike herpes simplex) but are otherwise ineffective.

12. **E**, Pages 1717–1718.

Scabies is caused by an intradermal mite and is associated with intense itching. The patients present with reddish papules on a mildly erythematous base with multiple excoriations. Children can get scabies involving the face, neck, and rarely the scalp, unlike adults. Crotamiton (Urax) is the drug of choice for children under 3, because of the potential neurotoxicity of Quell.

13. **E**, Page 1717.

Pediculosis is increasing annually, and in some schools pediculosis capitis has reached epidemic proportions. In children, the nits are white, while the adults' are dark. Most people do not require a second treatment unless they are reinfected. Household members should be examined but not treated unless nits are found.

14. **A**, Page 1720.

The FTA-ABS is the most sensitive and specific serologic test for syphilis. A false positive is defined as a positive VDRL but a negative FTA-ABS. The VDRL is positive in only 75% of cases of primary syphilis but nearly 100% of cases of secondary syphilis. Because it takes a certain period of time before any serologic test becomes positive, the dark field examination identifying spirochetes is the best way to diagnose primary syphilis.

15. **E**, Page 1710.

Most patients with acute urticaria have a benign course and even an extensive search for etiology is nonproductive. It is so common that a complete work-up for everyone would be prohibitively expensive.

16. **B**, Page 1714.

This is the typical picture of rubella. Measles presents as a fever, Koplik's spots on the buccal mucosal, then 2–3 days later a rash of the forehead and upper neck. Roseola is typified by a high fever for 3–4 days, then a rash that begins on the trunk and erupts as the fever fades. Rocky Mountain spotted fever begins on the wrists and ankles, with involvement of the palms and soles being particularly characteristic. Scarlet fever begins on the chest and has a sandpaper-type texture.

17. **C**, Page 1727.

The rash of meningococcemia occurs in 75% of cases and can be mimicked by viral infections or more rarely other bacterial illnesses. Chloramphenicol is the drug of choice in a penicillin-allergic patient (cephalosporins do not penetrate the meninges well enough). Many casual contacts, including hospital personnel, will become anxious when news of meningococcus ensues and will inappropriately request prophylaxis. Rifampin has a number of side effects, including hepatitis, and should only be given to direct household contacts and those immediately involved in the resuscitation, *not* casual contacts. Waterhouse-Friderichsen occurs occurs in only 10% of cases; if it is present, steroids should be used because adrenal shutdown is part of this syndrome.

18. **E**, Page 1703.

This patient has tinea versicolor, which responds well to topical antifungals. The fungal infections of the head (tinea capitis) or nails require oral griseofulvin. Topical steroids are used for contact dermatitis, which has more crusting and is seldom as widespread as this. Penicillin is used for impetigo, which is a pustular lesion. Lindane is used to treat scabies or pediculosis.

93
Stroke

1. **A**, Pages 1733–1734.
Although all listed risk factors are important in stroke, by far the most important predisposing factor is hypertension. The major risk factor is the development of atherosclerosis, which is generally the result of longstanding hypertension. In addition, intracerebral hemorrhage most often results from rupture of arterioles weakened by chronic systemic hypertension. Therefore, hypertension is the most important predisposing factor for the two major categories of stroke, hemorrhogic and occlusive.

2. **E**, Pages 1744–1745.
Patients with TIA have sudden focal symptoms of cerebral dysfunction that resolve within 24 to 72 hours. If these patients are not candidates for endarterectomy, aspirin or sodium warfarin (Coumadin) may be given for 3 to 6 months after the attack in an attempt to lessen the likelihood of future attacks or completed stroke, which are preceded by TIAs in about 75% of these patients. This patient's symptoms have progressed over a period of days and are not of sudden onset. Thus, a stroke or TIA is an unlikely cause. Hypoglycemia does not produce these symptoms, and diabetics on no medications are unlikely to suffer from these episodes. Finally, this patient's findings do not indicate a pontine hemorrhagic stroke, which produces acute onset of symptoms with early coma and pinpoint pupils and bilateral decerebrate posturing. Patients with subdural hematomas, on the other hand, have symptoms that develop slowly over days to weeks. The degree of headache, drowsiness, and confusion is often greater than the focal deficits seen. A CT scan can usually differentiate this condition from the others mentioned.

3. **A**, Page 1734.
Dysarthria, clumsiness, and weakness in one extremity and mild slurring of speech are a cluster of symptoms related to lacunar infarction of the pons. Cerebellar infarctions cause more ataxia than this patient presents with. Ruptured berry aneurysms usually produce headache, loss of consciousness, confusion, nausea and vomiting, and neck or back pain. These are not this patient's findings. Although migraine may be associated with a constellation of symptoms, a headache is a usual complaint, which, again, this patient does not have. Acute myocardial infarction is unlikely to cause these symptoms, although left arm and chest pain complaints are frequent.

4. **E**, Pages 1740–1741, 1745.
Patients with rheumatic heart disease and atrial fibrillation, and those with coronary artery disease and a history of recent myocardial infarction, are both likely candidates for embolic infarctions. Patients with deep venous thrombosis may be as likely to have embolic infarctions, but only in the presence of a cardiac septal defect. Patients on anticoagulation therapy are more likely to have hemorrhagic infarctions than embolic ones.

5. **E**, Pages 1735–1736.
Carotid artery disease is responsible for approximately 50% of patient's symptoms of transient unilateral loss of vision (amaurosis fugax). It is usually the result of platelet emboli from atheromatous plaques in that arterial system.

6. **D**, Pages 1737–1738, 1741.
This patient's symptoms are those of a cerebellar stroke. This would not be classified as an infarction if the symptoms resolved on their own. It would be a TIA. Remote trauma is unrelated to this event. Eye findings such as conjugate gaze palsy and ipsilateral fifth and seventh nerve dysfunction can occur over 1 to 3 days postinfarction secondary to the resultant edema, compressing the brain stem. This can be relieved by surgical decompression of the posterior fossa. Noncontrast CT scan can identify 37% of infratentorial infarctions if the study is performed as near to the acute event as possible.

7. **B**, Pages 1742–1743.
The peak age of incidence for subarachnoid hemorrhage from congenital aneurysm is age 35 to 65 years. Occasionally there are warning signs, but headache is the most common initial sign. This patients's symptoms are classic, including the leukocytosis and slight hyperthermia from meningeal irritation. The presence of a bruit over the eyeball, carotid artery, or mastoid of a young patient strongly suggests the presence of a cerebral arteriovenous malformation, which is the cause of 20% of subarachnoid hemorrhages. Although lumbar puncture plays an important role in making the diagnosis of subarachnoid hemorrhage, it is not the procedure of choice. Ergotamine alkaloids have no accepted place in the treatment of this disorder. CT scan can identify all mass lesions within the range of the resolution of the imager's capabilities. Currently, detection is good for lesions around 1 cm, but there is no study that is 100% sensitive.

8. **A**, Page 1743–1744.

This patient has hypertension and is in the appropriate age group for a stroke. Her other symptoms are also consistent with a hemispheric lesion. The fixed and dilated pupil, however, should alert the physician to the possibility of brain stem compression secondary to increased intracerbral pressure. Papilledema is often a late finding in patients with acute increases of intracranial pressure. Intravenous steroids, glycerol, mannitol, and hyperventilation are all treatment regimens used to decrease intracranial pressure. CT scan is the more appropriate method of diagnosis of increased intracranial pressure, since lumbar puncture might risk brain stem herniation.

94
Seizure

1. **C**, Pages 1751–1752.

Acetylcholine is an excitatory neurotransmitter, an excess of which can contribute to cellular excitability and hence seizures. All of the others are thought to be inhibitory or aid in the cessation of seizure activity.

2. **B**, Pages 1752–1755.

Supratentorial lesions have a 50% incidence of seizures, whereas the incidence is less than 3% with infratentorial tumors.

3. **D**, Page 1755.

Simple febrile convulsions are characterized by an initial onset at an age between 9 and 18 months. They tend to have no focal features, to last less than 15 minutes, to appear soon after a rise in temperature, do not occur in a series, and to have a high familial incidence. Febrile seizures that are long in duration, focal, or occur in a series are designated as complex.

4. **A**, Page 1758.

Simple partial seizures are usually brief, begin and end abruptly, and involve little or no alteration of consciousness.

5. **B**, Pages 1759–1760.

Convulsive status epilepticus in secondary epilepsy is probably related to the proposed major pathogenetic factors. On the other hand, stupor status is almost always seen in patients with primary epilepsy or chronic epilepsy of unknown cause.

6. **C**, Page 1761.

Syncope almost always occurs when the patient is upright (Strokes-Adams attacks are an exception). Syncope does not usually involve a postsyncopal headache, drowsiness, or mental confusion. It does

have a more gradual onset, and syncope is rarely associated with injuries from falling or with incontinence.

7. **D**, Page 1761.

Breathholding spells may represent stress reactions in children. The patient displays vigorous crying with hyperventilation followed by sudden apnea. The resultant hypoxia leads to cyanosis, loss of consciousness, muscle jerks, and finally relaxation.

8. **A**, Page 1761.

A is false because placing hard or wooden objects in the patient's mouth or forcing open the closed tonic jaw can produce dental or soft tissue injuries and possible tooth aspiration.

9. **B**, Page 1765.

In general, phenytoin is the preferred drug for status epilepticus. It should be used with great caution when bradycardia, cardiac conduction blocks, or cardiac failure is present, and it may be preferable to use phenobarbital in these patients. If anticonvulsant drug withdrawal is the suspected cause of status, then the withdrawn medication should be replaced. If chronic anticonvulsant therapy is needed in a child with a febrile convulsion, phenobarbital is the usual drug of choice.

10. **D**, Pages 1765–1766.

Phenobarbital should be used with caution in patients with myasthenia gravis. It is the drug of choice (after the initial diazepam) in the other three patient groups.

95
Vertigo and Syncope

1. **A**, Page 1773.

Disturbance in statokinetic system (which consists of semicircular canals, utricle, vestibular division of eighth cranial nerve and vestibular nuclei) causes true vertigo. Posterior columns are part of the proprioceptive system along with tendons, muscles, and joints. Eye muscles and the eyes constitute the visual system. The visual system, proprioceptive system, and statokinetic system constitute the equilibrium triad.

2. **C**, Page 1774.

Nystagmus is termed horizontal or vertical and named for its *fast* component. Fast components are either right or left— and up or down.

Differential characteristics for symmetric weakness

	Guillain-Barré syndrome	Myasthenia gravis	Botulism
Reflexes	Decreased	Intact	Intact or decreased
Pain	Uncommon	—	Paresthesias
Ascending/descending onset	Ascending	—	Descending
Fever	—	—	—
Proximal/distal onset	Distal	Proximal	Proximal
Eye involvement	Rare	Extraocular muscle weakness	Extraocular muscle weakness, pupillary changes
Gastrointestinal symptoms	—	Secondary to anticholinergics	Common

3. **D**, Pages 1775–1776.
   External auditory canal foreign body obstruction (or impacted cerumen) can cause true vertigo. It may be accompanied by hearing loss or tinnitus. Removal of obstruction is curative.

4. **C**, Pages 1779–1780.
   Otosclerosis is an autosomal dominant disease of stapedial immobilization. It is the most common cause of conductive hearing loss in adults and can produce recurrent or single attacks of vertigo or imbalance.

5. **C**, Page 1790.
   Aortic stenosis is the most common cause of syncope, but the mechanism is unknown. Theories include decreased cardiac output and hyperactive carotid sinus reflex.

6. **D**, Page 1796.
   All are true of vasovagal syncope. It may be associated with distention of esophageal diverticuli and other intestinal viscera, as well as endoscopic procedures.

7. **B**, Pages 1797–1798.
   This type of syncope results from a derangement of the glossopharyngeal nerve and its relationship with the carotid sinus reflex. Carbamazepine is helpful.

8. **D**, Page 1798.
   All are mechanisms of syncope associated with drug ingestion.

9. **B**, Page 1798.
   In the awake patient feigning unconsciousness choice *A* would be correct.

96
Weakness

1. **B**, Page 1803.
   Fever is uncommon with all three illnesses. Eye involvement is almost never present with Guillain-Barré, while extraocular muscle weakness is present initially with myasthenia gravis. Extraocular muscle weakness and pupillary changes occur in botulism. Reflexes are diminished with Guillain-Barré, variably affected with botulism, and intact with myasthenia gravis. Ascending paralysis is characteristic of Guillain-Barré, while descending paralysis occurs with botulism.

2. **B**, Pages 1803–1805.
   Guillain-Barré is characterized at its onset by symmetrical leg weakness, whereas the facial weakness may be asymmetric. The CSF reveals a protein count of greater than 400 mg/l and a cell count of less than 10/ml all of which are mononuclear.

3. **B**, Pages 1805–1806.
   Patients presenting with weakness, sweating, lacrimation, salivation, mioses, and tackycardia are suffering from cholinergic crisis due to overtreatment with acetylcholinesterase inhibitors. Worsening of symptoms with edrophonium is diagnostic. Atropine will reverse the muscarinic effects but has no effect on the neuromuscular blockade. Such patients may require ventilatory support until the acetylcholinesterase inhibitors wear off.

4. **B**, Pages 1805–1808.
   Botilism is caused by a toxin that prevents release of acetelcholine from nerve endings but has no effect on acetelcholine receptors. Infantile botulism is caused by spore growth within the gut. The spores can survive boiling for up to 2 hours. Eaton-Lambert syndrome is similar to myasthenia grovis and is associated with lung carcinoma. Acetylcholinesterase inhibitors usually do not reverse weakness, however. Tick paralysis is an ascending paralysis that develops over 1 to 2 days.

97
Adult Meningitis

1. **C**, Page 1812.
   Male sex will predispose one to meningitis along with the factors listed on page 218:

Table 97-1.

2. **D,** Pages 1814–1816.

Papilledema, as well as any focal neurologic deficit with the exception of lateral gaze ophthalmoplegia, is indicative of a mass lesion with increased intracranial pressure. Nuchal rigidity occurs with meningitis and seizures may also occur.

3. **A,** Page 1814.

Ophthalmoplegia may occur with bacterial meningitis. Table 97-2 below outlines indications for CT scan.

INDICATIONS FOR CT SCAN BEFORE LUMBAR PUNCTURE IN PATIENTS WITH SUSPECTED BACTERIAL MENINGITIS
Altered mental status
Papilledema
Focal neurologic deficit—excluding ophthalmoplegia
Subacute presentation with significant clinical suspicion of subarachnoid hemorrhage or other intracranial pathologic condition as principal diagnosis
Minimal or absent fever
History or evidence of head trauma—recent or remote
New-onset seizure

Table 97-2.

4. **B,** Pages 1815–1819.

Xanthochromia with a high protein count (greater than 150 mg/dl) is indicative of a traumatic tap. Xanthochromia with a low protein count indicates subarachnoid hemorrhage. Elevated bilirubin does not cause xanthochromia except in premature infants. Subdural hematomas do not cause xanthochromia.

5. **A,** Page 1820.

Penicillin G is indicated for all choices but *H. influenzae*, for which chloramphenicol plus ampicillin are indicated.

Table 97-3. Antimicrobial therapy for bacterial meningitis

Organism	Treatment of choice	Alternate treatment
Neisseria meningitidis	Penicillin G 5 million IU IV stat then 2 million IU IV q.2h.	Chloramphenicol 25 mg/kg IV stat then q.6h.
Streptococcus pneumoniae	Penicillin G 5 million IU IV stat then 2 million IU IV q.2h.	Chloramphenicol 25 mg/kg IV stat then q.6h.
Streptococcus pyogenes (A, B, C, G)	Penicillin G 5 million IU IV stat then 2 million IU IV q.2h.	Chloramphenicol 25 mg/kg IV stat then q.6h.
Haemophilus influenzae	Chloramphenicol 25 mg/kg IV stat then q.6h. *plus* Ampicillin 50 mg/kg IV stat then q.4h.	Cefotaxime* 2 g IV stat then q.4h. *or* Cefuroxime* 3 g IV stat then q.8h.
Staphylococcus aureus	Nafcillin 50 mg/kg IV stat then q.6h.	Vancomycin 20 mg/kg IV stat (not to exceed 1 g) then 10 mg/kg IV q.6h.
E. coli and other gram-negative enterics except *Pseudomonas aeruginosa*	Ampicillin 50 mg/kg IV stat then q.4h. *plus* Gentamycin 1.7 mg/kg IV stat then 1.5 mg/kg IV q.8h. (adjusted according to renal function) *plus* 5 mg intrathecally q.12h.	Cefotaxime* 2g IV stat then q.4h.
Pseudomonas aeruginosa	Carbenicillin 100 mg/kg IV stat then q.6h. *plus* Gentamycin 1.7 mg/kg IV stat then 1.5 mg/kg IV q.8h. (adjusted according to renal function) *plus* 5 mg intrathecally q.12h.	Carbenicillin 100 mg/kg IV stat then q.6h. *plus* Amikacin 7.5 mg/kg IV stat then q.12h. (adjusted to renal function) *plus* 15 mg intrathecally q.12h. *or* Cefoperozone* 3 g IV stat then q.6h.
Listeria monocytogenes	Ampicillin 2 g IV stat then q.4h.	Chloramphenicol 25 mg/kg IV stat then q.6h.

*Or equivalent third-generation cephalosporin.

218

Table 97-4. Initial antimicrobial therapy of meningitis when causative organism is unknown

Patients	Likely pathogens	Recommended treatment	Alternatives
Otherwise healthy adult < 40 years of age	S. pneumoniae N. meningitidis	Penicillin G 5 million IU IV stat then 2 million IU IV q.2h.	Chloramphenicol 25 mg/kg IV stat then q.4h.
Age > 40 years otherwise healthy	S. pneumoniae N. meningitidis H. influenzae Gram-negative enteric bacilli	Ampicillin 50 mg/kg IV stat then q.4h. *plus* Gentamycin 1.7 mg/kg IV stat then 1.5 mg/kg q.8h. (adjusted to renal function) *plus* 5 mg intrathecally q.12h.	Cefotaxime* 2 g IV stat then q.4h.
Recent neurosurgery, traumatic dural defect, V/P shunt	Gram-negative enteric bacilli S. aureus S. epidermidis S. pneumoniae	Nafcillin 50 mg/kg IV stat then q.6h. *plus* Amikacin 7.5 mg/kg IV stat then q.12h. (adjusted to renal function) *plus* 15 mg intracally q.12h. *plus* Cefoperazone* 3 g IV stat then q.6h.	Vancomycin 1 g IV stat then q.12h. *plus* Amikacin 7.5 mg/kg IV stat then q.12h. adjusted to renal function) *plus* 15 mg intrathecally q.12h.
Immunocompromised, intravenous drug abuser, alcoholic	S. pneumoniae N. meningitidis Gram-negative enteric bacilli L. monocytogenes H. influenzae S. aureus	Ampicillin 2 g IV stat then q.4h. *plus* Gentamycin 1.7 mg/kg IV stat then 1.5 mg/kg q.8h. (adjusted to renal function) *plus* 5 mg intrathecally q.12h. *plus* Nafcillin 50 mg/kg IV stat then q.6h.	Chloramphenicol 25 mg/kg IV stat then q.6h. *plus* Gentamycin 1.7 mg/kg IV stat then 1.5 mg/kg q.8h. (adjusted to renal function) *plus* 5 mg intrathecally q.12h. *plus* Nafcillin 50 mg/kg IV stat then q.6h.

*Or equivalent third-generation cephalosporin.

6. **B**, Page 1820.
Penicillin G is the most appropriate choice.

98
Approach to Violence

1. **E**, Pages 1827–1834.
All of these disorders may be manifest by violence. Depressed patients may deem themselves, and therefore everyone else, worthless, thus becoming violent. Substance abuses are prone to violence while intoxicated as well as during withdrawal or abstinence. Personality disorders and paranoia may present violently.

99
Suicide

1. **D**, Pages 1835–1838.
The suicide rates in younger persons have tended to increase in recent years. Suicide is the second leading cause of death for young adults in the 15- to 24-year-old group. The incidence of suicide rose from 10.6 to 12.4 per 100,000 from 1960 to the late 1970s. The present adolescent suicide rate has doubled in the past 10 years and tripled in the last 20. Risk factors for suicide include being male, white, and of middle age.

2. **B**, Pages 1838–1840.
Retterstol's Norwegian study of persons who had attempted suicide demonstrated that 80% of them were living in "full social functioning" without apparent illness and expressed satisfaction that their attempt had failed. Statements *C* and *D* are both just the opposite of what is true for suicide attempters. Treatment rendered in the emergency department is only exceedingly rarely a factor in determining whether a patient will attempt suicide again.

3. **D**, Pages 1838–1840.
An accident-prone person may have an unconscious suicide impulse. Common to the ED is a person in a one car accident who lost control for no apparent reason, as well as other accidental injuries such as falls or cutting oneself while at work. Although persons with psychotic depression and frank schizophrenia do attempt suicide, many attempters are not psychotic when they attempt suicide. They may be reacting to severe life stresses, have depressed personality traits, or be seeking, by their actions, to manipulate others. Answer *A* is incorrect because psychotics may not be depressed, but rather delusional when attempting suicide. Many patients form a suicide plan and call another person to inform them of their attempt. They may knowingly then take a sublethal overdose of drugs so that their plan will be unlikely to succeed.

4. **A**, Pages 1838–1840.

Aside from psychosis and alcoholism, each of which raises the risk of future suicide attempts, the psychiatric diagnosis itself is generally not a major determinant of suicide risk. Patients with attention-seeking behavior will in general choose less lethal methods of suicide as well as notify another person. Recent attempts and a feeling of helplessness greatly increase the risk of suicide.

100

Organic Brain Syndromes

1. **C**, Page 1851.

Although all of the answers may be appropriate at some point in this patient's evaluation, any person who presents in a delirious state with signs of meningismus and fever should have meningitis/encephalitis ruled out immediately. The amphetamines alone could be the cause for delirium and could precipitate paranoid schizophrenia. One might also suspect caffeine intoxication in this patient.

2. **D**, Page 1850.

Onset of behavioral symptoms after age 40 is frequently due to organic disorders. Delirium as defined by DSM-III criteria includes clouding of consciousness, perceptual disturbances, wake-sleep cycle disturbance, incoherent speech, increased or decreased psychomotor activity, disorientation, fluctuating symptoms, and evidence of an organic etiology.

3. **A**, Page 1847.

All of the following except phencyclidine withdrawal are associated with delirium. Of these, withdrawal from chronic use of drugs is the most common association today. Phencyclidine is associated with delirium and toxic psychosis in the acute rather than withdrawal state. Of the metabolic disorders, diabetes mellitus is most commonly associated with delirium.

4. **D**, Page 1846.

Periaqueductal petechial hemorrhages are found in Wernicke's disease. Hippocampal neuron degeneration is noted in anoxic encephalopathy, and cerebrocortical neuronal degeneration is found in anoxic, hypoglycemic, and hepatic encephalopathy. Cerebral edema can be found in acute alcohol intoxication and uremia. Increased rather than decreased astrocyte numbers are associated with uremia and hepatic encephalopathy.

5. **B**, Pages 1850–1851.

Asterixis and myoclonus are usually not found in functional syndromes such as dementia; rather they are associated with the organic syndromes of delirium.

6. **D**, Page 1857.

Evidence is lacking substantiating the use of acetylcholine precursors or degradation blockers alone or in combination. Medications with anticholinergic properties should be avoided since they may worsen confusion in demented patients and Hydergine should be avoided in patients with advanced SDAT. Therapy is primarily symptomatic and supportive.

7. **B**, Page 1855.

Although all patients should have reversible causes of dementia ruled out with appropriate historical, physical, neurologic, mental status, and laboratory evaluation; the most important of these is the mental status examination, and of these tests, the earliest affected is the short-term memory and concentration abilities.

101

Thought and Affective Disorders

1. **D**, Page 1866.

All the above responses may eventually be required in evaluation and treatment of patients, but often an agitated patient may be brought under control by taking a firm but nonthreatening stance. Encourage the patient to express her feelings by the use of such statements as "What is the matter" or "You seem upset."

2. **A**, Page 1874.

Lithium takes 1 week for improvement and several weeks for its full effect. Antipsychotic agents are quite useful during the full-blown manic episode and in severe cases the intramuscular use of haloperidol or thiothixene can be used. In this way, the patient's symptoms can be brought under control in a matter of hours. Lithium is best added to the treatment regimen as the patient is being brought under control and the antipsychotic is being tapered. The initial dose is usually 1500–1800 mg per day in divided doses with careful monitoring of lithium levels. At the time the therapeutic effect is reached the dose usually needs to be reduced to maintenance levels between 900 through 1200 mg per day. Lithium therapy should be initiated in an inpatient setting for patient compliance, education, and careful monitoring.

3. **E**, Pages 1863–1864.

Psychiatric interview is central to the assessment of a patient with a thought disorder. It should be initiated with open-ended questions to elicit the patient's explanation of the problem and should be nonjudgmental. At the same time the physician should be observing the patient's appearance, body language, and speech. The initial part of the interview should guide the physician to help confirm or rule out diagnoses according to DSM-III criteria. A brief mental status examination is important to see if there is evidence for organic mental disorder. The examination tests orientation, memory, cognitive function, affect, and general knowledge and could be done by asking a few questions. Although the interview is ideally accomplished in 15 minutes, it can be done in far less time, making it a technique that takes no longer than other common emergency procedures.

4. **C**, Page 1865.

A review of Table 101-1 shows that this patient exhibits seven features favoring a medical cause for his abnormal behavior, including (1) age of onset greater than 40, (2) apparent lack of past psychiatric history, (3) visual as opposed to auditory hallucinations, (4) medication to treat hypertension, (5) impaired cognitive function, (6) abnormal vital signs, and (7) incontinence of urine. A thorough medical evaluation starting with an accurate list of medications is indicated in this patient.

5. **B**, Page 1866.

In the psychotic patient, the treatment is aimed at reversing errors in information processing. Target symptoms such as agitation, hyperactivity, delusions, hallucinations, and bizarre speech and behavior are monitored in titrating doses of antipsychotic medication. Hypotension and oversedation are minimized by the use of high-potency agents but can still occur, necessitating careful monitoring of the patient during treatment. Extrapyramidal effects such as acute dystonic reactions are common and require the use of anticholinergic agents such as benztropine.

6. **C**, Page 1867.

The patient should not be admitted to the hospital against her will until prearranged protocols are followed and it is determined that the patient meets the requirements spelled out in the statutes according to state law. These procedures and conditions for involuntary commitment vary greatly by local and state, thus making a carefully planned written protocol a necessity to minimize legal and medical difficulties. Although the physician is caught in a double bind when treating the uncooperative patient, it is generally prudent to practice "good medicine" and treat the patient as a reasonable physician acting in the best interests of the patient would do. It cannot be overemphasized that the medical chart should reflect why the patient was involuntarily treated.

7. **B**, Page 1868.

According to DSM-III, if a depressive episode precedes psychiatric symptoms then a diagnosis of schizophrenia cannot be made. This has resulted in a less frequent diagnosis of schizophrenia and more frequent diagnosis of affective disorders. Similarly the presence of an organic mental disorder, from whatever cause, exludes the diagnosis of schizophrenia. Schizophrenia, schizophreniform disorder, and brief reactive psychosis have the same signs and symptoms during the acute phase of the illness. They are differentiated by their duration and ultimate prognosis. Schizophrenia requires at least a 6-month course of illness. Because of these more stringent criteria, it is not safe to assume that a diagnosis of schizophrenia made in the past is correct.

8. **C**, Page 1871.

This patient demonstrates the classic symptoms of akathisia, which is most often seen in middle-aged patients on the more potent antipsychotic medications between the first and tenth weeks of therapy. Akathisia is a state of motor restlessness characterized by a physical need to be moving constantly. The danger here is that the reaction can be mistaken for a decompensating psychosis leading to a vicious cycle in which more medication is given to treat a side effect caused by the same medication. The treatment is similar to that used in dystonic reacton utilizing anticholinergic, antiparkinsonian agents.

9. **A**, Pages 1872–1873.

It is estimated that 15% of all patients with a diagnosis of Primary Affective Disorder eventually kill themselves. Thus, the presence of high-risk factors such as: associated psychosis, a near-lethal attempt or plan, and continued active suicidal ideation almost always require admission. Other relative risk factors such as lack of future plans, unemployment, financial losses, adolescence, lack of secondary gain, and no decrease in symptoms after the psychiatric interview should be taken into account when making a disposition. Early pharmacologic studies on depressed patients led to the view that the depresion was caused by insufficient release of catecholamines and serotonin from central synapses in the brain. This, however, fails to explain the delay in therapeutic effect of antidepressants. According to DSM-III, to make a diagnosis of major depressive episode, the patient must have dysphoric mood and at least four of the following eight symptoms nearly every day for at least 2 weeks: problems with sleep, appetite, activity, interest, energy, guilt, concentration, and suicidal tendencies. The diagnosis is considered primary if it appears before other significant medical or psychiatric illnesses. Medications and substance abuse are common causes of depression (centrally acting antihypertensive agents, propranalol, cortical steroids, oral contraceptives, levodopa, traquilizers), are all capable of producing or agitating depression. Alcohol, amphetamine, and cocaine use are frequently associated with depression. Trazodone is virtually devoid of anticholinergic effects, making it safer for use in the elderly and safer in overdose cases. Its main side effect is sedation and a variety of neurologic complaints. Although controversial, if antidepressants were prescribed to a patient in an emergency department setting, this drug would have less potential for a fatal overdose.

102
Substance Abuse

1. **B**, Pages 1881–1882.

   Muscular weakness including quadriplegia, can be profound, especially with toluene inhalation. Without knowing the history of hydrocarbon abuse, it could be mistaken Guillain-Barré. Neurologic deficits are frequently reported in chronic abusers, including cerebellar and optic atrophy, peripheral neuropathies, and cerebral infarction secondary to cerebral vasospasm. Numerous authors have reported increasing incidence of sudden cardiac death in inhalant abusers of halogenated hydrocarbons, most notably freeon, found in aerosol cans, and TCE (trichloroethylene), found in typewriter correction fluid. Clinical observation and animal studies support a hypothesis of cardiac sensitization that, combined with excessive catecholamine release, induces fatal cardiac dysrhythmias. Renal abnormalities including oliguric renal failure, hematuria, proteinuria, and myoglobinuria are common with chronic toluene abuse and are generally reversible.

2. **A**, Page 1883.

   Chronic toluene produces hypokalemic, hyperchloremic *acidosis* that can be profound. Anion gap may be normal or elevated. Distal renal tubular acidosis has been observed in abusers and may contribute to these metabolic disturbances. The cause of hypokalemia is still unclear and may involve a redistribution of potassium similar to hypokalemic periodic paralysis. Both hypophosphatemia and hypocalcemia may be so profound as to result in tetany.

3. **C**, Pages 1884–1885.

   Occasionally, nitrous oxide exposure may result in death, but this is usually caused by anoxia. No direct cardiotoxic effects of nitrous oxide have been demonstrated. Hallucinations generated by nitrous oxide exposure cease as soon as exposure is terminated because the gas is rapidly cleared by the lungs. Chronic abuse may result in a myeloneuropathic syndrome, which may be confused with multiple sclerosis, diabetic neuropathy, alcoholic cerebellar degeneration, and peripheral neuropathy or subacute combined degeneration. This may be related to a disturbance of B_{12} metabolism observed with nitrous oxide toxicity, which can also cause megaloblastic hematopoetic changes. No bone marrow depression or aplastic anemias have been reported in association with nitrous oxide toxicity.

4. **C**, Pages 1887–1889.

   Nystagmus is the most common physical finding, vertical, horizontal, or rotary, and has been noted in 57% of cases overall. It does, however, occur in other intoxications as well, including ETOH. PCP is concentrated in gastric acid 30–50 times that of serum by a secretory phase in spite of the mode of intoxication. Clinical presentation of PCP intoxication is divided into three stages: stage I— patients are agitated or violent, but vital signs are normal; stage II—moderate intoxication hallmark tachycardia, hypertension, and only responsiveness to pain; stage III—completely unresponsive, depressed respirations, seizures, and death. Rhabdomyolysis with hyperactive state is often seen with increased CPK and myoglobinuria.

5. **C**, Pages 1889–1890.

   Alkalinizing the urine would slow PCP excretion. Acidification has been used and is theoretically advantageous, but in clinical experience has not proven to be efficacious. Most authorities recommend against acidification because it may exacerbate other properties of the overdose. Phenothiazines are not recommended because they can potentiate anticholinergic symptoms and lower seizure threshold and produce hypotension. Haldol is recommended for agitation, 5–10 mg IM. Gastric emptying and repeated charcoal administration is at least theoretically advantageous because of the gastric secretion of PCP from the serum, regardless of the route of administration. Hemodialysis has not been shown to be of any value in increasing PCP clearance.

6. **D**, Page 1893.

   High-flow oxygen is recommended to further saturate available hemoglobin and increase oxygen delivery to the tissues. Orthostatic hypotension is usually secondary to vasodilation and responds to crystalloid infusion and Trendelenberg position. On occasion, direct-acting vasopressors such as alpha agonists may be required. Methylene blue is the antidote for methemoglobinemia, acting as an electron carrier in the NADPH, requiring alternate pathway of methemoglobin reduction and quickly restoring oxygen carrying capability to hemoglobin. Thiosulfate is specific antidote for cyanomethemoglobin, converting it to thiocyanate in treatment of cyanide poisoning.

7. **E**, Pages 1901–1902.

Because of its inhibitory effect on gastric motility, seeds may be recovered even as late as 24 hours post-ingestion. Therefore, gastric emptying followed by charcoal is recommended in all cases despite a delay from the time of exposure. Physostigmine is theoretically advantageous since the belladonna alkaloids cause a pure anticholinergic poisoning. Since it acts to increase acetylcholine levels, physostigmine can precipitate a cholinergic crisis, including heart block and asystole. It is therefore recommended to reserve physostigmine for severe and potentially life-threatening anticholinergic complications. Valium may be used safely to calm agitated patient. Phenothiazines, however, may potentiate anticholinergic effects and are to be avoided.

8. **A**, Pages 1902–1904.

There is no documented cardiotoxicity of LSD; fatalities that do occur in general are secondary to perceptional distortions induced by the drug leading to suicides, homicides, or accidental deaths.

9. **C**, Pages 1907–1909.

Hypoglycemia may be seen in severe cocaine toxicity, of which this is a typical description. Cocaine may be cut with heroin or taken together as a "speedball" and Narcan should be administered as in any unresponsive patient. Physostigmine is reserved for specific anticholinergic poisonings. Although this case has certain features of anticholinergic poisoning (elevated temperature, tachycardia, and flushing), other features are more consistent with cocaine toxicity, namely hyperactive bowel sounds, pulmonary edema, and diaphoresis. Metabolic acidosis may be a prominent feature of serious cocaine toxicity and should be treated aggressively.

10. **D**, Pages 1908–1909.

Aggressive treatment of hyperthermia includes iced gastric and rectal lavage, cooling blanket or ice immersion. Abdominal x-rays may reveal presence of latex balloons filled with cocaine, called "body-packing," that cause fatal or prolonged cocaine toxicity. Saline diuresis will be necessary in severe cocaine toxicity complicated by rhabdomyolysis and myoglobinuria to prevent renal failure. There is no evidence of benefit from gastric emptying and oral charcoal in cocaine toxicity except in the rare case of ingestion. Most cocaine is nasally inhaled or intravenously infected.

103
Sexual Assault

1. **C**, Pages 1920–1921.

Sperm remain motile in the vaginal vault for 6 to 12 hours but can remain motile in the cervix for up to 5 days. The other answers are all true. A small volume of semen is discharged before a full ejaculation, which can cause pregnancy and be found in the vaginal vault.

2. **C**, Pages 1917,1922.

Many cases have been lost through faulty handling of the chain of evidence. It is incumbent on the examining physician to label the evidence so that it can be accurately identified later and to see that only the people so authorized receive such evidence. Only 2% of those accused of rape ar ever convicted. Many authorities suggest only a medical history as necessary from the patient and no history of the alleged event from the suspect. To do so increases the likelihood that you will be required to appear in court. A woman has the right to a medical evaluation without a legal examination if she so chooses. Likewise, no information or physical evidence can be released until she consents to do so.

3. **A**, Page 1923.

Vaginal adenosis and cancer in the female and penile and testicular lesions in males are well described in the offspring of mothers treated with DES during pregnancy. None of the other answers have been reported with any greater frequency.

4. **A**, Page 1921.

The toluylene blue dye test can identify clinically invisible tears in the vaginal mucosa. It must be remembered that the speculum exam can cause small lacerations and the toluene blue is spermatocidal so all samples for semen analysis should be collected first.

5. **E**, Page 1920.

Your evaluation of the sexual assault victims should address each of these issues. It should be noted that it is penetration of any body cavity that determines carnal knowledge, not ejaculation.

104
Adult Abuse

1. **B**, Page 1930.

Twenty-five percent of homicides are committed by relatives.

2. **B**, Page 1930.

Women are far more likely to be killed by intimates than men. There are at least 1,200 documented murdered wives and girlfriends annually in the United States, and estimates are that the number is much higher than that.

3. **C**, Page 1930.

The typically abused patient is isolated, young, and with few friends. She usually leaves her family at an early age and becomes financially dependent on her husband. She typically has a very low self-esteem and often develops the feeling that she deserves the abuse she gets.

4. **A**, Page 1931.

Older boys that witness domestic violence display aggressive antisocial behavior while older girls usually become withdrawn and anxious.

5. **C**, Pages 1931–1932.

Once the wife is beginning to sense positive overtones of reconciliation after abuse she is often unlikely to be responsive to any intervention. Learned helplessness is a separate theory of abuse that describes how abused wives may become extremely passive, may develop chronic fear, and may lose their ability to protect their own lives.

6. **B**, Page 1933.

The period immediately after the abuse is the time when appropriate intervention appears to be most effective. This is the period when emergency physicians have the greatest opportunity to achieve therapeutic intervention in wife abuse.

7. **C**, Page 1938.

Active neglect is defined as withholding necessities, confinement, and/or lack of supervision leading to physical harm.

8. **C**, Page 1939.

Neglect does appear to be more common with the most impaired elderly, whereas abuse is more common with the least disabled elderly. Usually the abused elderly are functionally dependent on the abuser and often live with them.

105
Acid-Base Homeostasis

1. **B**, Page 1954.

This is an acute process as evidenced by minimal renal compensation. Induction of CO_2 narcosis is unlikely in a patient with acute respiratory acidosis. Cardiac output and blood pressure are usually well-maintained during moderately severe acute respiratory acidosis.

2. **D**, Page 1964.

Respiratory compensation for metabolic alkalosis is triggered by chemoreceptors that sense the alkaline pH. $PaCO_2$ increases 0.6–0.7 mm Hg for every 1 mEq/L increase in the plasma HCO_3 concentration. It should be remembered that the body never overcompensates in acid-base disturbances, i.e., simple compensation for chronic respiratory acidosis will never produce an alkalotic pH.

3. **A**, Page 1964.

Low levels of mineral corticoids in Addison's disease decrease renal excretion of H+ ions, thus producing metabolic acidosis.

4. **B**, Page 1960.

Paradoxical CSF *acidosis* can occur due to diffusion of CO_2 produced by alkali therapy across the blood-brain barrier without comparable diffusion of HCO_3.

5. **C**, Page 1950.

Without hemoglobin, venous pH would be 4.5. Hemoglobin receives H+ forming Hg H+, freeing HCO_3 ion.

6. **B**, Page 1953.

Serum potassium is directly influenced by serum pH. K+ will rise 0.8 mEq/L for every decrease in pH of 0.1 units.

106
Fluid and Electrolyte Balance

1. **D**, Page 1970.

Hypertonic saline infusion will raise the ECF osmotic strength, which will then draw intracellular fluid until the osmolalities are equalized.

2. **C**, Page 1971.

K+ concentration in the cell is 140 mOsm/L and 4 mOsm/L in the ECF.

3. **B**, Page 1970.

The formula for estimating serum osmolality is 2(Na+) + glucose/18 + BUN/2.8 = 285–295 range.

4. **A**, Page 1971.

Alcohol is highly lipid soluble enabling it to rapidly penetrate cell membranes. Osmotic equalization is then able to take place without fluid shifts. This is not true for the other choices.

5. **E**, Page 1972.

Hyperventilation increases pulmonary losses, exercise and hypermetabolic state increase pulmonary and heat reduction losses, and low humidity facilitates cutaneous fluid losses. Assisted ventilation with humidification can contribute to fluid overload.

6. **A**, Page 1972.
Increased, not decreased, plasma osmolality will increase ADH secretion in order to withhold more free water and thereby normalize the osmolality. Hypotension, stress, and trauma have all been shown to increase ADH secretion.

7. **A**, Page 1973.
When inappropriately secreted, ADH will cause the kidneys to retain free water, leading to hyponatremia and a simultaneous nondilute urine. Normally you would expect a dilute urine in hyponatremia because the kidneys will seek to excrete the excess free water.

8. **D**, Page 1973.
Hyponatremia with dilute urine indicates the kidneys are reacting appropriately to a free water excess. Therefore, *D* is the most appropriate.

9. **D**, Page 1973.
Almost any pathologic state of the CNS can cause SIADH.

10. **B**, Page 1973.
The most prominent manifestations of SIADH are neurologic, most often consisting of dizziness or headache but ranging from apathy to disorientation. Neoplasms, especially bronchogenic carcinoma, are the most common causes of ectopic ADH secretion.

11. **D**, Page 1973.
Although this patient has SIDAH, it is not severe enough to warrant hypertonic saline, because he is asymptomatic except for the symptoms referrable to the tumor. Treatment is fluid restriction to decrease free water intake and is usually sufficient.

12. **A**, Pages 1973–1974.
Patients are usually able to maintain sufficient fluid intake to keep up with their losses and are thus usually asymptomatic except for polydipsia and polyuria.

13. **D**, Page 1974.
Only ADH replacement will correct this condition. Pitressin is available in oral, injectable, and inhalant preparations. Chlorpropamide has been shown to be useful in partial DI.

14. **A**, Page 1974.
Acetazolamide causes a metabolic acidosis because of its renal effects, but it does not cause DI. The others can cause nephrogenic DI by a direct action on the kidney.

15. **A**, Page 1974.
Aldosterone causes $Na+$ conservation and $K+$ excretion. This serves to maintain ECF volume.

16. **C**, Page 1974.
Choices *A* and *D* are early changes in dehydration. *C* is correct because both signs listed are changes found in more severe dehydration.

17. **A**, Page 1975.
Orthostatic hypotensive changes usually indicate a TBW deficit of at least 10%. Hypotension is usually associated with a blood volume deficit of at least 15–25% and an even larger interstitial fluid deficit.

18. **A**, Page 1975.
Fluid losses from burns have a low $Na+$ content leading to hypernatremic dehydration. Insensible losses from the skin are greatly increased.

19. **D**, Page 1975.
Aldosterone conserves $Na+$, thus hypoaldosteronism leads to hyponatremia.

20. **B**, Page 1975.
Sweat $Na+$ concentration ranges from 5 to 50 mEq/L.

21. **D**, Page 1976.
Hypernatremia causes brain dehydration, not edema. Subsequent decreased brain volume can lead to subdural and subarachnoid hemorrhages from tension on bridging veins. Thrombosis of venous sinuses may occur.

22. A, Page 1976.
If water replacement is too rapid, the plasma will become hypotonic relative to the brain, leading to cerebral edma and seizures. Additionally, the intravascular volume will expand too rapidly, which may lead to CHF, especially in elderly patients.

23. A, Page 1978.
Hyperlipidemia can cause a pseudohyponatremia because the lipids will displace a portion of the plasma water, therefore there will be less $Na+$ in a given volume, but the tonicity will be normal.

24. **D**, Pages 1978–1979.
More than 10 drugs have been shown to cause hyponatremia. If the onset of hyponatremia is gradual, a patient may be only mildly symptomatic as low as 110 mEq/L. Aldosterone secretion increases in response to hyponatremia. Hemiparesis or unilateral Babinski's sign can be caused by hyponatremia. CSF pressure increases because of cerebral edema.

25. **B**, Page 1979.
Aggressive treatment is indicated when any but the mildest of neurologic symptoms is manifested. Central line monitoring is needed also to guard against fluid overloading. This is especially indicated in elderly people.

26. A, Page 1981–1982.
Any process that increases the volume of fluid passing through the distal tubules increases the total amount of $K+$ secreted by increasing the chemical gradient for $K+$ across the tubular membrane. Decreased $Na+$ delivery to the distal tubule will decrease the chemical gradient for $K+$ as well. Discontinuing diuretic therapy will decrease fluid delivery to the distal tubule. Alkalosis will increase the intracellular $K+$ and deliver less $K+$ to the kidney.

27. **A**, Pages 1982–1983.

Pardoxical aciduria is caused by hypokalemia, not hyperkalemia, because the kidneys will preferentially save K+ and excrete H+, forming a more acidic urine.

28. **A**, Pages 1984–1985.

DKA leads to total body K+ deficit, because the acidosis causes K+ efflux from cells and is then excreted by the kidneys.

29. **D**, Page 1989.

Hyperglycemia by itself cannot lead to K+ transit across cell membranes. Insulin is required for the coupled passage of glucose and K+ into cells.

30. **B**, Page 1984.

As mentioned earlier, K+ excretion is directly proportional to the Na+ delivery at the distal tubule. As the GFR falls in renal failure, less Na+ is delivered to the distal tubule. Aldosterone secretion from all mechanisms results in K+ excretion.

31. **C**, Page 1984.

Chemotherapy for lymphomas and other tumors results in hyperkalemia caused by the massive cell lysis and release of K+.

32. **E**, Page 1985.

This effect averages a 0.5 mEq/L elevation for the normal person, but it can be much more for patients with burns, soft tissue injuries, and neuromuscular diseases such as multiple sclerosis, Parkinson's disease, tumors, and muscular dystrophy.

33. **D**, Page 1986.

In order, choice *C* occurs first above 6 mEq/L, then *A* as the K+ approaches 8, and *B* as the K+ rises above 8.

34. **D**, Page 1986.

Various heart blocks, injury patterns, and pericarditis can develop in hyperkalemia.

35. **B**, Page 1986.

This patient needs immediate therapy and the most rapid intervention is with Ca gluconate, which does not alter the K+ concentration but has a direct effect on the myocardium. The other choices will decrease the K+ and are preferred for less urgent situations.

36. **A**, Page 1987.

Kayexalate exchanges Na+ for K+, thus ridding the body of excess K+ but can cause Na+ overload and subsequent CHF. Rebound hyperkalemia does not occur. Hypokalemia without EKG changes is unlikely to be the cause. Bicarbonate therapy is an unlikely cause since it is used only in the initial phase of treatment.

37. **C**, Page 1987.

Florinef is the drug of choice for this condition. However, if this patient were experiencing severe symptoms, emergency therapy including 20 ml of 10% calcium gluconate IV should also be employed.

38. **D**, Page 1987.

All GI fluids, including gastric, have 2 to 3 times the K+ concentration of plasma, therefore excessive losses of any GI fluid can lead to hypokalemia. GI losses can lead to a secondary hyperaldosteronism from renin-angiotensin activation in the presence of decreased plasma volume. Hypoaldosteronism then leads to further renal and colonic K+ secretion. Over 50% of the patients with villous adenoma get hyperkalemia since these tumors secrete a watery mucus high in potassium.

39. **D**, Pages 1987–1988.

Addison's disease is an absence or deficiency in mineralocorticoid secretion. A lack of aldosterone activity on the kidneys will cause increased K+ resorption and often lead to hyperkalemia. Glucocorticoid excess in Cushing's syndrome can lead to hypokalemia because glucocorticoids have some mineralocorticoid activity.

40. **A**, Page 1988.

Aldactone contains spironolactone, which blocks the distal tubule Na+/K+ exchange site. It is at this site where the K+ is lost because of the increased Na+ load delivered to the distal tubule by the other diuretics. This then greatly curbs K+ loss for those on aldactone.

41. **B**, Page 1990.

In hypokalemia the kidneys will preferentially save K+ and excrete H+, even though that leads to a metabolic alkalosis. Or in other words, to correct for the hypokalemia, K+ is transported out of cells in exchange for Na+ and H+. This also occurs in the renal tubule cells, leading to a paradoxical aciduria, because their relative intracellular acidosis causes them to be more inclined to excrete H+ and save HCO_3.

42. **E**, Page 1991.

Although Lasix should cause concern in that it must be stopped in a patient who is hypokalemic, the presence of hypokalemia will potentiate the toxic cardiac effects of digoxin.

43. **E**, Page 1992.

Alkalosis from any cause can lead to symptoms of hypocalcemia, because H+ and Ca++ compete for the same protein-binding sites in the plasma. With a lack of H+ in alkalosis there is less competition for Ca++ at the binding sites. The bound Ca++ is not physiologically active.

44. **A**, Page 1992.

A lower albumin level makes fewer sites available for Ca++ binding, thus decreasing total Ca++ while having no effect on the free ionized fraction.

45. **A**, Page 1995.
Colon carcinoma infrequently causes osteoclastic bone destruction or ectopic PTH production. The other cancer sites are the three most common causes of hypercalcemia in malignancy.

46. **E**, Pages 1997–1998.
Ca++ and digitalis have the same relative effect on the myocardium. Thus when elevated, they potentiate the toxic effect of each other.

47. **D**, Page 1999.
The treatment of choice for any Ca++ level above 15 is emergent forced saline diuresis, which means both Lasix and as much normal saline as the patient can tolerate to maintain a urine output of 500 ml/hour or more. Insulin has no place in therapy for hypercalcemia.

48. **D**, Pages 2000–2001.
Choices *A* and *B* are incorrect because hypocalcemia by unknown mechanisms and blood transfusions cause it by complexing with citrate in bank blood. Parathyroid adenomas cause hypercalcemia.

49. **A**, Page 2002.
Hypocalcemia causes hyperexcitability of neurons, not hypoexcitability. Chvostek's sign is correct as noted and Trousseau's sign is carpopedal spasm following 3 minutes of tourniquet-induced arterial occlusion of the arm.

50. **C**, Pages 2002–2003.
Your clinical suspicion in this case is certainly sufficient to require IV Ca++ therapy.

51. **B**, Pages 2004–2005.
Hypermagnesemia causes hypotension, not hypertension, because it relaxes vascular smooth muscle. Hypomagnesemia occurs in 25% of alcoholics from malnutrition and excessive urinary losses caused by alcohol diuresis.

52. **A**, Page 2006.
Initially, Mg levels are elevated in half of DKA patients, probably from dehydration, but with insulin therapy an intracellular shift similiar to that of K+ often occurs leading to hypomagnesemia. Hypophosphatemia occurs by basically the same mechanism.

53. **A**, Page 2007.
Magnesium sulfate is the drug of choice. Too high a dose can lead to hypotension.

54. **C**, Page 2009.
It is very important to give half of your total K+ replacement as K-phosphate, which will adequately replace the phosphate deficit in most situations. Blood levels should be monitored.

55. **E**, Pages 1973, 1979–1980.
Hyponatremia is first evaluated in terms of total body water, which in this case is clinically excessive. Renal failure can be further differentiated from CHF, cirrhosis, and nephrotic syndrome by having a urine sodium greater than 20 mEq/L. Treatment involves water restriction.

56. **D**, Page 1980.
The initial step in the differentiation of hyponatremia etiologies is the state of the total body water.

57. **E**, Page 2002.
In the treatment of hypocalcemia when an IV cannot be established, it may be given IM in the gluceptate or gluconate forms. However, the calcium gluconate should not be given to infants because of the risk of sterile abscess formation.

107
Endocrine Disorders

1. **D**, Page 2025.
Blockade of the peripheral adrenergic hyperactivity of thyroid crisis is perhaps the most important factor in reducing morbidity and mortality.

2. **Beta Blockers**, Page 2025.
Beta blockade is currently the method of choice for staunching the peripheral manifestations of thyroid storm. Intravenous propanolol can reduce dysrhythmias, hyperpyrexia, tremor, palpitations, restlessness, and anxiety. Dose: 1–2 mg bolus every 10–15 minutes until desired effect is obtained.

3. **C**, Page 2024.
Thyroid storm is a clinical diagnosis and a medical emergency.

4. **B**, Page 2025.
The three most common precipitating factors of myxedema coma in those with underlying hypothyroidism are exposure to cold, infection, and congestive heart failure. In one study less than 10% of patients did not have exposure to cold as the primary precipitating event. Although the precipitating factors (see table in textbook) should be diligently searched for, many times they will be unidentified.

5. **D**, Pages 2028–2029.
The FTI (product of TT_4 and T_3 RU) is an indirect measure of FT_4 (free T_4)—it is this unbound hormone that is metabolically active and is at a low level in hypothyroidism. Low FT_4 releases its inhibition on the anterior pituitary and causes increased serum TSH.

6. **B**, Pages 2029–2030.
In all cases of hypothyroidism levothyroxine (T_4) is usually preferred over triiodothyronine (T_3) because it has a more gradual onset of action—T_4 must first be converted to T_3 in vivo. Theoretically this may reduce the chance of cardiac complications seen with intravenous administration of thyroid hormone, which is probably the single most important factor in survival for patients in myxedema coma. At present T_3 is not available commercially for intravenous use.

7. **A**, Pages 2032–2033.

In primary adrenocortical insufficiency the lesion is in the adrenal gland itself. Decreased glucocortical production produces hypoglycemia (seen in both primary and secondary adrenocortical insufficiency) and elevated ACTH (seen only in primary adrenocortical insufficiency and caused by disinhibition on the hypothalamic-pituitary axis). In primary adrenocortical insufficiency aldosterone production can also be interfered with (not seen in secondary adrenocortical insufficiency) and thus the Na+ and K+ abnormalities can be commonly seen.

8. **B**, Pages 2030–2031.

It has been found that over 90% of the adrenal gland must be destroyed before signs of insufficiency develop. Thus there is significant reserve for all but catastrophic destruction of the gland.

9. **D**, Page 2031.

The probability of hypothalamic-pituitary-adrenal axis suppression depends on the frequency, strength, and schedule, as well as the duration of steroid therapy. The degree of suppression cannot be predicted accurately even with consideration of these factors. Recovery of the HPA axis following discontinuation of therapy may take up to 1 year.

10. **E**, Page 2034.

Treatment of hypoglycemia in suspected acute adrenocortical insufficiency should be immediate. For symptomatic hypoglycemia (perspiration, tachycardia, weakness, nausea, vomiting, headache, convulsions, coma) or low serum glucose levels, intravenous glucose (1–2 amps D50W) is preferred. If intravenous access is unobtainable, subcutaneous glucagon (1–2 mg) may be used. The major causes of mortality and morbidity in this disease are secondary to either hypoglycemia or hypotension.

11. **C**, Pages 2033–2034.

The 48-hour ACTH stimulation test can not only diagnose adrenocortical insufficiency but also differentiate primary from secondary causes. The 8-hour ACTH stimulation test is of course faster (24-hour urine 17-hydroxysteroid level confirms this diagnostic test) but may have an unacceptably high false-positive rate.

12. **A**, Page 2034.

Although much more potent, dexamethasone has similar in vivo glucocorticoid properties as cortisol (equal hydrocortisone). Since therapeutic and diagnostic procedures should proceed simultaneously in suspected acute adrenocortical insufficiency and since hydrocoritisone hemisuccinate will falsely elevate serum cortisol levels, thus making diagnostic tests inaccurate, IV dexamethasone is the agent of choice under these conditions. Unlike situations where hydrocortisone (with its mineralocorticoid properties) can be used for replacement, Florinef (strict mineralocorticoid effects) must be used with dexamethasone to prevent salt loss.

108
Diabetes

1. **D**, Page 2039.

Diabetes is a disorder of all those listed above.

2. **C**, Page 2039.

One-half of all children with diagnosis of diabetes mellitus will die of renal disease 25 years after the initial diagnosis, not cardiac disease. The rest of the statements are true.

3. **C**, Pages 2039–2040.

Very low levels of insulin, not moderate levels, are required to inhibit intracellular lipolysis. The other statements are true.

4. **D**, Page 2040.

D is false. Glucagon causes increase in blood glucose, whereas insulin lowers blood glucose. Thus, their effects are antagonistic, not synergistic. *A, B,* and *C* are true.

5. **C**, Page 2040.

A is false because Type I diabetics are classically younger, nonobese patients with low levels of insulin, not poor peripheral sensitivity to insulin. *B* is false because Type II diabetics have poor peripheral sensitivity to insulin and may, in fact, have elevated insulin levels. *D* is false because Type I diabetics are not treated with oral agents, and Type II diabetics many times need insulin to control hyperglycemia.

6. **D**, Pages 2041–2042.

Acidosis causes falsely elevated K+, thus 0.8 mEq/L K+ must be subtracted for each 0.1 decease in pH during DKA. *B* is ture. Generally Beta-hydroxybutyrate will not be measured, so anion gap calculations can be helpful to assess contribution of organic acids, i.e., ketones to the anion gap. *A* is true. *C* is true.

7. **A**, Page 2043.

It is most classically seen with Type I diabetics. *B, C,* and *D* are all true.

8. **D**, Page 2043.

All are commonly seen in patients with DKA.

9. **D**, Page 2044.

Narcotic overdose may cause coma but will not present with other physical findings and history consistent with DKA. *A*, *B*, and *C* are consistent with DKA.

10. **D**, Pages 2045–2046.

All are true.

11. **A**, Pages 2044–2046.

A is false—pregnancy and DKA is extremely critical and thus aggressive early treatment is critical. *B* is true, and *C* is true. *D* is true—cerebral edema may occur following infusion of 0.45 normal saline because of the rapid reduction in hyperosmolality. Most authors now recommend 0.9% initially.

12. **A**, Pages 2045–2046.

You do not use D5W in resuscitating DKA patients. 0.9% normal saline is preferrable over 0.45% normal saline. Do not add dextrose until initial fluids have been given and blood sugar is approximately 250 mg/dl.

13. **C**, Page 2045.

20 ml/kg of 0.9% normal saline over the first hour is correct initially.

14. **C**, Pages 2045–2046.

pH should only be corrected with bicarbonate if below 7.1. The pH should not be corrected above 7.20 with bicarbonate. *A* is true—acidosis may be protective secondary to the 2,3 DPG deficiency and may actually increase oxygen delivery to the peripheral tissues. *B* is true. *D* is true.

15. **C**, Page 2046.

Initial therapy should be IV volume replacement, which will reestablish vascular volume and help begin to correct the acidosis. Insulin should be started, but fluid replacement is more vital initially. Glucose and K+ replacement are important as resuscitation continues. Bicarbonate therapy is not an initial step.

16. **C**, Page 2046.

You don't want to drop the glucose quickly with high-dose insulin because this may precipitate cerebral edema. Average doses of 10–15 units regular insulin per hour is common therapy. *A*, *B*, and *D* are all true.

17. **A**, Page 2045.

B, *C*, and *D* are all incorrect since rebound alkalosis does not occur, and rebound *hyper*glycemia is not a problem. Rather, *hypo*glycemia can be precipitated with large insulin doses.

18. **D**, Page 2047.

19. **B**, Pge 2047.

Blood glucose can be expected to be greater than 600 mg/dl, osmolarity greater than 350 mOsm/L, and no significant acidosis.

20. **C**.

21. **D**, Page 2048.

All of the above statements are true.

22. **A**, Page 2048.

Patients can become comatose and may be asymptomatic, but the most common presentation is listed in choice *A*.

23. **D**, Page 2049.

All of the choices listed above are true.

24. **D**, Page 2049-2050.

All of the listed areas can be affected by prolonged diabetes.

25. All are areas of change occurring to help regulate glucose control.

109
Alcohol-Related Disease

1. **C**, Page 2065.

There are probably 12,000,000 alcoholics in this country and more than 200,000 alcohol-related deaths each year.

2. **C**, Page 2065.

Addiction is a behavioral pattern of compulsive and overwhelming desire for alcohol use with a consistent tendency to relapse after withdrawal. Physical dependence is an altered physiologic state that necessitates the continued consumption of alcohol to prevent a withdrawal syndrome.

3. **A**, Page 2065.

The primary pathway for alcohol breakdown is through alcohol dehydrogenase. With chronic alcohol exposure the microsomal ethanal oxidizing system can be induced to increased activity.

4. **B**, Page 2066.

In a nonalcoholic, fine motor control is affected at even the low levels of blood alcohol. Chronic drinkers can function at much higher alcohol concentrations because of tolerance.

5. **B**, Page 2067.

Fructose has the potential effects of nausea, vomiting, and abdominal pain. In addition, potential dangerous lactic acidosis, hyperglycemia, and osmotic diuresis may result. It has not been shown to precipitate alcohol withdrawal.

6. **B**, Page 2067.

Minor withdrawal is exhibited by anxiety, irritability, insomnia, and tremor. Major withdrawal is exhibited by fever, diaphoresis, disorientation, and hallucinations. Delirium tremens is the extreme type of major withdrawal exhibited by gross tremor, profound confusion, fever, frightening visual hallucinations, and mydriasis and is quite rare.

7. **C**, Page 2070.

In patients with known previous withdrawal seizures, seizures may occur despite adequate benzodiazepine therapy. Superior seizure prophylaxis can be attained by adding phenytoin with a loading dose of 19 mg/kg orally to be maintained at 300 mg/day for 5 days.

8. **C**, Page 2071.

Alcohol intoxication will decrease cardiac output in both alcoholics and nonalcoholics with preexisting cardiac disease. Supraventricular dysrhythmias, specifically atrial fibrillation, ventricular dysrhythmias, and ventricular tachycardia, have been documented in alcoholics after heavy drinking.

9. **B**, Page 2072.

As with viral hepatitis the severity of alcoholic hepatitis can be assessed readily in the emergency department by the prothrombin time.

10. **A**, Page 2073.

Wernicke's encephalopathy consists of ocular motor disturbances, usually nystagmus, and ocular palsies as well as abnormal mentation and ataxia. This results in part from thiamine deficiency. However, although ophthalmoplegias and nystagmus usually respond to thiamine, the mental changes of Wernicke's encephalopathy are usually irreversible.

11. **C**, Page 2074.

The objectives of treatment to prevent acute renal failure in rhabdomyolysis is to obtain a urinary pH greater than 6.5 and maintain a diuresis of 300 ml or more per hour.

12. **A**, Page 2074.

As in the general population *Streptococcus pneumoniae* is still the most common organism causing pneumonia.

13. **A**, Pages 2075–2076, Table 109-3.

Malnutrition, vomiting, and diarrhea are major contributors to these electrolyte abnormalities.

14. **D**, Page 2077.

Alcoholic ketosis usually occurs in severe chronic alcoholics after an interval of heavy drinking followed by 1 to 3 days of protracted vomiting, decreased food intake, and abstinence. They are symptomatic with tachypnea, dehydration, ketonuria, and little to no glucose urea and because the ketone bodies in alcoholic ketoacidosis are mainly beta hydroxal, then nitroprusside reagent test may be negative.

15. **D**, Page 2077.

Iron deficiency anemia is very common among alcoholics and, as in the general public, is usually secondary to blood loss from the gastrointestinal tract.

110
Tricyclic Antidepressants

1. **A**, Page 2090.

Classic cardiac changes include QRS and QT prolongation and conduction defects such as bundle branch block (predominantly the right). PR prolongation rather than shortening is also a common finding.

2. **D**, Pages 2090–2091.

In this case one cannot rely on her history for several reasons, including drug-induced amnesia or mental alteration, deliberate misinformation, and plain ignorance. Her lack of early symptoms should not cause you to undertreat this patient. A significant number of patients without early symptoms go on to develop serious cardiac complications or coma. On the other hand, early anticholinergic symptoms are just as unreliable in predicting the same complications. Therefore, definitive treatment should be instituted prior to the return of the toxicologic studies, and the patient cannot be discharged until observed without any signs of toxicity for 4–6 hours.

3. **A**, Page 2091.

Due to delayed gastric emptying secondary to the anticholinergic effects of the tricyclics, emesis or gastric lavage can be productive up to 24 hours. Physostigmine can be helpful in treating CNS symptoms but is by no means always indicated and should be given slowly over 1 minute rather than pushed. Sodium bicarbonate is indicated for cardiac not CNS symptomatology. It is the drug of choice for supraventricular and ventricular tachycardia.

4. **C**, Page 2093.

Bicarbonate is the drug of choice, and most arrhythmias can be ameliorated by maintaining a slightly alkalotic pH. If life-threatening tachyarrhythmias persist, phenytoin has at least the theoretical advantage of improving cardiac conduction without depressing myocardial contracility; however, there are insufficient data on clinical efficacy. Lidocaine and bretylium can be used with caution. Physostigmine and beta blockers have been recommended in the past but have been associated with fatal side effects such as worsening conduction defects and profound hypotension.

5. **B**, Page 2092.

Valium gives the best response with the least side effects; phenobarbital is second. Alkalinization is of no use in CNS manifestations.

6. **D**, Pages 2087–2088, 2091–2092.
Physostigmine has been used in the past because it can reverse the anticholinergic side effects of tricyclic antidepressants. However, this is only one of the toxic effects of tricyclic antidepressant overdose and rarely are the anticholinergic effects a cause of death. In addition, physostigmine itself can *enhance* such problems as seizures, myocardial depression, conduction defects, and cardiac arrest.

111
Tranquilizer Overdose

1. **C**, Page 2099.
Although the benzodiazepines are involved in more overdoses than any other drug, it is very difficult to die from these drugs when taken alone. Phenothiazines have a high therapeutic index while lithium has a low index, which is why most overdoses from this drug are incidental to routine therapy. Most tranquilizer overdoses involve women, lower socioeconomic groups, and the minimally educated.

2. **D**, Page 2105.
The ferric chloride test is very specific for phenothiazine ingestion and should be considered in suspected cases (salicylates also produce a positive test).

3. **D**, Page 2105.
Benadryl is extremely effective in rapidly resolving all dystonic reaction secondary to phenothiazines.

4. **B**, Page 2106.
Thioridazine and lithium are exceptions to the above scenario due to their ability to display serious delayed toxicity, and such patients usually warrant admission for observation.

5. **D**, Page 2105.
Dystonia, a frequent event in young people experimenting with phenothiazines or butyrophenones, is an idiosyncratic rather than a dose-related event.

6. **D**, Page 2105.
Phenothiazine, being radiopaque, can appear on x-ray films of the abdomen. In phenothiazine overdose cases, induced emesis may be a problem because of the antiemetic effect of these drugs. Gastric lavage can be valuable even hours after ingestion because of decreased gastric motility. Phenothiazines produce quinidine-like ECG changes with prolongation of PR and OT intervals. Phenothiazines are not dialyzable. Acidifying the urine decreases phenothiazine reabsorption.

7. **D**, Page 2099.
The benzodiazepines themselves are involved in more

overdoses than any other class of drug. However, there are extremely few well-documented reports of death solely from the ingestion of benzodiazepine. Serious poisoning, following even large overdoses, is extremely rare.

8. **D**, Page 2099.
The phenothiazine group has a high therapeutic index: maximum tolerated dose per kilogram/minimal curative dose per kilogram. Although a number of deaths have been reported in the literature, overall this is an uncommon event.

9. **C**, Page 2105.
Most overdoses from lithium are incidental to therapy, rather than deliberate or accidental, because this agent has a very narrow of safety. In both acute and chronic toxicity, patients must be admitted to the hospital to be observed for symptom progression. Hemodialysis should be performed in severe cases. In patients with normal renal function, osmotic and saline diuresis increases renal lithium.

10. **D**, Page 2105.
Epinephrine is a potent beta-1 stimulatory agent. It can cause peripheral vasodilatation when its alpha activity is diminished by phenothiazines, which are potent alpha blockers. This further exacerbates the blockade-induced vasodilatation and hypotension.

11. **E**, Page 2106.
Benzodiazepines and the phenothiazines are not dialyzable, while meprobamate and lithium are dialyzable with hemodialysis.

112
Sedative-Hypnotics

1. **B**, Page 2121.
Meprobamate has a significant renal clearance with as much as 10% active drug excreted unchanged in the urine. The others listed have minimal renal clearance and the risk of hypotension and pulmonary edema far outweighs the minimal effect of forced diuresis.

2. **C**, Page 2120.
Chloral hydrate causes CNS depression rather than excitation. It is well known as a mucosal irritant and causes a variety of dermatologic manifestations. The cause of cardiac arrhythmias is unknown, but both supraventricular dysrhythmias have been documented. Aqueous hemodialysis and/or charcoal hemoperfusion both produce high clearance rate of the active metabolite trichloroethanol, which accounts for the majority of life-threatening effects of chloral hydrate.

3. **D**, Pages 2121–2122.

The active ingredients in Sominex include scopolamine, which produces anticholinergic effects and methapyrilene, an antihistamine that tends to produce a paradoxical CNS excitation rather than depression in children. The antihistamines may also produce anticholinergic symptoms. Fatalities have been reported in children, but not in adults.

4. **B**, Page 2109.

Of all the sedative hypnotic agents, barbiturates are responsible for the majority of deaths, mainly due to their abuse potential.

5. **A**, Pages 2112–2113.

Hypothermia rather than hyperthermia is caused by barbiturate overdose via depression of the pontine thermoregulatory center.

6. **D**, Page 2113.

This cutaneous phenomenon is found in 4–6% of barbiturate overdose cases and in 50% of overdose deaths.

7. **A**, Page 2114.

Choice A is correct because it is imperative in barbiturate overdose to monitor the CVP and wedge pressures while fluid volume is being given because these patients are prone to pulmonary edema. Dopamine and norepinephrine are second-line therapies and MAST trousers are insufficient.

8. **C**, Pages 2112–2115.

Phenobarbital has the lowest pKa, therefore is most susceptible to alkaline diuresis as mentioned above.

9. **B**, Page 2117.

Choices A and D are more frequent with barbiturate overdose and coma; nystagmus and ataxia are common to other drugs as well. Only hypertonicity and hyperreflexia are generally unique to methaqualone overdose.

10. **A**, Page 2117.

Forced diuresis is not appropriate because it will not increase drug elimination and because hepatic degradation is the primary mechanism for its disposal. Such therapy may lead to further hypotension.

113
Narcotics

1. **E**, Pages 2126–2128, Table 113-1.

Methadone and diphenoxylate are metabolized much more slowly than the other narcotics.

2. **D**, Pages 2129–2131.

Hypotension caused by narcotic overdose is not due to myocardial depression but to vasodilatation. Significant hypotension is usually not caused by nar-

cotics alone and one must be alert to other etiologies, especially mixed ingestions.

3. **B**, Page 2130.

Since pulmonary edema is not seen in therapeutic dosages, it is thought not to be idiosyncratic or a hypersensitivity phenomenon. Cardiac depression does not occur, nor do the pulmonary wedge values increase. Thus, since it is seen in all fatal cases, hypoxic damage and intense vasoconstriction is the most plausible hypothesis.

4. **C**, Page 2131.

A metabolite of Demerol, morperidine has marked excitability effects on the CNS that can lead to seizure activity. Propoxyphene likewise is more likely than the narcotics to cause seizure activity.

5. **A**, Page 2131.

This reaction is due to histamine release soon after ingestion or injection.

6. **E**, Page 2132.

The lack of any agonist activity makes it extremely safe to give in quantity to patients who have taken large doses of narcotics or who have mixed ingestions.

7. **D**, Pages 2129–2131.

Pinpoint pupils are classic for narcotic overdose and are present in 90% of cases.

8. **A**, Pages 2134–2135.

Pentazocine, propoxyphene, and codeine have all demonstrated resistance of naloxone.

9. **B**, Page 2133.

Naloxone dosage in text.

10. **D**, Page 2133.

One must avoid recurrent respiratory depression especially in long-acting narcotics such as methadone by using a continuous infusion but in a low enough dose to avoid withdrawal symptoms. IM naloxone has a prolonged effect but is unreliable.

11. **E**, Page 2127.

Morphine fails to cross the maternal blood-brain barrier well while crossing the placenta and the fetal blood-brain barrier due to its immaturity. Thus, the child in utero may be profoundly depressed while the mother may not be affected.

12. **A**, Page 2127.

This factor helps to explain the erratic course often seen in propoxyphene overdoses and at least partially explains its resistance to naloxone.

13. **C**, Page 2131.

In supine patients morphine has no effect on the heart rate, heart rhythm, or blood pressure, even in the presence of respiratory depression.

14. **C**, Page 2134.
    Due to the fat-soluble properties of propoxyphene, late recurrence of symptoms is possible, requiring an extended observation period for those who have displayed symtpoms.
15. **B**, Page 2135.
    Diphenoxylate is the main constituent in Lomotil and is so toxic to children under 2 years of age that it should never be prescribed for them. As little as 7.5 mg (3 tablets) has caused respiratory arrest in young children.
16. **A**, Pages 2130, 2135.
    No cases of pulmonary edema have been associated with pentazocine.
17. **D**, Page 2134.
    Death is common at doses of 35 mg/kg.
18. **B**, Page 2133.
    With a child the initial dose should be 0.01 mg/kg administered intravenously.
19. **D**, Page 2137.
    Very rarely is it absolutely necessary to administer narcotics to patients developing abstinence syndrome. It is more of a psychosocial problem rather than a medical problem and should be treated with an established addiction control program.

114

Salicylates and Acetaminophen

1. **C**, Page 2142.
    Absorption of commercial products is quite variable and depends largely on tablet dissolution. Enteric-coated tablets resist gastric secretions and dissolve in the alkaline small intestine. Absorption time may then lag, resulting in peak levels 6 to 9 hours after ingestion. While most nonenteric-coated products are rapidly absorbed, other factors such as pylorospasm or formation of a concreted mass in the stomach may also delay absorption.
2. **C**, Page 2143.
    The uncoupling of oxidative-phosphorylation prevents the energy derived from the Krebs cycle from being used for ATP synthesis. Instead, energy dissipates in the form of heat, resulting in potentially lethal hyperthermia. The hypermetabolic state resulting from inefficient phosphorylation leads to increased utilization and demand for glucose. Hepatic gluconeogenesis and lipid metabolism then results in hyperglycemia, glucosuria, and ketosis. Hyperglycemia also results from adrenal stimulation and release of epinephrine and cortisol. In addition, salicylate inhibition of dehydrogenase enzymes in the Krebs cycle results in impairment of aerobic glycolysis and a shift toward the anaerobic metabolic products, lactic and pyruric acids. These products contribute to anion gap metabolic acidosis. Although there is increased metabolic production of CO_2, the direct stimulating effects of salicylate on the medullary respiratory center more typically result in hyperventilation and respiratory alkalosis.

3. **D**, Page 2143.
    Respiratory alkalosis is usually the only disturbance seen in adults and older children and results from direct stimulation of the respiratory center in the medulla. This serves as an important protective mechanism as the resulting rise in pH further ionizes salicylate and prevents passage across lipid membranes into tissues. This explains the grave prognosis for the patient who develops acidemia. Children under 2 years of age commonly develop metabolic acidosis due to the accumulation of organic ions in the blood. Therefore, they will often present with a mixed disturbance of respiratory alkalosis and metabolic acidosis.
4. **B**, Page 2144.
    A number of factors contribute to potassium loss. Vomiting results in loss of potassium. Direct effects on the renal tubules promote increased urinary excretion of potassium. Potassium is lost from intracellular stores by changes in membrane permeability that result in passive efflux. The uncoupling action of salicylate also inhibits the active transport system used to maintain ionic gradients across cell membranes. This results in intracellular accumulation of sodium and water and further loss of potassium. The net result is rapid potassium depletion.
5. **A**, Page 2143.
    For an unknown reason, diabetics more often have a decreased glucose rather than an elevated glucose in response to salicylate overdose. Nondiabetics, on the other hand, are more often hyperglycemic following a salicylate ingestion.
6. **B**, Page 2143.
    Initially, salicylates stimulate the respiratory center in the medulla causing a respiratory alkalosis.
7. **C**, Page 2146.
    This test is an extremely sensitive indicator of the presence of salicylates. Add a few drops of 10% ferric chloride to a few drops of urine; it is positive if it turns violet or purple. It should be remembered that the presence of phenothiazines will turn this solution pink.

8. **A**, Page 2148.

Ipecac is preferred in this patient because she is alert and able to protect her airway and emesis is more effective in removing gastric contents. The IV should have dextrose in it due to the potential for delayed hypoglycemia, and K+ should be in the initial IV because patients are almost always K+ depleted. Isotonic saline or LR is needed for plasma expansion and should be given liberally to rehydrate and maintain a high urine flow.

9. **E**, Page 2148.

Blood levels at this time are not reliable; serial levels will tell you where the peak occured. A second level drawn 2 hours later will help determine if the salicylate level is declining or rising.

10. **D**, Pages 2148–2149.

If there is not sufficient K+ present, the kidneys will not be able to adequately alkalinize the urine no matter how alkalotic you make the patient with bicarbonate. This is because the kidneys will not have the K+ to excrete in exchange for H+, which would alkalinize the urine.

11. **E**, Page 2145.

It is important to keep in mind the possibility of chronic salicylate ingestion, particularly in the elderly patient. Salicylates are used over long periods of time to treat a variety of conditions including rheumatoid arthritis, TIAs, minor pain, and fevers. Inadvertent toxicity is not common but is often unrecognized in its initial presentation. It may mimic a variety of conditions or may present as confusion, hallucinations, seizures, hyperthermia, or dehydration. A mixed respiratory alkalosis and "anion-gap" metabolic acidosis is common, as are hypernatremia, hyperglycemia, ketonemia, and hypokalemia. Serum salicylate levels bear little correlation with the severity of intoxication in chronic ingestions.

12. **A**, Page 2147.

To confirm the diagnosis and estimate the severity of toxicity, a blood salicylate level should be drawn 6 hours or more after ingestion. Referring to a Done nomogram will function as a prognostic guide to the potential severity of intoxication based on the serum level and the interval since ingestion. The nomogram is applicable only to single-dose ingestions. When a reliable history is available, the ingested dose can be used as a rough predictor of a potentially toxic or lethal ingestion.

13. **E**, Pages 2148–2149.

Alkalinization of the urine should be considered in all patients with a salicylate level in excess of 35 mg/dl or in which clinical symptoms of salicylate are present. Therapy is aimed at achieving a urine pH in 7.5 to 8.0 by administering 1–2 mg/kg $NaHCO_3$ over 1–2 hours, then adjusting dosage based on serum pH.

Potassium depletion must be corrected prior to alkalinization since the kidneys are unable to produce alkaline urine in the face of a potassium deficit. Forced alkaline diuresis, however, affords no advantage over alkaline diuresis and risks fluid overload and cerebral edema. Rehydration is important in maintaining adequate circulatory volume and renal perfusion. 5% dextrose will help to avoid hypoglycemia. Gastric emptying with airway precautions and administration of activated charcoal will help to prevent further salicylate absorption.

14. **A**, Pages 2151–2152.

Barbiturates induce the cytochrome P-450 microsomal enzyme system that leads to an accelerated breakdown of acetaminophen resulting in depletion of hepatic glutathione stores. When present in sufficient quantity, glutathione is able to form readily excretable conjugates of the acetaminophen metabolized, but when overwhelmed, alternate pathways lead to toxic intermediate metabolites that cause hepatic necrosis by destruction of hepatocyte membranes. Alcohol may actually have hepatoprotective effects by its inhibition of the P-450 pathway.

15. **A**, Page 2153.

These ranges are not absolute, obviously, and the plasma half-life should be determined for borderline cases.

16. **D**, Page 2152.

Although diaphoresis is an initial finding, tremors and confusion are not. Most consistently, anorexia, nausea, and vomiting are seen without CNS or mental status changes.

17. **B**, Page 2153.

Forced diuresis is ineffective because the renal excretion is not dependent; therefore an insignificant amount is excepted in the urine. Charcoal therapy is controversial because it binds Mucomyst and thus might inhibit its absorption. Hemodialysis has not been shown to be particularly effective but is not contraindicated.

18. **B**, Page 2154.

This sulphur containing compound has the typical taste and smell of "rotten eggs." Dilution in a soft drink will make it more palatable. The maintenance dose is 70 mg/kg q 4 hours for 72 hours.

19. **B**, Page 2153.

Plasma APAP levels cannot be interpreted if measured less than 4 hours after ingestion due to continued and possibly delayed absorption. This level is nontoxic but needs to be repeated at 4 hours. While plasma APAP half-life is a useful prognosticator, it is usually not available, and single levels can be used utilizing the Rumack nomogram to predict toxicity. Children seem to be less susceptible to liver toxicity but should be treated according to the same guidelines as those used for adults.

20. **C**, Page 2155.
This is a potentially toxic ingestion of APAP as part of a multi-drug overdose. Treatment should consist of gastric emptying, administration of activitated charcoal, and cathartic. N-acetylcysteine can be given after re-lavage with water or saline until clear. In this case, the delay in obtaining APAP levels would require initiation of N-acetylcysteine treatment prior to the return of the serum level. Activited charcoal is not withheld in multidrug overdoses.

115
Hallucinations

1. **E**, Pages 2118, 2158.
Glutethimide is a sedative hypnotic that does not cause agitation. All of the other choices must be considered. The acute psychosis seen with either cocaine or LSD may be indistinguishable from true psychiatric disease.
2. **D**, Pages 2160–2161.
A. muscaria requires supportive care only. Atropine is contraindicated because it often worsens the anticholinergic effects already present. Valium may worsen the periods of deep sleep and further confuse the clinical picture. Admission to pediatric ICU is not needed unless anticholinergic effects, seizures, or mixed ingestion are present. Intubation and nasogastric lavage are not needed, nor is ipecac since ingestion was 2 hours previously.
3. **B**, Page 2163.
There are no reported deaths from marijuana use. All of the others are associated with intravenous use of marijunana.
4. **D**, Page 2169.
PCP is excreted mostly by the liver, and urine acidification will precipitate or worsen myoglobinuric renal failure. Continuous nasogastric suction, after gastric lavage, is recommended due to the ion trapping of the PCP in acidic gastric juice.
5. **B**, Pages 2169–2170.
Rhabdomyolysis and myoglobinuric renal failure are most common. The others are other medical complications of PCP toxicity.

116
Stimulants

1. **D**, Page 2179.
Phenothiazines may cause paradoxical hyperthermia

and they lower the seizure threshold. Phentolamine blocks both the alpha and beta adrenergic effects. Lidocaine or propranolol are used for ventricular dysrhythmias. Forced diuresis aids excretion and acidification of the urine decreases renal reuptake of drug.
2. **A**, Pages 2176, 2178–2179.
Cocaine causes CNS stimulation then depression with respiratory failure. Acute toxic psychosis resembles paranoid schizophrenia and is often seen in borderline patients. Urine drug screen is positive for l-benzoylecgonine for 24-36 hours after use. Propranolol is recommended by many authors for all toxic cardiac effects and for CNS stimulation.
3. **A**, Page 2177.
Chronic fatigue does not differentiate the two. The physical findings listed are commonly seen complications in stimulant abuse.

117
Corrosives

1. **C**, Page 2185.
Nasogastric or orogastric aspiration or lavage is almost universally condemned after alkali ingestion.
2. **C**, Page 2183.
Alkalis are the offending agents about 10 times as often as acids, reflecting their availability in the home and the level of patient tolerance.
3. **A**, Page 2185.
The risk of gastric intubation is exceedingly small with acid ingestions. Esophageal injury is shallow because of a firm protective eschar formed by coagulative necrosis that delays caustic damage. Dilution of concentrated acid with an equal volume of water results in a temperature rise of 80°C; also water added to concentrated acid may cause boiling and explosive steam and is therefore not recommended. Syrup of ipecac is contraindicated. Prophylactic antibiotics and steroids are not advocated at this time. Blind nasotracheal intubation is to be avoided.

118
Hydrocarbons

1. **C**, Page 2189.

   The more viscous hydrocarbons, such as lubricating oil, grease and diesel oil, are poorly absorbed from the GI tract and are best left there. The less viscous compounds should be removed with either emesis or gastric lavage. Left lateral decubitous position is recommended to prevent aspiration.

2. **E**, Page 2190.

   Respiratory distress and multiple types of pulmonary complications often occur despite a history inconsistent with aspiration. Metabolic acidosis is common due to its toxic effects on cellular machinery leading to anaerobic metabolism and lactic acidosis. Neurologic dysfunction varies from agitation to obtundation.

3. **B**, Pages 2189–2190.

   While all of these are potential results of certain types of hydrocarbon exposure, most cases of acute toxicity follow inhalation or aspiration of the substance, even after oral ingestion.

119
Acute Iron Poisoning

1. **B**, Page 2193.

   Iron is converted from the ferrous to the ferric form in the GI cells. It is taken up by transferrin and is extracted by the bone marrow for hemoglobin synthesis. It is also stored in hepatocytes and reticuloendothelial system, of which the bone marrow is a part, as hemosiderin. Absorption does proceed by first order kinetics.

2. **E**, Page 2194.

   Self-explanatory.

3. **D**, Page 2194.

   Anion gap metabolic acidosis can be present in iron toxicity. Hypoglycemia is present as is a leukocytosis and prolonged PT leading to coagulopathy when hepatic damage has occurred.

4. **D**, Pages 2194–2195.

   Patients can have hepatic necrosis and failure but this Stage IV is "relatively rare." However, patients frequently present in Stage I with vomiting, often bloody, as well as bloody diarrhea or in Stage II with no symptoms or improvement of perviously observed symptoms. Patients don't usually present with coma but in severe cases this can develop.

5. **B**, Page 2195.

   Serum iron levels greater than 300 ug/dl are "cause for concern" but the opposite is not true. A first voided urine may be normal after deferoximine challenge since it may represent residual urine in the bladder.

6. **C**, Page 2196.

   The patient's airway should be secured before any lavage or emesis is done. In this patient an intact gag reflex was not yet sought or noted. Bezoar removal initially is not a priority. Phosphage solutions are not recommended for lavage in iron poisoning.

7. **E**, Table 119-4, Page 2198.

   All of the listed answers can be used to further assess this patient and determine the steps to take for treatment.

8. **B**, Page 2196.

   Deferoxamine binds the ferric form of iron. It acts both intra- and extracellularly. 9.35 mg of elemental iron is bound by 100 mg of deferoxamine. Ferrous sulfate contains 22% elemental iron or 72 mg of elemental iron. If 15 tablets are available the total elemental iron is 1080 mg. A ratio can be set up:

   $$\frac{9.35}{100} = \frac{1080}{X}$$

   $$9.35\,(X) = 108,000$$

   $$X = \frac{108,000}{9.35}$$

   $$X = 10.5g$$

9. **B**, Pages 2194 (Table 119-1), 2198 (Table 119-4).

   Moderate to severe toxicity involves ingestion of greater than 20 mg/kg of elemental iron. In example B, 6 tablets of ferrous sulfate contain approximately 420 mg of elemental iron. A 30-lb toddler (or 14 kg) would have to ingest 280 mg or more of elemental iron for moderate to severe toxicity.

120
Fever of Unknown Origin

1. **C**, Pages 2203–2204.

   Febicle infants less then 60 days of age have a 3.6% incidence of occult bacteremia; 75% have no source of infection. In addition, bacteremia may occur in the absence of fever. Patients having temperature above 41.1°C have a 25% incidence of bacteremia.

2. **C**, Pages 2206–2207.

   The following laboratory results may indicate serious bacterial infection: greater than 500 band cells/mm^3, C-reactive protein greater than 10 mg/l, erythrocyte sedimentation rate greater than 5mm/hour, WBC count greater than 15000/mm^3, and PMN leukocyte count greater than 10000/mm^3.

121
Acute Bacterial Meningitis

1. **B**, Pages 2213–2214.

   In older infants, *H. influenzae* type B accounts for over one-half of the cases of meningitis. This species, *S. pneumoniae*, and *N. meningitidis* account for 70% of the documented cases of bacterial meningitis in the pediatric age group.

2. **B**, Page 2216.

   Chemoprophylaxis for all family members and intimate contacts of a child with meningococcal disease is an accepted mode of therapy to prevent secondary cases. Rifampin, the current drug of choice may significantly decrease the risk of a meningococcal secondary spread which typically occurs within 2 to 3 days of the index case.

3. **C**, Pages 2216–2217.

   A cerebrospinal fluid examination is mandatory in a child who appears ill and has nuchal rigidity. However, there are many conditions besides meningitis that can cause nuchal rigidity, for example, mumps parotitis. When one of these diagnoses is established in a child who is not otherwise ill, has no alteration of his sensorium, and lacks other manifestations of an intracranial infection, individual evaluation regarding the need for a lumbar puncture is acceptable. Brief generalized seizures with postictal somnolence and an absence of neurologic abnormalities in children age 6 months to 5 years in the context of a febrile illness are common occurrences. However, if any of the above-mentioned conditions exist, or if the child is outside the usual age range for febrile seizures, a lumbar puncture should be done.

4. **D**, Pages 2217–2220.

   In the newborn, no single antibiotic has bacteriocidal activity against all the possible organisms commonly encountered, and thus ampicillin is typically combined with an aminoglycoside.

5. **B**, Pages 2217–2220.

   In patients over 2 months of age, in the absence of evidence suggesting the presence of unusual organisms, a combination of ampicillin and chloramphenicol is advocated. In the past, ampicillin alone was used, but with the emergence of ampicillin-resistant strains of *H. influenzae* (in up to 30% of cases), it is now necessary to administer chloramphenicol concurrently until sensitivity studies are available.

6. **E**, Page 2220.

   Seizure activity should be initially terminated with diazepam followed by diphenylhydantoin intravenously. Phenobarbital should be avoided if possible to prevent hypotension and lethargy. The dose is 10 to 15 mg/kg, not 50.

7. **B**, Page 2220.

   Although MAST trousers and volume expanders are possibilities, MAST trousers are rarely available and initial hydration with D$_5$LR at 20 ml/kg is usually a sufficient volume expansion trial. Methylprednisolone 30 mg/kg, though controversal, may be used.

122
Ear Infections

1. **B**, Pages 2223–2224.

   Streptococcus pneumoniae is the most common pathogen, although *Hemophilus influenzae* may predominate in some locales.

2. **A**, Pages 2224–2225.

   Newborns are at the greatest risk for gram-negative enteric pathogens. For this reason, tympanocentesis should be considered. *S. pneumoniae* and *H. influenzae* remain the most common pathogens in neonates.

3. **A**, Page 2227.

   Though fluid from the external auditory canal is found in suppurative otitis media with drum perforation, it can also be found with otitis externa. Hyperemic tympanic membranes are a nonspecific finding as is tenderness on otoscopic examination. Acute suppurative otitis media is characterized by the finding of bulging tympanic membranes.

4. **B**, Page 2225.

   Aspiration of the middle ear effusion for organism identification is necessary in all newborns and immunosuppressed patients (because of the wide spectrum of infecting organisms). It is also indicated for severe otalgia and fever persistently present after 3 days antibiotics, two consecutive treatment failures, orotitis onset during antibiotic therapy.

5. **D**, Page 2226.

   Though *S. pneumoniae* is the most common etiologic agent in otitis media (25% to 50%), the cause of recurrent otitis is usually *H. influenzae*. *S. pyogenes* accounts for 1% to 6% of otitis media and *N. catarrhalis* is also known to cause otitis media. *P. aeruiginosa* is most commonly associated with otitis externa.

123
Croup and Epiglottitis

1. **B**, Pages 2232–2233.
   Botulism produces no fever, whereas fever is present with Ludwig's angina, croup, and epiglottitis.
2. **C**, Pages 2229–2231.
   For a child with a clinical croup without intrinsic laryngeal disease home management with humidified or cool air is advocated. Sedation, steroids, and antibiotics are unacceptable outside the hospital setting.
3. **B**, Pages 2232–2234.
   Epiglottis is clasically present in children 3 to 7 years of age. Croup, acute spasmodic laryngitis, and foreign body obstruction are classically present in children 6 months to 3 years of age.
4. **A**, Pages 2229–2232.
   Croup, which is a common name for acute laryngotracheobronchitis, is characterized by a barky cough, nontoxic appearance, low grade fever, and typically a recumbent child. The etiologic agent is usually a virus.
5. **C**, Pages 2232–2234.
   Airway protection is paramount in acute epiglottitis with progressive obstruction. Should intubation be indicated, nasotracheal is preferable to orotracheal, and tracheostomy is preferable to cricothyroidotomy. Forced bag-mask ventilation is an acceptable temporary ventilation technique should intubation or tracheostomy be unavailable.
6. **B**, Pages 2232–2234.
   Soft tissue x-rays are used primarily to identify epiglottitis. Croup will cause a pencil-point narrowing of the subglottic airway in frontal and lateral projections. (Figs. 123-1 and 123-2).

124
Asthma and Bronchiolitis

1. **B**, Pages 2242–2244.
   A PEFR greater than 65% of predicted value indicates that an adult or older child may be safely discharged. Isoetharine is a very short-acting bronchodilator. Metaproterenol is longer acting and may be given prior to discharge. A normal pCO_2 is an ominous sign that indicates respiratory decompensation.
2. **D**, Pages 2244–2245.
   Adrenal suppression may occur in patients receiving steroids, not in patients experiencing their first asthma attack. Tension pneumothorax, pneumomediastinum and ventilatory failure all may complicate asthma.

3. **C**, Pages 2245–2246.
   Patients with $PaCO_2$ over 40 and PaO_2 under 70 on O_2 should be admitted to the ICU. Bronchiolitis generally occurs in infants less then 1 year of age. A trial of epinephrine is generally indicated since patients often respond. Pneumomediastinum may occur in 5% of asthma patients.

125
Pneumonia

1. **A**, Pages 2251–2253.
   Normal children younger than 5 years of age may experience 6 upper respiratory infections and perhaps a single episode of pneumonia yearly. Most cases of pneumonia under 5 years of age are viral. A work-up for pneumonia is indicated if the child shows signs of cough, fever, and rales or more commonly tachypnea.
2. **B**, Pages 2251–2253.
   Neonates have minimal or nonspecific symptoms with pneumonia. Productive cough would be unlikely in this age group. Lethargy, poor feeding, decreased muscle tone, and fever may be the only clues in a very sick infant.
3. **D**, Pages 2251–2254.
   All choices represent situations in which the patient may deteriorate rapidly if not identified early.
4. **C**, Page 2253.
   Viral pneumonias do not progress to bacterial superinfection in previously healthy children, therefore antibiotics are not indicated.
5. **A**, Pages 2252–2254.
   Pneumonia can be caused by many etiologic agents. However, clamydial pneumonia is unique in that it is usually seen at 3 to 12 weeks of age in a child who is afebrile, coughs without whooping, and has eosinophilia. Conjunctivitis is associated with 50% of cases.
6. **D**, Pages 2254–2256.
   If respiratory distress is noted in a child with pneumonia, hydration and humidified oxygen are necessary. In addition, the tracheobronchial tree may need assistance with clearing, which antitussive agents would impair.
7. **A**, Page 2256.
   Most uncomplicated bacterial pneumonias in children over 1 year of age are caused by *Streptococcus pneumoniae*. The drug of choice is penicillin, with improvement in 1 to 2 days expected. Though not the therapy of choice, erythromycin or amoxicillin are acceptable alternatives in ambulatory patients.

126
Diarrheal Disease

1. **B**, Page 2261.
   Yersinia is unique in its predilection for winter months. Abrupt diarrhea is common to *Vibrio*, enterotoxigenic and enteroinvasive *E. coli*, and *Shigella*. Most infectious diarrheas are self-limiting associated with abdominal cramping. Enteropathogenic *E. coli* and *Salmonella* stools are typically green in color and may contain blood but usually not mucus.
2. **B**, Pages 2260–2261.
   Shigella enteritis is characterized by infrequency of vomiting.
3. **D**, Page 2260.
   Salmonella enteritis is well characterized in *D*. Typically these children are seen after home remedies have failed.
4. **A**, Page 2260.
   Rotavirus accounts for 70% to 80% of winter episodes of diarrhea.

5. **A**, Page 2262.
   Antibiotics decrease both the amount of diarrhea and the duration of infectivity.
6. **C**, Page 2262.
7. **B**, Page 2262.
8. **A**, Page 2262.

127
Cardiac Disease in Children

1. **C**, Page 2272.
   Midface hypoplasia, short palepbral fissure, and VSD are all components of the fetal alcohol syndrome. See Table 127-1 below.

Table 127-1. Selected clinical syndromes associated with congenital heart disease

Syndrome	Features	Cardiac anomalies*
Congenital rubella	Deafness, cataracts, hepatosplenomegaly, purpura	PDA, PS, VSD, CA
DiGeorge syndrome (thymic/parathyroid deficiency)	Mandibular hypoplasia, deformed ears, short philtrum	Aortic atresia, hypoplastic left ventricle
Fetal alcohol syndrome	Midface hypoplasia, short palpebral fissures	VSD
Fetal dilantin syndrome	Hypertelorism, hypoplastic nails	PS, AS, CA, PDA
Fetal trimethadione syndrome	Upslanting eyebrow, simian crease	Septal defects, tetralogy of Fallot
Holt-Oram	Hypoplastic fingerized thumb	ASD
Hurler's syndrome	Mental retardation, skeletal anomalies	Mitral or tricuspid stenosis or regurgitation
Kartagener's syndrome	Situs inversus, sinusitis, bronchiectasis	Defects in cardiac septation
Klinefelter's syndrome	Mental retardation, gynecomastia, small testes	VSD
Laurence-Moon-Biedl syndrome	Mental retardation, obesity, hypogonadism, polydactyly, retinitis pigmentosa	PDA, TGV, PS
Marfan's syndrome	Tall habitus, long fingers ectopia lentis	AI, PI, aortic dissection
Multiple lentigenes syndrome	Multiple lentigenes, hypertelorism, deafness	PS
Noonan's syndrome	Small stature, hypertelorism, low set ears	Valvar PS
Osteogenesis imperfecta	Blue sclera, lax joints, brittle bones, deafness	AI
Supravalvular aortic stenosis (William's syndrome)	Small nose, full lips, hypoplastic nails, ± hypercalcemia in infancy	AS
Trisomy 13 (Patau's syndrome)	Holoprosencephaly, mental retardation, polydactyly, omphalocele	VSD, PDA, ASD
Trisomy 18 (Edward's syndrome)	Mental and physical retardation; micrognathia, cleft palate, flexed fingers, rockerbottom feet	VSD, ASD, PDA
Trisomy 21 (Down's syndrome)	Mongoloid slanting eyes, cataracts, simian crease, hypotonia, macroglossia	Endocardial cushion defects (AV canal), PDA
Turner's syndrome (gonadal dysgenesis)	Webbed neck, shield chest, short stature, increased carrying angle of elbows	Coarctation of the aorta, PS
Vater association	Vertebral anomalies, anal atresia, tracheoesophageal fistula, radial dysplasia, renal anomalies	VSD

AI, aortic insufficiency; *ASD*, atrial septal defect; *AS*, aortic stenosis; *CA*, coarctation of the aorta; *PDA*, patent ductus arteriosus; *PI*, pulmonary insufficiency; *PS*, pulmonary stenosis; *VSD*, ventricular septal defect.

2. **A**, Page 2273.

Coarctation of the aorta is the only congenital cardiac anomaly of those listed that is characteristically acyanotic.

3. **D**, Pages 2272–2274.

Failure to thrive is the most common and constant finding in cases of significant cardiac disease. Cyanosis, congestive heart failure, and associated dysmorphic features all suggest cardiac disease but are inconstant findings.

4. **A**, Pages 2281–2284.

Tetralogy of Fallot is characterized by obstruction of right ventricular outflow, dextroposition of the aorta, ventricular septal defect, and right ventricular hypertrophy. Ebstein's anomaly is characterized by anomalous tricuspid valve, tricuspid insufficiency, and right atrial enlargement. Truncus arteriosus is characterized by single arterial truck for both systemic and pulmonary circulation. Eisenmenger's syndrome is characterized by pulmonary hypertension and any septal defect.

CLASSIFICATION OF CARDIAC DISEASE IN CHILDREN

Presence or absence of cyanosis

X-ray study evaluation of pulmonary blood flow as increased, decreased or normal

ECG criteria for ventricular hypertrophy

I. Cyanotic
   A. With decreased pulmonary flow and right ventricular hypertrophy
      Tetralogy of Fallot
      Severe pulmonary stenosis
      Pulmonary atresia with or without ventricular septal defect
      Pulmonary vascular obstruction (Eisenmenger's syndrome)
      Ebstein's anomaly
   B. With decreased pulmonary flow and left ventricular hypertrophy
      Tricuspid atresia
      Pulmonary atresia with hypoplastic left ventricle
   C. With decreased pulmonary flow and combined, left, or right ventricular hypertrophy
      Transposition of the great vessels with pulmonic stenosis
      Truncus arteriosus with hypoplastic pulmonary arteries
   D. With increased pulmonary flow and right ventricular hypertrophy
      Hypoplastic left heart syndrome with aortic atresia
      Transposition of the great vessels
      Total anomalous pulmonary venous return
   E. With increased pulmonary flow and combined, left, or right ventricular hypertrophy
      Single ventricle
      Tricuspid atresia with transposition
      Transposition of the great vessels with ventricular septal defect
      Truncus arteriosus
      Pulmonary vascular obstruction with bidirectional shunt

II. Acyanotic
   A. With normal pulmonary flow and right ventricular hypertrophy
      Mitral stenosis
      Pulmonary stenosis
   B. With normal pulmonary flow and left ventricular hypertrophy
      Coarctation of the aorta
      Aortic stenosis
      Mitral regurgitation
      Myocarditis
      Endocardial fibroelastosis
   C. With increased pulmonary flow and right ventricular hypertrophy
      Atrial septal defect with pulmonary hypertension
      Ventricular septal defect with pulmonary hypertension
      Patent ductus arteriosus with pulmonary hypertension
   D. With increased pulmonary flow and left ventricular hypertrophy
      Ventricular septal defect
      Patent ductus arteriosus
      Arteriovenous fistulae

Table 127-2.

128
Child Abuse

1. **C**, Pages 2289–2292.
   Homicide accounts for 1 in 20 deaths under the age of 18 and is the only cause of death in that age group to have risen in recent years. 50% of fractures in children less than 1 year of age are due to abuse. Shaken baby syndrome often causes subdural hematomas when the dural bridging veins are ruptured by violent shaking. Polle's syndrome is Munchausen's syndrome by proxy.
2. **B**, Pages 2299–2301.
   25% of women and 10% of men have been victimized by sexual abuse during their childhood. 10% of all childhood injuries may be the result of child abuse. Head trauma is the most common cause of death. The incidence of venereal disease is high in cases of child sexual abuse; therefore antibiotic prophylaxis is indicated.

Comprehensive Review

1. **D**, Chapter 8, Page 160.
   Hypotension will ensue for blood loss greater than 25%. It is important to treat these patients aggressively since they can go into shock quite rapidly because their compensatory efforts fail around the 25% blood loss.
2. **B**, Chapter 8, Pages 173–174.
   Subclavian line is difficult to insert and hazardous, especially in a child less than 10-kg weight.
3. **D**, Chapter 9, Pages 180–181.
   Epinephrine is a neurotransmitter released from the adrenal medulla in response to sympathetic stimulation mediated by a decrease in mean blood pressure. Norepinephrine is released from nerve endings in the heart and great vessels from a similar stimulus.
4. **A**, Chapter 10, Page 222.
   Positive identification of the honey bee is easiest since it is the only stinging insect that leaves its stinger at the site of injury.
5. **B**, Chapter 20, Page 413.
   Posterior nosebleeds are rare in children and young adults and when diagnosed neoplasm must be excluded as an etiology. Benign angiofibromas are occasionally encountered in males and squamous cell carcinoma has been discovered, although usually in an older population. A Water's view of the sinuses exhibits a mass if present.
6. **C**, Chapter 21, Page 422.
   The initial description of oozing blood suggests venous injury and with sudden decompression air embolism must be suspected. If he does not improve with the maneuver, thought must be given to pericardiocentesis of right ventricle to remove air. If *A* was present he should have significant respiratory distress, deviated trachea, and unilateral decreased breath sounds in addition to deteriorating vital signs. *B* is a possibility but unlikely as a cause of sudden deterioration. *D* should be done but not until air embolism is corrected if present.
7. **C**, Chapter 24, Page 496.
   Interpretation of a widened mediastinum and obscuration of the aortic knob are the most reliable radiographic indications to proceed to aortography to detect aortic rupture.
8. **D**, Chapter 27, Page 557.
   The most common fetal injury reported at birth is skull fractures, strongly associated with maternal pelvic fractures late in the third trimester when the head is fixed. Fetal death is uncommon, unless mother dies or goes into shock.
9. **B**, Chapter 28, Page 563.
   Although 10–15% of pelvic fractures have associated bladder injuries, the overwhelming majority are associated with a full bladder.
10. **B**, Chapter 30, Pages 588–589.
11. **C**, Chapter 30, Pages 588–589.
12. **A**, Chapter 30, Pages 588–589.
    Though each poison has its own unique characteristic, these three should be of interest. The bitter almond odor of cyanide poisoning is detectable by only 30–50% of the population and is often masked by smoke odor on clothing. The rotten egg smell of hydrogen sulfide can be fatigued if in low concentrations and the red-brown-copper colored gas of nitrogen oxide should be recognized immediately because of its lethality!
13. **E**, Chapter 31, Pages 612–613.
    First degree frostbite is characterized by erythema and swelling. Second degree implies blister or bleb formation. Third degree is full thickness with gangrene of the skin and subcutaneous tissue but not loss of body part. Fourth degree is complete necrosis with loss of body part. This patient has at least second degree frostbite, but it may take weeks or even months to determine the exact extent of the injury.
14. **B**, Chapter 38, Page 669.
    At the extremes of life, hypothermia is often associated with fulminant sepsis.
15. **A**, Chapter 100, Page 1847.
    Physostigmine is a cholinesterase inhibitor and therefore reverses cholinergic blockage that is associated with neurotransmitter dysfunction and memory impairment.

16. **D**, Chapter 110, Page 2091.

Without a gag reflex, you cannot trust the patient to protect his own airway during gastric lavage. Intubation will prevent life-threatening aspiration. This is especially true in tricyclic antidepressant ingestions, where mental status can deteriorate abruptly before ipecac can take effect.

17. **E**, Chapter 112, Page 2118.

The pupils are usually dilated and unreactive rather than pinpoint and unreactive.

18. **B**, Chapter 113, Page 2133.

Initial management of narcotic overdose should be aimed at correcting hypoxia and hypoglycemia. Naloxone is then given initially as 0.4 mg IV. If no response, give 2 mg IV and repeat every 3–5 minutes to a total of 10 mg. If no response is noted after this, it is probably not primarily a narcotic overdose. However, if some response is noted, up to 10–15 mg of naloxone may be required to fully antagonize an overdose of pentazocine. Naloxone resistance has also been noted in codeine and propoxyphene overdoses. Lasix is contraindicated for narcotic-induced pulmonary edema because it can lead to severe hypotension.

19. **B**, Chapter 114, Page 2141.

Ingestion of oil of wintergreen causes a disproportionately large number of salicylate-related deaths due to the lack of awareness of its toxicity and its high concentration of methyl salicylate. The potentially lethal dose in 2-year-olds is roughly 1 teaspoon.

20. B, Chapter 18, Page 371.

The goal is to have three immunizations of dT plus Hyper-Tet if it is a "dirty wound." Hyper-Tet is not recommended for clean wounds, regardless of immunization status. Hyper-Tet is recommended for all dirty wounds unless patient has had three prior tetanus immunizations. If the patient had had no prior immunizations, he should receive 0.5 ml dT now, again in 4 to 6 weeks, and again in 6 to 12 months plus Hyper-Tet if indicated.

21. **A**, Chapter 20, Page 397.

The cribriform plate is located along the superior aspect of the nasal cavity. When fractured and associated with a dural tear, this results in CSF rhinorrhea.

22. **D**, Chapter 106, Page 1979.

Demeclocycline in daily doses of 600 to 1200 mg can be effective, as can lithium.

23. **A**, Chapter 106, Pages 1990–1991.

Hyperkalemia can cause first degree heart block, but it does not cause flattened T waves or QT prolongation. Rather it causes just the opposite. Hypocalcemia can cause the changes in this patient, but not hypercalcemia. Hyponatremia and hypernatremia have primarily neurologic effects and are unlikely causes

of EKG changes.

24. **D**, Chapter 106, Pages 2005–2007.

Hypomagnesemia causes neuromuscular irritability and all the signs consistent with hypocalcemia. It is probably more likely in an alcholic patient, 25% of whom have hypomagnesemia.

25. C, Chapter 106, Page 1976.

In hypernatremia the goal is to correct the osmolarity halfway toward normal over 24 hours. Too rapid a water replacement may precipitate cerebral edema, especially in children.

26. **D**, Chapter 78, Page 1471.

This patient has the classic presentation for mesenteric vascular occlusion. While x-rays are seldom diagnostic, gas in the bowel wall, if found, is highly suggestive of this disease. Free air beneath the diaphragm suggests a perforated viscus. Distention of the small bowel with air fluid levels would suggest a small bowel obstruction. Calcifications in the epigastric area would most likely be chronic pancreatitis. Blurring of the psoas shadows is a nonspecific finding that can be due to retroperitoneal bleeding.

27. **B**, Chapter 78, Page 1474.

Intussusception is typified by increased mucus production that is mixed with blood. It typically involves a child who may not appear acutely ill. The expected physical finding is a sausage-shaped mass usually in the right side of the abdomen. Diagnosis is by barium enema, which is also therapeutic in 50–75% of cases.

28. **D**, Chapter 78, Page 1471.

Gas in the bowel wall or portal venous system is considered relatively specific for intestinal infarction. It is a subtle finding but of immense diagnostic importance and is usually seen in the transverse colon.

29. **A**, Chapter 78, Page 1474.

Intussusception is most common during the first year of life. It is typified by intermittent pain initially followed by the typical signs and symptoms of a small bowel obstruction. Early in the course, the patient may appear quite comfortable between attacks and have no physical or laboratory abnormalities. Pyloric stenosis is characterized by projectile vomiting more than pain. Sigmoid volvulus or incarcerated hernias would have constant rather than intermittent pain. Hirschsprung's disease presents as increasing constipation with abdominal distention.

30. C, Chapter 78, Page 1441.

Trophzoites are rarely found in the stool. The diagnosis is best made by a liver scan to identify an abscess and serology to correctly identify the etiology.

31. **E**, Chapter 77, Page 1449.

This patient has pancreatitis, probably due to cholelithiasis. The ultrasound can give information about the head of the pancreas and is the method of choice to diagnose gallstones. Antibiotics are not helpful unless there is clear evidence of infection and cimetadine has not proved to be useful. Endoscopy without ERCP is not helpful, and in acute pancreatitis ERCP can increase pancreatic inflammation. This patient will require surgery, but preferably as an elective procedure after 24–48 hours of stabilization.

32. **E**, Chapter 77, Page 1452.

The amylase:creatinine ratio uses a spot serum amylase and creatinine and a spot urine amylase and creatinine to determine the amount of amylase cleared by the kidneys. A ratio of less than 3 is normal, while a ratio greater than 5 indicates pancreatitis with the exception of burns and diabetic ketoacidosis. Macroamylasemia is a nonpathologic condition in which the circulating amylase molecule is larger than normal. Because of its increased size, less is cleared by the kidney, which results in a higher circulating amylase level but a lower than normal amylase to creatinine clearance.

33. **A**, Chapter 77, Page 1442.

Minor elevations in alpha-fetoprotein can be seen in some patients with acute hepatitis. Elevation over 500 ng/cc is virtually diagnostic of a malignant hepatoma.

34. **E**, Chapter 74, Page 1336.

All of these disorders can mimic coronary ischemia. Reviewing old tracings and looking for reciprical changes are helpful to correctly differentiate these disorders from true coronary ischemia.

35. **C**, Chapter 62, Page 1130.

This patient's symptoms began after starting a new drug. Cimetadine is known to impair hepatic degradation of theophylline and increase serum levels. Nausea is a major symptom of theophylline toxicity.

36. **E**, Chapter 72, Page 1293.

Kerley B lines are 1-cm long horizontal markings appearing above the diaphragms near the chest wall. They are believed to represent interstitial edema or dilated lymphatics. While they can be caused by viral infections, pulmonary fibrosis, etc., they correlate most closely with congestive heart failure.

37. **B**, Chapter 63, Pages 1153–1154.

Narcotic overdose, unless accompanied by aspiration, is a pure defect in ventilation. The P_{CO_2} is the best gauge to ventilation. There should not be a large A-a gradient and the patient is hypoxic only to the extent that CO_2 replaces O_2 in the alveoli.

38. **A**, Chapter 69, Pages 1236–1239.

One negative 12 lead does not effectively rule out the possibility of acute myocardial infarction. More history along with serial EKGs and cardiac enzymes would be necessary. Mitral valve prolapse frequently first diagnosed between the ages of 20–40 often presents as atypical nonexertional chest pain. Dizziness and fatigue are commonly associated findings; however, if syncope is present the patient is at greater risk for significant dysrhythmias. Aortic stenosis can also present with left-sided chest pain and syncope. The murmur described is a murmur typical for aortic stenosis. Generally, most patients are not seen with symptoms until the fourth or fifth decade of life. Mitral stenosis presents with dyspnea on exertion, orthopnea, and hemoptysis rather than chest pain or syncope. The associated murmur is diastolic and heard best at the apex.

39. **C**, Chapter 90, Page 1675.

Total electrical alternans is the beat to beat change in size of the P and QRS complexes. It is rare, but when present is diagnostic of cardiac tamponade. It is usually seen with neoplastic pericarditis.

40. **A**, Chapter 89, Page 1653.

This patient presents with all of the pentad of thrombotic thrombocytopenia purpura, which consist of: (1) thrombocytopenic purpura, (2) microangiopathic hemolytic anemia, (3) fluctuating neurologic signs, (4) renal disease, and (5) fever. This disease is often not recognized and untreated has 80% mortality. Therapy is controversial and includes corticosteroids, splenectomy, exchange transfusion, and antiplatelet agents such as aspirin and Persantine.

41. **B**, Chapter 85, Page 1594.

A previously healthy woman of child-bearing age with sudden vascular collapse has a ruptured ectopic pregnancy until proven otherwise. While all of the listed answers can cause profound hypotension, a ruptured ectopic pregnancy is more common than all the others combined.

42. **C**, Chapter 78, Page 1461.

This patient has the triad of small bowel obstruction—abdominal pain, vomiting, and prior surgery. The x-ray film demonstrates multiple air fluid levels, which would be expected with a mechanical small bowel obstruction. It may be impossible to differentiate adynamie ileus from mechanical bowel obstruction with x-ray studies alone.

43. **A**, Chapter 63, Pages 1168, 1153.
44. **B**, Chapter 63, Pages 1168, 1153.
45. **C**, Chapter 63, Pages 1168, 1153.
46. **E**, Chapter 63, Pages 1168, 1153.

47. **D**, Chapter 63, Pages 1168, 1153.

The patient with a pulmonary embolus will have a PO_2 less than 80 more than 88% of the time. You would expect a low PCO_2 in respiratory alkalosis caused by increased ventilation in an attempt to correct the hypoxia. Asthmatic attacks will start out with hypoxia and hypocarbia, but as the attack progresses and respiratory muscles tire the patient will begin to retain CO_2. These patients require urgent intervention and sometimes intubation. Patients with chronic bronchitis are always hypoxic and hypercarbic. The clue that this is a chronic condition is the near normal pH in spite of a significantly increased PCO_2. Another patient with decompensating COPD may actually have a PCO_2 lower than another patient's baseline. Again, the pH is the way to tell if the CO_2 retention is acute or chronic. Gastric aspiration can be a form of the adult respiratory distress syndrome and is associated with severe hypoxia and a respiratory alkalosis.

48. **C**, Chapter 70, Page 1251.

This patient has hypertensive encephalopathy and immediate reduction of the diastolic pressure of 90 to 100 is mandatory. While an acute cerebral hemorrhage can cause seizures and increased blood pressure, it does not do so to this level. Likewise, a diabetic that seizes should be given $D_{50}W$, but this patient's urgent problem is his marked hypertension, which is not elevated with hypoglycemia.

49. **A**, Chapter 76, Page 1416.

Boerhaave's syndrome is spontaneous esophageal perforation that usually occurs after forceful vomiting. There is acute collapse, with chest and abdominal pain. Left pleural effusion occurs in 90% and most have mediastinal emphysema. None of the other answers listed would have a pleural effusion except pancreatitis, and that disease has a more gradual onset.

50. **B**, Chapter 76, Pages 1407–1408.

Pyloric stenosis typically affects the first born male. It typically is manifested when the child is 3 to 5 weeks old but can be delayed as long as 6 months. The initial complaint is projectile vomiting and weight loss. The pathognomonic finding is an "olive" palpable in the epigastrium in 70% to 90% of patients.

51. **A**, Chapter 76, Pages 1420–1422.

This patient demonstrates air under both diaphragms. This is caused by perforation of an ulcer over 90% of the time. The other listed entities can all cause free air in peritoneal cavity but do so much less often.

52. **E**, Chapter 77, Page 1442.

Patients on birth control pills can develop asymptomatic hepatic cell adenomas, which can spontaneously rupture and cause signs of hypovolemia. An ectopic pregnancy must be considered, but with a normal pelvic exam, no vaginal bleeding or amenorrhea, this diagnosis is less likely. The normal amylase helps to exclude pancreatitis. It is likewise unusual for acute pancreatitis. It is likewise unusual for acute appendicitis to cause this much volume loss.

53. **D**, Chapter 73, Page 1306.

Normally the wedge and pulmonary artery diastolic pressure are equal. When the pulmonary artery diastolic is greater than the wedge pressure, the cause is elevated pulmonary vascular resistance. The most common cause of sudden elevation of pulmonary vascular resistance is pulmonary emboli.

54. **A**, Chapter 71, Page 1270.

55. **B**, Chapter 74, Page 1293.

56. **E**, Chapter 71, Page 1284.

57. **D**, Chapter 95, Page 1792.

58. **C**, Chapter 64, Page 1236.

Any patient with unexplained atrial fibrillation should have thyroid studies done, especially if there is a rapid rate resistant to digitalization. Constrictive pericarditis should be considered in any patient with signs of right-sided failure, a small heart on x-ray, and mild left-sided failure. People have been treated for years for hepatomegaly and ascites believed to be caused by liver disease, which proved to be from constrictive pericarditis. A young woman presenting with chest pain, palpitations and shortness of breath may not be hysterical. Prolapse of the mitral valve should be considered and the typical midsystolic click with a late systolic murmur listened for carefully. An echocardiogram is the best way to confirm the diagnosis. Most athletes who die suddenly have IHSS. It is usually a malignant arrhythmia rather than outflow tract obstruction that causes death. In cases of WPW in supraventricular tachycardia, the antegrade conduction is through the AV node, whereas retrograde conduction is over the accessory bypass tract and the QRS appears normal. After they are converted to a sinus rhythm when antegrade conduction occurs over both the normal and bypass tracts, the typical delta wave is seen.

Notes

Notes